Language, Discourse, Society

General Editors: **Stephen Heath, Colin MacCabe** and **Denise Riley**

Selected published titles:

Reena Dube
SATYAJIT RAY'S *THE CHESS PLAYERS* AND POSTCOLONIAL THEORY
Culture, Labour and the Value of Alterity

John Anthony Tercier
THE CONTEMPORARY DEATHBED
The Ultimate Rush

Erica Sheen and Lorna Hutson
LITERATURE, POLITICS AND LAW IN RENAISSANCE ENGLAND

Jean-Jacques Lecercle and Denise Riley
THE FORCE OF LANGUAGE

Geoff Gilbert
BEFORE MODERNISM WAS
Modern History and the Constituency of Writing

Stephen Heath, Colin MacCabe and Denise Riley (*editors*)
THE LANGUAGE, DISCOURSE, SOCIETY READER

Michael O'Pray
FILM, FORM AND PHANTASY
Adrian Stokes and Film Aesthetics

James A. Snead, edited by Kara Keeling, Colin MacCabe and Cornel West
RACIST TRACES AND OTHER WRITINGS
European Pedigrees/African Contagions

Patrizia Lombardo
CITIES, WORDS AND IMAGES

Colin MacCabe
JAMES JOYCE AND THE REVOLUTION OF THE WORLD
Second edition

Moustapha Safouan
SPEECH OR DEATH?
Language as Social Order: a Psychoanalytic Study

Jean-Jacques Lecercle
DELEUZE AND LANGUAGE

Piers Gray, edited by Colin MacCabe and Victoria Rothschild
STALIN ON LINGUISTICS AND OTHER ESSAYS

Geoffrey Ward
STATUTES OF LIBERTY
The New York School of Poets

Moustapha Safouan
JACQUES LACAN AND THE QUESTION OF PSYCHOANALYTIC TRAINING
(*Translated and introduced by Jacqueline Rose*)

Stanley Shostak
THE DEATH OF LIFE
The Legacy of Molecular Biology

Elizabeth Cowie
REPRESENTING THE WOMAN
Cinema and Psychoanalysis

Raymond Tallis
NOT SAUSSURE
A Critique of Post-Saussurean Literary Theory

Laura Mulvey
VISUAL AND OTHER PLEASURES

Ian Hunter
CULTURE AND GOVERNMENT
The Emergence of Literary Education

Denise Riley
'AM I THAT NAME?'
Feminism and the Category of 'Women' in History

Mary Ann Doane
THE DESIRE TO DESIRE
The Woman's Film of the 1940s

Language, Discourse, Society
Series Standing Order ISBN 0-333-71482-2
(*outside North America only*)

You can receive future titles in this series as they are published by placing a standing order. Please contact your bookseller or, in case of difficulty, write to us at the address below with your name and address, the title of the series and the ISBN quoted above.

Customer Services Department, Macmillan Distribution Ltd, Houndmills, Basingstoke, Hampshire RG21 6XS, England

The Contemporary Deathbed

The Ultimate Rush

John Anthony Tercier

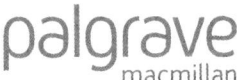

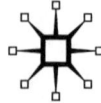

© John Anthony Tercier 2005

All rights reserved. No reproduction, copy or transmission of this publication may be made without written permission.

No paragraph of this publication may be reproduced, copied or transmitted save with written permission or in accordance with the provisions of the Copyright, Designs and Patents Act 1988, or under the terms of any licence permitting limited copying issued by the Copyright Licensing Agency, 90 Tottenham Court Road, London W1T 4LP.

Any person who does any unauthorized act in relation to this publication may be liable to criminal prosecution and civil claims for damages.

The author has asserted his right to be identified as the author of this work in accordance with the Copyright, Designs and Patents Act 1988.

First published 2005 by
PALGRAVE MACMILLAN
Houndmills, Basingstoke, Hampshire RG21 6XS and
175 Fifth Avenue, New York, N. Y. 10010
Companies and representatives throughout the world

PALGRAVE MACMILLAN is the global academic imprint of the Palgrave Macmillan division of St. Martin's Press, LLC and of Palgrave Macmillan Ltd. Macmillan® is a registered trademark in the United States, United Kingdom and other countries. Palgrave is a registered trademark in the European Union and other countries.

ISBN-13: 978–1–4039–4628–7
ISBN-10: 1–4039–4628–0

This book is printed on paper suitable for recycling and made from fully managed and sustained forest sources.

A catalogue record for this book is available from the British Library.

Library of Congress Cataloging-in-Publication Data

Tercier, John Anthony, 1953–
   The contemporary deathbed : the ultimate rush / John Anthony Tercier.
     p. cm. – (Language, discourse, society)
        Includes bibliographical references and index.
        ISBN 1–4039–4628–0 (cloth)
   1. CPR (First aid)–Social aspects. 2. Death. I. Title. II. Series.

RC87.9.T45 2005
616.07′8–dc22   2004056786

10 9 8 7 6 5 4 3 2 1
14 13 12 11 10 09 08 07 06 05

Printed and bound in Great Britain by
Antony Rowe Ltd, Chippenham and Eastbourne

This book is dedicated to Paul Hirst and Dorothy Porter

Contents

Acknowledgements	ix
List of Abbreviations	x
Foreword	xi
Introduction	1
Part One The Paradigms	**7**
1. Death-with-Dignity: The Fantasy	9
2. Cardiopulmonary Resuscitation: The Protocol	24
CPR	24
The structure of protocol	37
3. The Royal Humane Society: The Method	49
The Royal Humane Society	50
The Method	72
Part Two The Techniques	**95**
4. Defibrillation: *Scintilla Vitalis*	97
Defibrillation	98
Living and life	106
5. Mouth-to-Mouth: The Lips of a Corpse	124
Artificial and rationalizations	127
6. External cardiac compression: Beating a Dead Horse	154
External cardiac compression	154
Protocol and ritual	162

Part Three The Fantasies	**187**
7. The Media: Getting it Right?	189
Mediated death	190
The pornography of death	210
8. Conclusion: Modern Living/Modern Dying	219
Notes	245
References	263
Index	281

Acknowledgements

Figure 2.1 Tachycardia Algorithm, p. 45. Reproduced with permission, *Advanced Cardiac Life Support* © 1997, Copyright American Heart Association.

List of Abbreviations

ABCD	airway-breathing-circulation-defibrillation
ACEP	American College of Emergency Physicians
ACLS (ALS)	advanced cardiac life support (advanced life support)
AED	automated external defibrillator
AHA	American Heart Association
ATLS	advanced trauma life support
BHF	British Heart Foundation
BLS (BCLS)	basic life support (basic cardiac life support)
CPR	cardiopulmonary resuscitation
ECC system	emergency cardiac care system
ECG (or EKG)	electrocardiogram
EEG	electroencephalogram
ELS	emergency life support
EMS	emergency medical services
ER	emergency room
FBAO	foreign body airway obstruction
GSW	gunshot wound
ICU	intensive care unit
ILCOR	International Liaison Committee on Resuscitation
IPPV	intermittent positive-pressure ventilation
IV	intravenous infusion
JAMA	*Journal of the American Medical Association*
MVA	motor vehicle accident
NALS	neonatal advanced life support
NSR	normal sinus rhythm
PAD	public access defibrillation
PALS	paediatric advanced life support
PEA	pulseless electrical activity
POV	point of view
RHS	Royal Humane Society
VF	ventricular fibrillation
VT	ventricular tachycardia

Foreword

There is one thing that we all know. We do not know when and we do not know how, but we do know that we are going to die. This knowledge is continually disavowed, particularly in contemporary society, but it can never be completely denied. It must be supposition, but a reasonable one, that we all have semi-conscious fantasies of our death: the car crash, cancer, a terrorist bomb. Much of these fantasies will inevitably be informed by the audio-visual representations of death that we consume ever more greedily in the developed world, a consumption in inverse ratio to our declining direct experience of death itself. There can be no question, however, of the most dominant conscious image of modern death; it is a staple of every hospital soap and the well-rehearsed scene begins with a heart attack, a cardiac arrest. This is the signal for frenzied activity by the hospital staff and even more frenzied camera activity by the director as electrodes are applied to the patient's chest in an attempt to restart the heart. The scene is required by its poetics to end with a long, steady shot of the electrocardiograph representing the heart beat pulsing into life or finally terminating in the flat line of death.

It is this scene that is the starting point of John Tercier's brilliant analysis of the contemporary deathbed. For the most striking fact in a book that produces striking facts like a demented magician with a surplus of rabbits is that this cardiopulmonary resuscitation (CPR) procedure is very marginal indeed to a patient's chances of life or death. Yet it occupies a central place in both the general and the medical imaginary of death.

Tercier's explanation of this phenomenon is in large part historical. Much of his book traces the history of this technique from its origins in the attempt to resuscitate victims of drowning to its contemporary form as a comprehensive protocol for maintaining the circulation of oxygenated blood in emergency circumstances. It is a commonplace of recent developments in the history of medicine and science that it is impossible to maintain a simple history in which advances in scientific knowledge are simply applied to the treatment of patients. But I know of no account of the history of medicine that makes as clear the extent to which our phantasmatic representations and investments in the body are written deep into what are supposedly rational histories. Tercier's study of CPR is an exemplary account of a detailed history of applied science – in this case medicine – which leaves us in no doubt whatsoever that the treatment of patients has as much to do with unconscious fears and desires as it has with the development of rational knowledge.

Tercier's book is exemplary because it demonstrates clearly and elegantly that even a recent and specific medical procedure (CPR was first elaborated in 1960) carries within it the most complicated of histories and the most fundamental of fantasies.

The history is simply fascinating. Dull would he be of soul who could read Tercier's account of 'The Institution for Affording Relief to Persons apparently dead from Drowning' (which would become the Royal Humane Society) without being moved to wonder at how complicated is the history of human institutions. Tercier, moving effortlessly from contemporary accounts of drowning to the development of chemistry, shows how the practical desire to revive the drowned in London in the eighteenth century must be linked to both the complicated attempts to understand human life in the new metropolis and to the history of science. Then, to complicate matters further, at exactly the moment when theoretical science and practical philanthropy had given the firmest of bases to mouth-to-mouth resuscitation, theoretical science provided an analysis which meant that a proven therapeutic technique was abandoned. By the 1770s Lavoisier had identified Priestley's 'dephlogisticated air' as oxygen and had given a fundamentally accurate account of respiration, which made clear the centrality of oxygen to human life. But if in a first moment this was used to support the development of mouth-to-mouth techniques which had been developed medically since the 1740s, by 1812 the Humane Society considered the technique harmful and it was banished from its protocols. Thus the most effective means of immediately introducing oxygen into a patient's lungs was banished from medical practice for 150 years. At one level the reason for this is simple: a better understanding of respiration produced the knowledge that the exhaled breath of the rescuer contained higher proportions of carbon dioxide and lower proportions of oxygen. But what is puzzling is that this knowledge was used to support a manual ventilation therapy, which was clearly less effective than mouth-to-mouth resuscitation.

Explanations of this history to date have concentrated on the inadequacy of early nineteenth-century scientific method, but Tercier's explanation takes us well outside any simple understanding of science. First and most evidently, Tercier considers the whole question of our deep psychological aversion to practising mouth-to-mouth resuscitation. However – and here is the originality of his argument – he is not willing to stop with this apparently satisfactory explanation. Rather, he asks what it was about manual ventilation, the replacement therapy, which made it so satisfactory an adjunct to death. The answer he finds is in the violence that it applies to the dying body, for Tercier finds at the centre of our rational treatment of the dying and the dead not a protocol for the saving of life but a ritual for the aversion of death. What makes manual ventilation so attractive a therapy is that it builds into our treatment of the dying some of the most permanent and primitive features of our attitudes to death, in which fear and anger are as important as sympathy and kindness.

In demonstrating that in order to understand both the history and contemporary practice of CPR we must have recourse as much to anthropology and psychology as to scientific and technological progress, Tercier shows, with exemplary scientific rigour, that questions of the body and death can never simply be questions of biology and chemistry. Our therapeutic protocols are also symbolic rituals.

If Tercier had simply achieved the impressive and detailed demonstration of this thesis, then his book would already be a major contribution to our understanding of death. But there is more. Unlike most historians of science and medicine Tercier is a doctor and one who has practised in accident and emergency wards where death is a common occurrence. The book is punctuated by accounts of such deaths. The historical discourse of the book looks for general patterns of explanation of the death bed; the brief prose descriptions attempt to capture the intensity of particular deaths. In the dialectic between the two, a dialectic as much of form as of content, Tercier achieves something rich and strange.

Colin MacCabe
London Consortium
December 2004

Introduction

Saving a life is the ultimate rush.[1]

In the opening scene of the movie, Bringing Out the Dead, *it's night. The flashing red lights of an ambulance are reflected in a black street shiny with rain. The ambulance pulls up to the open door of an apartment building. Paramedics, one thin and pale, the other fat and sweating, haul open the back doors of the ambulance and pull out equipment. The paramedics labour up the dark narrow stairs to the top floor. The door to the apartment is open. An elderly woman in a nightdress points towards the bed. A grey-haired man is lying crosswise on the bed. At the head of the bed, a young woman is giving mouth-to-mouth and the occasional chest compression. A man, kneeling at the foot of bed says: 'It's my Dad. We were just watching TV. And he started punching his chest.' The thin paramedic approaches the bed, leans over the old man. Ear next to nose, listening for breath. At the same time, he checks for a carotid pulse. The paramedics grab the old man by his arms and legs and move him from the bed to the floor. The old man's eyes are rolled back in his head. His arms flop loosely. The thin paramedic kneels at the old man's head. His left hand opens the old man's mouth by pushing down on the stubble-covered chin. He feels for breath. Opens an orange bag. Pulls out the laryngoscope. The fat paramedic slaps electrodes onto the grey-haired chest; sweat drips from the paramedic's chin. The daughter sheds quiet tears. The son gazes anxiously towards bed. The defibrillator is turned on and beeps twice. Thin paramedic attaches an ambubag to ET tube. He turns to daughter. 'I need you to squeeze this once every three seconds.' Sound of defibrillator charging up: 'Breeeeeeeeeeeeeep.'*

2   The Contemporary Deathbed

> Defibrillator paddles are rubbed together to spread the electrode paste. 'Clear! Clear.' 'ZAP!!!' The old man's body convulses. Wife flinches. Daughter shakes her head and looks away. Defibrillator recharges: 'Breeeeeeeeeeeeeeep.' Gasp and tears from daughter. 'Clear! Clear.' 'ZAP!!!' Chest convulses. Daughter screams: 'No more. Please stop.' More tears. 'Breeeeeeeeeeeeeeep.' 'Clear! Clear.' 'ZAP!!!' Body arches and flops back with a thud. Daughter in tears. Bends down to embrace father. The thin paramedic pops the top off an amp of epinephrine. Inserts a needle into IV line. The fat paramedic begins chest compressions. 'One-thousand-one, one-thousand-two, one-thousand-three...' The thin paramedic looks towards the cardiac monitor. A flat green line wavers across the screen.
>
> (Bringing, 1999)

How do we picture ourselves dying? A 'death with dignity' – the darkened room, the family gathered around the bedside, a few murmured farewells, and then an exit 'gentle into that good night'? Essentially, it's a nineteenth-century death: a tubercular death ameliorated by opium, a death that has come to be labelled the 'good death'. Or is it in the lights-flashing, siren-wailing, chest-pumping maelstrom of an ambulance hurtling towards the ER?[2] Certainly, in the last ten years, the two most robust vehicles of popular culture, film and television, have opted for the latter. In films such as *Flatliners* and *Bringing Out the Dead*, and in television shows such as *ER* and *Casualty*,[3] we are confronted, almost nightly, with a technological whirlwind of death.

In this book, I shall give an account of the dominant mode of death in the twenty-first century: the death commonly enacted in our hospitals and portrayed on our TV screens: the hi-tech death of the ER (emergency room) and ICU (intensive care unit). This mode of death is fashioned by a resuscitative protocol: CPR (cardiopulmonary resuscitation).[4] CPR is often presented as modern medicine triumphant. The general public holds the belief that CPR produces survival rates of 50–75 per cent (Schonwetter et al., 1991, p. 295; Mead and Turnbull 1995, p. 39; Diem, Lantos, and Tulsky, 1996, p. 1578; Gordon, Williamson, and Lawler, 1998, p. 780). Unfortunately, in real life, over the last 30 years, overall survival rates for out-of-hospital cardiac arrest have been more in the range of 1.3–6.3 per cent (Nichol et al., 1999, p. 517; Pell, 2003, p. 1375; van Alem, 2003, p. 1312). Given these somewhat disappointing results, why does CPR hold such a prominent place in the medical armamentarium? And why has it become such a powerful icon within popular culture? Why do we continue to fantasize about the 'good' death as the death-with-dignity, while at the same time instituting more and more elaborate versions of its opposite number, and then broadcast them over television and cinema screens?

Analyses and critiques of the modern deathbed have come primarily from the social sciences. Over the last 50 years society's attitudes towards death, our 'denial' of death, and our hopes for a 'good' death have been well documented by authors such as Ariès (1981), Gorer (1965), Illich (1976), Kübler-Ross (1973), and so on. We are accused of being 'unable to accept death and thus unable to deal with the physical, psychological and spiritual approach of death' (Annas, 1994, p. 1240). Death has become 'medicalized', and we lament our unnatural relationship with it (Gorer, 1965; Illich, 1976; Ariès, 1981; Elias, 1985; Baumann, 1992; Baudrillard, 1993; Timmermans, 1999). We castigate ourselves for turning away, hiding from death, refusing to talk about it, abandoning the dying and denying our own mortality. We look back with envy to a golden age when death was a part of everyday life.

Voices have emerged attempting to reverse this trend – to 'revive' the role of death in life (Walter, 1994, pp. 3–4). Social scientists such as Norbert Elias (1985) and Stefan Timmermans (1999), physicians such as Elizabeth Kübler-Ross (1973) and Cicely Saunders (1990) and the general public, through the non-fiction genre of 'pathography',[5] concentrate on demonstrating why our present modes of dying are bad and what must be done to make them better. They seek to rationalize the deathbed in the form of the death-with-dignity. Over the last century, medicine has learned much about the physiology of death and the social sciences much about the psychology of loss. Medicine, though perhaps a little slow on the uptake, has taken in these critiques of modern death and made considerable progress through the inclusion of families, religious mentors and ethicists; through the implementation of advance directives, living wills and do-not-resuscitate (DNR) orders; and through a better understanding of palliative care technologies. And yet, we continue to beat people to death, or less dramatically, we continue to inflict heroic medical procedures on the hopelessly moribund, robbing them of dignity in the last moments of their lives. For a number of years now, medical personnel, while pumping on the chests of the dying, have been asking themselves, 'Why are we beating a dead horse?'

It is odd that in the growing body of thanatological literature there is relative silence from those in clinical medicine – paramedics, nurses, physicians – who see hundreds, even thousands, die. The specialty of palliative care and medical involvement in the hospice movement have, to some extent, given the clinician a voice (Kübler-Ross, 1973; Saunders, 1990; de Hennezel, 1998). But, by and large, those who deal with death every day, on the streets and in ERs and ICUs, remain silent. When they do speak, it is to each other. When they write, it is in odd little walled-off sections at the back of medical journals, wedged in between 'Book Reviews' and 'Correspondence'.[6] What they write is seldom analytical, but more in the mode of the lay pathography: short impressionistic reflections on mortality (Grim, 2000; Huyler, 2000). There are exceptions, but they are few (Nuland, 1994; Mims, 1999). Few attempt to explain why, given our dissatisfaction with the modern deathbed, we have such difficulty changing it (Walter, 1994; Seale, 1998). The intention of this book is not to defend the status quo but to attempt to explain it – explain why it is that we continue to beat a dead horse.

I shall begin with a short examination of what is currently considered the 'good' death – the death-with-dignity – and then go on to look at what is usually presented as its opposite number – the hi-tech death, as determined by the CPR protocol. I will explore the history of resuscitative protocols, from their origins in eighteenth-century instructions for the resuscitation of the drowned employing mouth-to-mouth ventilation, chest compressions and electrical shocks; through the nineteenth century, when each of these techniques went out of favour; to the late twentieth century, when they re-emerged as CPR. I hope to show that the somewhat tortuous course of resuscitation over the last 300 years is the result not only of the history of medical therapeutics, not only of the enduring needs of the psyche at the deathbed, but also of the occult relations between scientific protocol and religious ritual. I shall then move on to look at the role of the media in constructing contemporary fantasies of death, which in turn influence the realities of dying. Finally, I shall look at some of the problems that these relations engender in our treatment of the dying.

I should like to insert a caveat here. This book is meant to be neither a polemic against nor propaganda for CPR. It would be easy to interpret it as either. As we will see in the following chapters, CPR *does* work – for those things that it works for. On the other hand, we continue, apparently against our better judgment, to practise the protocol in situations of obvious futility. My object is not to lay blame, but to seek out why.

I should also like to make an apology. I suspect that what follows may not be easy reading. Not because its concepts are complex or its language difficult (at least I sincerely hope not), but because it deals with issues about which most people have very deep convictions. To those readers who have had a personal and traumatic experience of another's death, I apologize now, for there is no way I can avoid intruding on certain sensibilities; it is the nature of the topic. I can only beg that if I offend, the reader will forgive my clumsiness.

Finally, I should like to acknowledge my debt to Professors Paul Hirst and Dorothy Porter. The book would not have been possible without their comments, critiques, and support. I would like to acknowledge The Francis Fund at the University of California San Francisco. I also wish to recommend two excellent texts. Clive Seale's *Constructing Death: The Sociology of Dying and Bereavement* (1998), though dealing primarily the death-with-dignity (what I term 'the other paradigm'), was invaluable for its insights on the social construction of the deathbed. Stefan Timmermans' *Sudden Death and the Myth of CPR* (1999) was a great help in that it guided me towards many of the issues raised by the paradox of CPR.

Part One
The Paradigms

1
The Death-with-Dignity: The Fantasy

> Anyone can stop a man's life, but no one his death; a thousand doors open onto it.
>
> (Seneca, *Phoenissae* 1. 152)

It must have been about one in the morning when I was called. The sixteen-year-old girl with lymphoma on 4 West was in a lot of respiratory distress. The lymph nodes in her mediastinum had become so enlarged that they were now pressing upon her trachea, obstructing it so that she had to fight for every breath. She had had radiation, which had shrunk them for a while, but only for a while. When I arrived at the nursing station, the charge nurse told me they had put her on maximum oxygen, but with little effect. The patient was agitated and anxious because of her inability to get enough oxygen. I pushed open the door to the girl's room and took a few steps in. My eyes had not yet adjusted to the dim nightlight, when suddenly a figure leapt from the bed. Startled, I jumped. It was the girl's mother, a short, middle-aged woman. She began to apologize, afraid she had been caught breaking some rule. I tried to reassure her, but she remained upset and apologetic. I went over to the bed. Her daughter was awake and conscious, picking and pulling at the ties of the hospital gown. Too breathless to speak, she looked terrified. I took the mother outside the room and explained that we really had few options: I could intubate her, put her on a respirator and perhaps prolong things another couple of weeks; I could do nothing and perhaps she would last a few days; or I could give her morphine to ease the choking sensation and anxiety, but the morphine might stop her breathing entirely. The mother asked whether the morphine would make her comfortable enough to be able to talk. I said I thought so. I started with a small dose, and as it took effect, the girl ceased fidgeting and began to breathe easier. The mother sat in a straight back chair beside the bed and murmured to her daughter. I went out to the nursing station and grabbed a cup of coffee. In fifteen minutes, the mother came out, and said that her daughter was asleep. I checked the girl – and it was merely sleep. I told the mother that when her daughter awoke, if she seemed distressed, to ring the call bell, and I would give more medication. I left. In two hours, I returned; the mother leapt out of the bed, apologized. The girl was again distressed. I gave the morphine. She spoke with her mother. She slept. The leap, the apology, the medication, a little talk, then sleep – this same pattern repeated itself through the night at increasingly shorter intervals. At about 07:30 when I was getting ready to go off, I slipped back in to check on them. Mother and daughter were both asleep in the bed. The mother turned and saw me, but this time did not leap out of bed, did not apologize; she remained lying next to her daughter cradling her head. The girl was dead, and had been for some time.

A thousand doors

As unique as each death is, fantasies of the 'good' death tend to coalesce around identifiable cultural scripts, deathbed discourses or, in the terms I have chosen, paradigms.[1] In this book, I shall follow current literature in maintaining that, despite the enormous variability found in the dying process, two deathbed paradigms have come to dominate contemporary Western culture. One is the well recognized 'death-with-dignity', a cultural item that has been subject to intense scrutiny over the last 40 years. The other is what I have chosen to label the 'hi-tech death' – the breathless, chest-pumping, electricity-sparking explosion of resuscitative activity that occurs on city streets and in hospital ERs.[2]

In the literature of grief and mourning, these two paradigms are often presented as being in opposition to each other (Gorer, 1965; Illich, 1976; Ariès, 1981; Seale, 1998; Timmermans, 1999).[3] The death-with-dignity is presented as the good death, threatened by the violence of the hi-tech death. The hi-tech death is modernity gone awry, led astray by a misguided belief in progress. An increasingly technologically dependent, bureaucratized healthcare system is accused of ignorance, even the active mutilation, of the psychological, social and spiritual dimensions of dying. The hi-tech death is condemned for favouring technique over compassion, hospital over home and the patriarchal power of the physician over the feminine nurturing of the family. It is the 'bad' death. 'Modern medicine has made living better, but ... made dying much worse' (Klinkenborg, 1994, pp. 94–5).

A short history of the deathbed

The classic history of death is Philippe Ariès' *The Hour of Our Death* (1981), which describes dominant deathbed paradigms in Western culture since the Middle Ages. His schema has come under much criticism in the 20 years since its publication. However, it remains a point of reference for most of the literature examining the deathbed. It is in its broad sweep, in most authors' opinions, valid (Houlbrooke, 1989, p. 148; J. Davies, 1994, p. 26; Walter, 1994, p. 116; Campany, 1996, p. 94; Seale, 1998, p. 7). Ariès delineates five models of death, corresponding to succeeding historical eras:

1. 'The tame death', stretching from antiquity to the sixteenth century, was medieval Catholicism's great ritual edifice of the sacramental deathbed (Ariès, 1981, pp. 5–94). The Christian West, for most of its history, constructed biological death not as an ontological end, but as the beginning of a journey to a transcendent and, it was hoped, better world. There was no erasure of being, the soul continued on in heaven – or hell – forever. This was a measured death: social death, that is, the cutting of ties to the living, took place over a lifetime. It might be said to have started at the moment of birth, as consciousness of death was a life-long affair. Sociality even extended beyond biological death, for the living could continue to affect the fate of the dead through their prayers and the dead to affect the fate of the living through their intercessions as saints (D. Davies, 1997, p. 7). In this happy disjunction of biological, social and spiritual death, the finality of death could be legitimately denied (Houlbrooke, 1989, p. 148).[4]
2. 'The death of self' is located by Ariès in the sixteenth and seventeenth centuries (1981, pp. 95–202). It was the Protestant deathbed of declarations of faith, examinations of conscience, settling of accounts and preparation of the soul for heaven. The Reformation closed down purgatory and cut the ties between the living and the dead. Henceforth, it was one's behaviour in this life that determined one's fate after death. Any effort by the living to alter the fate of the dead by prayer, ritual, good works or the purchase of indulgences

was probably in vain. Thus, although ontological death was still forestalled, social death and biological death began to coincide.
3. 'The remote death' Ariès assigns to the eighteenth century (1981, pp. 297–408). The scientific revolution, rationalism and secularism weakened both Catholic and Protestant ritual structures and began to define death as a biological and medical phenomenon. In so far as the reality of the soul began to be questioned (and this was a minority belief), biological and ontological death began to coincide. In this paradigm, the living have no influence over the dead, not least because there is no place for the dead to be, but even more because, for the dead, there is no 'to be'. At the same time, the Enlightenment's revised view of nature (and God's and man's respective places in nature) was chipping away at established religion's political, economic and intellectual hegemony. Most doctors continued to believe in God, and priests continued to bless the dying; but there was now the possibility of examining life and death empirically, understanding both through the exercise of reason. Furthermore, it became permissible to materially affect the dying process through actions based on acquired knowledge (R. Porter, 1993, pp. 1449–68). It was becoming permissible to meddle with death. Though largely unable to reverse the dying process, the eighteenth-century physician could at least attempt to make it bearable through the use of opium, generally available in the West since the sixteenth century (R. Porter, 1999, p. 286). Opium provided unprecedented control over the processes of biological and social death. Through the judicious use of narcotics, one could in many circumstances make them coincide.
4. 'The Romantic death' of the nineteenth century was made possible by a weakening of the belief in eternal damnation and by the effective medical management of pain (Ariès, 1981, pp. 409–58). The good death became a calm, dignified leave-taking, which could be used as an example of man's respectful deference to the laws of nature. A will was written and final bequests bestowed, pious instructions given to survivors, forgiveness sought, blessings dispensed, promises of reunion made, and last words spoken. The business of the deathbed became just that: the tidying and tying up of unfinished business. The process of dying was reconstructed into something no more distressing than a final, peaceful sleep. This Romantic ideal of the Victorian deathbed – the darkened room, the family at the bedside, a few quiet farewells and a drifting off into eternal sleep, modelled on the tubercular death ameliorated

by opium – became the death-with-dignity. In its ideal form, this death was a perfect coincidence of social and biological death, and, although not ruling out ontological continuity, did not necessarily rely on it. The more religious forms of the death-with-dignity still clung to the hope of life everlasting. Its more secular forms found comfort in relief from pain and strife.

5. 'The invisible death' is the twentieth-century death, hidden within institutions, banished not only from vision but also from speech (Ariès, 1981, pp. 559–601). This disappearance of death is blamed on its medicalization. In the nineteenth century, the position of the physician at the deathbed was consolidated through improvements in therapeutic technique, an expanding pharmacopoeia and advances in pathophysiology. These technical advances coincided with an acceleration in the construction of the bureaucratic superstructure that was to become the operational basis for the modern state. In medicine, this was reflected in the growth of hospitals and dispensaries; and in death, by the regularization of death certificates, post-mortems and the storage and disposal of dead bodies (K. Arnold, 1997, pp. 14–24). Throughout the nineteenth and twentieth centuries, as the physician's control and authority over the process of dying increased, death was moved out of the familiar environs of the home to become institutionalized in the hospital and the morgue.[5]

The medicalization of death may be seen as a part of the secularizing process that made the world modern. The move from the care of the soul to the care of the body, from priest to doctor, from home to hospital, from post-mortem religious ritual to ante-mortem medical protocol, from redemption to revival was not the work of the last 50 years but of the last 300. That the secularization of life should be accompanied by the secularization of death should come as no surprise: to live in the modern is to die in it also. In the ideal modern death, biological, social and ontological death not only coincide but are meant to occur in such an instant that, perhaps, the whole business can be ignored, allowed to slip past unnoticed. Hence the invisibility of death.

The death-with-dignity

> When we think of our death, we imagine ourselves surrounded by loving friends, the room filled with a serene quietude that comes from nothing more to say, all business

finished; our eyes shining with love and with a whisper of profound wisdom as to the transiency of life, we settle back into the pillow, the last breath escaping like a vast 'Ahh!' as we depart gently into the light.

(Levine, 1988, p. 8)

Underpinning this image of the ideal death are certain aspirations: the death is under the control of the dying person; they are conscious until very near the time of death; they are surrounded by friends and relatives without being an undue burden on them; the death has meaning for the dying person and matters to others; the death occurs quickly and the pain is bearable; the dying person is treated with respect; the death is 'accepted' by survivors and society. Afterwards, there are rituals and public practices for comforting friends and families (Timmermans, 1999, p. 27). This nexus of desires has come to be thought of as a dignified death. Douglas Davies defines the 'dignity' expected in a death-with-dignity:

> It is often said in contemporary society that many people are not afraid of death but are afraid of the process of dying and of the pain they may suffer at the end of an illness. The word so often used is 'dignity,' as when people speak of wanting to 'die with dignity.' This can be interpreted to mean that wish to retain that status and sense of identity, which they had developed throughout their life. They do not wish to be reduced to some suffering individual, lacking all control and increasingly devoid of their sense of self-worth. (1997, p. 80)

As already stated, the death-with-dignity, in its mode of performance, borrows heavily from the romanticized image of the nineteenth-century tubercular death ameliorated by opium. However, TB is no longer the main villain in the piece. The dignified death of the late twentieth century is modelled primarily on the cancer death and, to a lesser extent, on death from AIDS.[6] It is these particular pathological processes that have become the dominant (albeit by no means exclusive) modes of death within the hospice and palliative care ward. Access to the death-with-dignity is determined not only by cultural preference but by the physical realities of any particular dying process. Cancer and AIDS, like TB, allow the time necessary to cultivate the growth of self-awareness and acceptance of death that are central to the death-with-dignity paradigm. Furthermore, access to the facilities, personnel and technology that enable such a death is limited to a small, albeit influential, section of Western society.[7] Nevertheless, the death-with-dignity remains the ideal in most literature dealing with the good death. 'We ... cling to an image of our final moments that combines grace with a sense of closure' (Nuland, 1994, p. 8). Yet, the deathbed, the locale of this scenario, is a place few of us have visited.

Denial and medicalization

Modern society's denial of death and medicine's institutionalization of the deathbed are blamed for death's removal from daily life; grief is denied its due place in the psychology of the individual and mourning in the social relations of culture (Walter, 1994, p. 122; D. Davies, 1997, p. 38; Seale, 1998, p. 53). Beginning in the 1950s, there began to be speculation that something had gone 'wrong' with death. In *The Pornography of Death* (1965), Geoffrey Gorer maintained that death in the late twentieth century had become as taboo a subject as sex in the late nineteenth. Jessica Mitford's indictment of the funeral industry, *The American Way of Death* (1963), was presaged by Evelyn Waugh's comic novel, *The Loved One* (1948). David Sudnow, in *Passing On: The Social Organization of Dying* (1967), and Ivan Illich, in *The Limits to Medicine* (1976), described the process of the medicalization of death and the abandonment of the dying patient by family and medical staff. Norbert Elias, in *The Loneliness of the Dying* (1985), charted how the civilizing process drew a veil over the animal truths of human existence. Jean Baudrillard, in *Symbolic Exchange and Death*, argued that 'little by little the dead cease to exist. They are thrown out of ... symbolic circulation' (1993, pp. 126–87). Zygmunt Baumann, in *Mortality and Immortality*, suggested that whereas people in traditional societies ate their enemies, incorporating them into the life of the living, modern society vomits them out, designating them as 'Other' (1992, p. 131). Philippe Ariès concludes *The Hour of Our Death* (1981) by blaming the invisibility, impoverishment and 'unnaturalness' of death in the twentieth century on the realization of modernity's secularization project.

During the 1960s, a social movement arose aimed at countering what was perceived as medicine's death-denying hegemony. The publication of Elisabeth Kübler-Ross's *On Death and Dying* (1973) is seen as a turning point in the revival of modern society's interest in death.[8] The founding of St Christopher's Hospice in South London by Dr Cicely

Saunders in 1967, generally taken to be the beginning of the modern hospice movement, was an important step in returning a measure of control over the dying process to the dying patient. Tony Walter has labelled this movement back to the deathbed 'Revivalism' – its aspiration being to 'revive' death in social discourse and return it to everyday life. It is presented as a way of rationalizing the deathbed and restoring dignity to death (1994, pp. 3–4). As used by Walter, the term covers a broad area – hospices, palliative care, grief counselling, 'thanatology', the humanist and New Age funeral and even, to some extent, euthanasia.[9] Though each of these movements is distinct and sometimes in opposition to the others, they have many members in common and an 'open' orientation towards death.

In general, the Revivalist movement, through the promotion of the death-with-dignity, seeks to counter the invisibility of death and what it perceives as modern medicine's abuse of the dying patient. It is, to a large extent, a reaction against inappropriate, overzealous medical interventions, of which my main subject, CPR, is held to be the prime offender. Revivalism in its various forms seeks not to cure, but to palliate – that is, control – pain, anxiety, fear and suffering so as to allow the patient to die 'in character'. In this schema, the dying person is the focus of both the dying process and the mourning that follows. They are allowed to die in the way they choose and their choice is made a visible part of life: their own and that of survivors. The grief of the bereaved is not hidden away, but acknowledged and allowed to take its natural course. The Revivalist movement sees in the denial and invisibility of modern death a gap between private experience and public discourse, which it seeks to correct by turning private experience into public discourse (Walter, 1994, p. 24). This publicizing of the private is presented as a form of therapy, a means of 'healing' through discourse, that is, therapeutic discourse.

Therapeutic discourse

Douglas Davies writes of the importance of 'words against death' (1997, p. 21). Words may be used in consolation to share the burden of pain. They may be part of the rituals that are enacted around the deathbed. They may help give meaning to what appears to be an otherwise meaningless act. They are seen as encouraging a conscious awareness of death, countering denial and invisibility. They lead to the acceptance of death, a necessary precursor to a death-with-dignity. The model used is that of therapy, specifically psychoanalytic therapy. This mode of therapy, the 'talking cure', has been accepted, more or less, by popular culture as a valid means of dealing with psychological and social stress. It is, crudely put, talk – talk that binds the dying, the bereaved and society into a 'caring community', which will sustain the dying, the bereaved and society through the difficult process of loss. The therapeutic discourse that constructs the death-with-dignity becomes the last chapter of an inner journey translated into a coherent narrative of a life lived heroically. It is through this self-shaping discourse that the victim becomes the hero of their own life and 'the chief mourner presiding over their own death' (Seale, 1998, pp. 47, 92–110). The death-with-dignity inscribes the final chapter of the deceased's life, and furthermore writes a dramatic chapter in survivors' life narratives.

Grief is the term used to describe the feelings of the bereaved; mourning, their behaviour (Hertz, 1960, p. 77; Freud, 1984b, pp. 251–67; Freud, 1985b, p. 57–89; Durkheim, 1995, p. 397). Walter maintains that grieving has replaced mourning. Bereaved individuals are encouraged to share their sorrow with one another in emotive discourse, rather than engage in specified behavioural patterns set down by formal social rules. In short, discourse replaces ritual: 'If traditional mourning rituals converted feelings into socially prescribed behavior, then bereavement counseling does the opposite: it translates behavior into feelings' (Walter, 1994, p. 137).

> If modern death is a private affair, and revival encourages the sharing of personal feeling, then neither is conducive to ritual, for ritual is rooted in community and in socially approved, not individually expressed emotion, in symbol more than in memory, in action as much as in talk. The neo-modernist, especially the expressivist, seeks not ritual but talk.... Ritual action around the body and within the community is replaced by talk in a group of strangers facilitated by a psychotherapist. (Walter, 1994, pp. 177–8)

Freud saw religion's prime purpose as being a defence against death (1985c, pp. 43–159). Religion provided a comprehensive and comprehensible narrative by which people could perceive their individual biographical situations as a part of a cosmic order. Science, which has taken over from religion the task of constructing order, when given the task of explaining the deeper mysteries of life and death, is neither so comprehensive nor so comprehensible. With religious ritual discounted and scientific reason deemed inadequate to the task of constructing the self, the modern self is, supposedly, constructed through a continuous conversation with the other. Through discourse, the self expresses itself and in that expression brings its own self into being. Ritual, though paid lip service by the Revivalist movement, is relegated to the role of an adjunct to therapeutic discourse. Its purpose becomes to help people 'open up' and discuss their feelings so that they, and importantly their survivors, might write the final chapter of their life's story and complete the project of the construction of self.[10]

Traditional, modern, post-modern death

Walter points out that Revivalist writers eulogize traditional modes of death. Revivalism longs for a past Golden Age where man had a 'natural' relationship with death. Alienation from nature and from the spiritual is blamed for the crisis of modern death. If we could but learn from the traditions of the past, then much of the anxiety and pain engendered by death and loss might disappear. A return to the wisdom and purity of the past would restore balance to our dealings with death. In a case of ontogeny repeating phylogeny, Revivalism asserts that primitive, unlike modern, cultures know how to *do* death better. Societies that live close to nature are more in tune with a 'natural' way of death, one that is dignified and peaceful.[11]

The death-with-dignity, aspiring to the 'naturalness' of the traditional deathbed and shaped by the dying person, in a culture of individualism that values a unique life uniquely lived, is characterized as 'postmodern'. In the postmodern, individuals are free to appropriate the traditions of the past, free to 'pick and mix' – to pick from an eclectic combination of disparate cultural objects and mix them into their own cocktail of meaning. The postmodern, then, is not a rejection of the modern or of tradition, but a mixing of them without the sense of inconsistency that would shame the true modernist. Revivalist models reject those elements of primitive death that do not fit their assumptions of a Golden Age, while remaining free to use modern medical and pharmacological techniques. This, Walter maintains, is an instance of the 'double coding' which is characteristic of postmodernity, a combination of the modern with an evocation of an imagined tradition (1994, p. 42). But this combination of modern techniques (pain control and therapeutic discourse) with the evocation of an imagined tradition (extended family and death as a passage through sleep to a new awakening) contains a paradox – in that a strong valorization of a traditional form of death heavily dependent upon community and the traditions of community is coupled with praise of personal autonomy, the very thing that has undermined traditional community (Seale, 1998, p. 115).

These tensions surface as contradictions in the exercise of therapeutic discourse. Therapeutic discourse, in its attempt to provide individual solutions to individual deaths, is accused of drifting towards anomie: degenerating into relativistic and relatively meaningless psycho-babble (Walter, 1994, p. 161). In its more institutionalized forms, therapeutic discourse turns into an overly prescriptive algorithm for grieving that becomes as coercive as the medical model it set itself to correct (Seale, 1998, pp. 178–98). These tensions also become apparent in the self-consciously constructed mortuary rituals that Revivalism frequently advocates, which, unfortunately, find difficulty in freeing themselves from parody (Giddens, 1991, p. 38).

Sherwin Nuland offers a possible 'scientific' alternative to both religious ritual and Revivalism:

> I have written this book [*How We Die: Reflection's on Life's Final Chapter*] to demythologize the process of dying. My intention is not to depict it as a horror filled sequence of painful and disgusting degradations, but to present it in its biological and clinical reality, as seen by those who are witness to it and felt by those who experience it. Only by frank discussion of the very details of dying can we best deal with those aspects that frighten us the most. It is by knowing the truth and being prepared for it that we rid ourselves of the fear of the terra incognita of death that leads to self-deception and disillusions. (1994, p. xvii)

Though Nuland's image of the deathbed as scientific and rationalist is quite different from what he characterizes as the sentimentality of the Revivalists' death-with-dignity, his aim is not that different. Nuland also hopes to foster an acceptance of death, not through the sharing of emotions, as in the Revivalist case, but rather through the sharing of facts. This 'medical' discourse gives precedence to biological fact as the basis for a form of existentialism that sees death as the end of existence in any form and, accepting it as such, rewards one with an 'authenticity of being' that is construed as a dignified acceptance of the inevitable.

In practice, therapeutic and medical discourses mix with each other. Physicians, hospice nurses, grief counsellors, psychologists and chaplains are expected to share both emotions and facts in the process of talking the dying and the bereaved through death. What might be seen as making their interventions 'scientific' and not 'religious' (even in the case of the chaplain) is their commitment to the therapeutic model, both medical and psychological. In this model, though disease may be the cause of death, loss, if not death, becomes, like disease, amenable to therapeutic manipulation. The aim of this therapy is the culmination of the modernist project of the construction of 'self' in the coincidence of social, biological and ontological death. Discourse, through the sharing of feelings and the facing of facts, attempts to pull social death forward to the moment of biological death. Medical therapeutics, including resuscitative protocols, attempts to forestall biological death until social death can catch up to it. And both therapeutic discourse and medical therapeutics hope to facilitate the change in being that is taking place by fostering its acceptance.

Therapeutic discourse and medical therapeutics seek to control nature, the nature of our psychic identities and the nature of our animal bodies, coordinating social and biological death, so that ontological death – that is, the translation of being into memory, which is the purpose of mourning in the modern – may occur as quickly and easily as possible, leaving survivors to get on with their lives. Therapeutic discourse, whether sharing emotions or sharing facts, and medical technology, whether the manipulation of opiates or the shock of the defibrillator, aspire to a death so momentary in its coincidence of the biological, the social and the ontological, that perhaps the loss engendered by death might slip past unnoticed. This rationalized death, which aims to tie up death, grief and mourning at the moment of one's last breath, is in its way less a denial of death than a denial of loss. The eternity of extinction for the victim and loss for the survivor becomes masked by an attempt to remove death from time, to make it an instantaneous event. I should emphasize that these are not invalid manoeuvres; the construction of death by culture is arguably the oldest and most consistent characteristic of humanity (Burkert, 1983, p. 3). However, the threat of extinction and the pain of loss are not so easily repressed.

Death denied?

We know that as we live, so shall we die. Though we know the fate that awaits us, while busy living it is difficult to maintain the plausibility of existence while contemplating extinction. Apprehensive of death, it seems necessary that we deny it in order to get on with the business of life. Malinowski (1962, p. 97) observed that religion was in the business of keeping the meaninglessness of suffering and the terror of death at bay. He maintains that denial is a precondition for survival. Constantly preoccupied with thoughts of our own death, participation in society and culture would lose meaning. Religion attempts to hide the reality of death from its members by, if not exactly denying death, certainly denying, through the promise of an afterlife, the possibility of extinction.

The denial of the finality of loss is probably less an affliction of modernity than a characteristic of the human psyche or, at the very least, of social function. Perhaps the charge brought against the medicalization of death in the modern world should be less that of denial, which some would argue is universal, than invisibility. As Seale points out, denial, the psychological repression of death's inevitability, is not the same as death's invisibility, its institutional sequestration (1998. p. 70). The two are all too frequently conflated. Oddly enough, the most effective way of denying death may not be by hiding it. Though invisibility may help us ignore the fact of death, it does little to rescue us from the fear of extinction and the reality of loss. Perhaps that is where the problem lies. In traditional cultures, denial of the finality of death is not an ignoring of death, but rather the opposite. Denial is an active process. Traditional societies deny the finality of extinction and inevitability of loss not by hiding from death, but by giving the impression that death is under control through the public construction of death by ritual (Malinowski, 1974, pp. 51–9). Public ritual is a means of establishing and demonstrating control over death (D. Davies, 1997, p. 16). It is argued that institutional sequestration of death, removing death from the public stage, is less a denial of death than a neurotic repression of it, preventing the very thing it is condemned for fostering – death's necessary and salutary denial (Seale, 1998, p. 70).

Death invisible?

There can be little argument that dying has become institutionally sequestered over the last 50 years. However, to maintain that death has become invisible in contemporary culture is to deny the evidence of our own eyes. Accused of hiding death, we seldom shut up about it. We are encouraged by psychologists, grief counsellors and TV talk show hosts to talk our way through grief. From the DIY of Gill and Fox's *The Dead Good Funerals Book* (1997), to Baudrillard's postmodern semiotics in *Symbolic Exchange and Death* (1993), bookstore shelves groan under the burden of writings on death, dying, grief and mourning. Ken Arnold points out that medicine has become preoccupied with death:

> What in the 1960s was regarded as the 'last taboo' is indeed now emerging as a central issue in almost every medical field. A glance at present-day medical journals reveals that issues such as abortion, selective feticide, terminal care, brain death, transplantation, resuscitation, persistent vegetative state, withdrawal of treatment, euthanasia, physician-assisted suicide and bereavement, fill increasing columns of type. The same issues have a high public profile in today's news ... (1997, p. 6)

However, it is in the popular media where death has really flourished. In spite of our lack of experience with the real thing, we are spectators to more deaths than any prior generation – though these deaths are but seen in the flickering shadows of the television and film screen. In the chapters that follow, I will explore this paucity of experience and surplus of representation, but for the time being it is enough to point out that though we see death, we do not touch it and, so the fear is, are not touched by it.

The contemporary deathbed *is* very different from those that have gone before. Religious ritual has declined. Existential anxiety finds little release in fantasy. For many, the soul persists only as the dim ghost of memory. Biological death is sequestered behind closed doors. Social death is imposed prematurely in retirement villages and nursing homes. The aspiration for instantaneous extinction attempts to mask perpetual loss. The physical real-life experience of the deathbed is replaced by representations of it on television and movie screens. As true as these things are, the contention that death has disappeared from cultural discourse is nonsense: 'All this sounds like a society obsessed with death, not one that denies it .... Death and our feelings about death are no longer taboo but a new radical chic' (Walter, 1994, pp. 1–2).

The limits of modern death

The great religious ritual edifices of the past, which offered shelter to the dying and the bereaved, have fallen into disrepair. 'The melancholy, long, withdrawing roar' of the 'Sea of Faith' has left us stranded on 'the naked shingles of the world' (M. Arnold, 1954, p. 406). One can chart an historical transition in modes of deathbed behaviour from ritual through medical protocol to therapeutic discourse, roughly parallel to manipulations of the soul, the body and the psyche, by religion, medicine and psychology.

> From ancient Egypt onwards, death has been represented as a journey, but the nature of the journey has changed. For centuries, the prayers of the living helped transport the soul of the dead. In the modern era, the doctor helps the dying complete its passage as painlessly as possible. In late-modern death, counselors and doctors and nurses trained in psychology help the dying person to reach Kübler-Ross's final stage of 'acceptance,' while other experts help bereaved people to pass through 'the grief process.' A spiritual journey became a physical one, which in turn is becoming emotional .... The soul is transported through ritual. The body is processed towards death by medical technology and pharmacology. And the psyche is moved towards acceptance (of dying) or resolution (of grief) through talk and through expressing feelings. (Walter, 1994, pp. 57–8)

Today, despite good intentions from all quarters, neither medicine's protocols nor psychology's discourse appear to have been entirely successful in manufacturing the 'good' death. That therapeutic discourse is faltering under the emotional burden of death, I hope the above discussion has at least indicated. Whether the medical protocol of CPR is an appropriate technique for dealing with the failing physiology of the dying body is something that I shall question in the next chapter. What place ritual might still have in our construction of death will be explored in the chapters following that.

2
Cardiopulmonary Resuscitation: The Protocol

At an introductory lecture to an ACLS Provider Course, I was told: 'Hi I'm Jerry.... I want you to introduce yourself to your neighbour on either side of you.... shake hands and say, "I'd rather be here than anywhere else."... Now that you know each other, you trust each other, you know us, all securities are met .... People die don't they? It's part of life. There are three phases to life – pre-arrest, arrest, and post-arrest. What causes death? We're talking about premature death. Father, husband, child; these people can be saved. It only takes the push of a button to save a life.... It's something you can do. You can bring the patient back, right in front of the family. There's no words to describe the feeling you get when you save someone's life .... Within the healthcare system, ACLS has become the "standard of care" and you are not only expected to apply it, and apply it correctly when you are confronted by a cardiac arrest, but you are legally liable if you do not. Of course, that is only in the hospital or as part of your job, if you are a paramedic, fireman, lifeguard, or anyone else who is considered to have a "duty of care". Are people in the grocery store, at the post office, in the line at the bank expected to give medical care? As a private individual walking down the street on a Sunday morning, you are under no legal obligation to provide resuscitation, but CPR is part of mankind's effort to assist their fellow man. It's part of our nature.... Everyone can be taught CPR; people learn it off the TV.... The American Heart Association is "Fighting for Your Life".'

Cardiopulmonary resuscitation

Resuscitative protocols, though varying in content depending upon circumstances, are all based, to greater and lesser extents, on the originary and still dominant resuscitative protocol of CPR – CardioPulmonary Resuscitation. In the early 1960s, the union of airway manoeuvres, mouth-to-mouth ventilation and external cardiac compression into a single life-saving protocol brought CPR into being. This protocol showed great promise and quickly became standard practice within hospitals (Lombardi et al., 1994, p. 678; Cummins et al., 1985, p. 114; Eisenberg, 1997, p. 30). CPR has, over the last 40 years, become the medical, legal and media standard for behaviour in the face of sudden death.

> Early cardiopulmonary resuscitation (CPR) improves survival for victims of out-of-hospital cardiac arrest. Over the past 25 years, clinical research has consistently validated the standard 'abc' sequence of modern CPR that is, airway patency – or opening, breathing – via MMV [mouth-to-mouth ventilation] and circulation – via chest compression. Based on both the success of CPR in the clinical setting and the physiological principles governing circulation and respiration, the established AHA [American Heart Association] protocol for CPR entails a MMV [mouth to mouth ventilation] sequence of 10–12 breaths per minute, with each breath followed by five chest compressions.[1] Although swift provision of defibrillation[2] – the process of electronically restoring heart rhythm – is recognized as the most significant determinant of successful resuscitation, conventional CPR can extend the window of time available for providing such treatment. In cities such as Seattle and Houston, where a multitude of citizens have been trained in CPR, the performance of immediate resuscitation efforts by bystanders has pushed the survival rates above 40 per cent in cases where a victim's collapse is witnessed and rapid defibrillation is subsequently delivered by the local EMS.[3] (Laurent, 1997)

Over the last 200 years, the traditional demographic of death, characterized by relatively high infant mortality rates and short life spans, has changed markedly. In 1750 the average Frenchman lived to about 27 years, the average Englishman to 36 (R. Porter, 1999, p. 281).[4] In 1996 in the USA, life expectancy at birth was 73.8 years for white males, 79.6 years for white females, 66.1 years for black males and 74.2 years for black females (CDC, 2004). However, in parts of sub-Saharan Africa life expectancy is still as low as 40 years. In first world countries, heart disease is the leading cause of death, accounting for about 30 per cent of deaths. Heart disease is followed closely by cancer (prostate, lung and colon in males; and breast, colon and lung in females). Most of these deaths (84 per cent) are in people over the age of 65 ('From', 1997, p. 1263; Neumar and Ward, 1998, p. 36). Deaths under the age of 40 account for only 6 per cent of all deaths. In this age group, the leading cause of death (63 per cent) is trauma (motor vehicle accidents, drowning, fire, homicide and suicide) (Guyer, Marti and MacDorman, 1997, p. 905). Death in the West has become almost entirely a 'disease' of the elderly. Living longer, each individual is encountering death later in their own lives and in the lives of others. As birth rates have dropped, families have decreased in size and the individual has become more isolated within society, and each person is exposed to fewer 'significant' deaths. It is now, thankfully, rare for a mother to bury her child, a teenage boy his sister, a working man his nursing wife. It is no longer uncommon to have no experience of the loss of a family member until one is well past the age of 40.

Based on these remarkable changes in the demography of death, one might think that sudden, premature or unnatural death would have become less of an anxiety. However, and perhaps somewhat paradoxically, by successfully pushing death into old age and the dying into institutions, medicine has increased the number of unexpected and 'unnatural' deaths. In our youth-oriented culture, with medical technology continually pushing back the threshold of old age, even the elderly are no longer considered senescent enough to be fit candidates for death. The category of 'natural' death, though much praised, is seldom invoked for any but the exceptionally ancient. Almost all death has come to be considered unnatural and unexpected.

Sudden death is formally defined as 'death within 24 hours of symptom onset in a previously functional individual' (Neumar and Ward, 1998, p. 36). Seventy-five per cent of sudden death (excluding trauma) is attributed to cardiovascular disease (Neumar and Ward, 1998, p. 36). There are about 450,000 deaths in the USA each year from out-of-hospital cardiac arrest (*American*, 2002). More generally, sudden death is equated with a death that is unexpected, premature, accidental or unnatural.[5] Sudden, unexpected death occurs to the wrong person in the wrong place at the wrong time in the wrong way for the wrong reason. The sudden death, as an unnatural death, is always constructed, in fantasy, if not in fact, as a potentially reversible death: physically, psychologically and morally. The unnatural death *qua* unnatural embraces hope, and the possibilities of prevention, reversal or justice. It is against the injustice of sudden death that the fantasy of resuscitation operates:

> [Those who die] from potentially reversible conditions imposed by the arbitrary mischances of Nature, before they have time to live full lives, should receive the benefits of emergency resuscitation, if there

is a chance that life with human mentation can possibly be restored. (Safar, 1977, p. 297)[6]

Sudden death becomes a call to action.

ABCD

> Matt (30), from Cambridge, realised the value of emergency life support skills when he saved the life of a passer-by in the street. He learned CPR when he trained as a policeman and it was not long before he used his skills in the streets of Cambridge. 'I was on patrol when I saw the lady collapse. I checked to see if she was breathing, and then we took turns to give chest compressions and mouth to mouth. The ambulance crew arrived a few minutes later and shocked her with a defibrillator. I later heard that she had survived and was recovering well.
>
> (British Heart Foundation, 2001)

CPR aims to prevent sudden death from cardiac arrest by maintaining the cardiac, respiratory and neurological systems until definitive treatment can correct whatever defect is responsible for their failure. At the core of CPR is the American Heart Association's ABCD mnemonic:

Airway: Manoeuvres to remove obstructions in the respiratory tract.[7]
Breathing: Artificial ventilation, for example, mouth-to-mouth, providing air to the lungs and thus oxygen to the blood.
Circulation: External cardiac compressions, preserving circulation of blood by maintaining the pumping action of the heart.
Defibrillation: Electrical shocks to restart the stalled heart, reversing abnormalities of cardiac rhythm preventing the circulation of blood. Defibrillation was, prior to the early 1990s, restricted to ACLS providers.
(American, 1994, p. 1–4)

CPR is a generic resuscitative protocol and is subsumed within both Basic Life Support (BLS) and Advanced Cardiac Life Support (ACLS).[8] Further refinements have produced different versions of the resuscitative protocol to deal with age specific and causal variations in cardiac arrest, for example:

NALS = Neonatal Advanced Life Support
PALS = Paediatric Advanced Life Support.
ATLS = Advanced Trauma Life Support.

Though there are significant differences among the above, they are all based on the fundamental techniques of CPR aimed at maintaining lung, heart and brain function. The latest recensions of CPR, BLS and ACLS are set out in *Guidelines 2000* published by the AHA.[9]

Cardiac arrest

> *Barry Wilkinson, from Devon was keeping fit at his local leisure centre when he found out how important emergency life support skills really are. He was using the rowing machine when he had a heart attack and collapsed. Fortunately, staff were on the scene within seconds with a British Heart Foundation funded defibrillator. Staff used their CPR training to keep him alive before shocking his heart back into a normal rhythm. Barry says; 'I can't remember anything, but if the staff weren't trained in life support skills I wouldn't be here today.'*
>
> (British Heart Foundation, 2001)

CPR is used to treat cardiac arrest. Cardiac arrest is the loss of cardiac activity as evinced by lack of pulse, breath and consciousness. Cardiac arrest results in the loss of circulation to the vital triad of head, heart and lungs. Loss of circulation to the brain:

- for ten seconds, results in a loss of oxygen supply causing unconsciousness;
- for 2–5 minutes, in the depletion of glucose, glycogen and adenosine triphosphate (ATP) stores in the brain cells;
- for greater than 4–5 minutes, in irreversible loss of neurological function, that is, brain death.

This pattern of loss is then repeated in the heart, followed by the other organs of the body, and finally the organism as a whole. All death, at some point, is triggered by loss of heart or lung or brain function, and then a combination thereof.

Cardiac arrest may be primary or secondary. In primary cardiac arrest, commonly termed a 'heart attack', the heart itself is the site of the initial malfunction. Primary cardiac arrest is most commonly due to atherosclerotic coronary artery disease. The coronary arteries supply the heart with blood. Narrowing of them is caused by a decades-long build-up of intra-arterial plaque. This may then be complicated by a rapid sequence of sudden plaque rupture, platelet adhesion and an occluding thrombus (blood clot). The arterial obstruction leads to areas of heart muscle suffering decreased levels of oxygen (myocardial ischaemia), which may result in cell death (myocardial infarction [MI]). Myocardial ischaemia also causes irritability in the electrical system controlling the heart's rhythm. Abnormal rhythms (arrhythmias) may be generated, some of which are incapable of maintaining the circulation of blood and thus are quickly fatal.

Arrhythmias are classified according to their characteristic electrical pattern on the electrocardiogram (ECG) (Einthoven, 1950, p. 275). The most common fatal arrhythmias are ventricular fibrillation (VF), ventricular tachycardia (VT), pulseless electrical activity (PEA) and asystole, though there are others.[10] The most common lethal arrhythmia is ventricular fibrillation, which is best treated by defibrillation. As already pointed out, heart disease is the chief killer in the developed world, accounting for about 30 per cent of all deaths. According to the AHA, of the 1.5 million Americans who suffer heart attacks annually, 300,000–500,000 will die, half of those within the first hour of the attack (Stratton and Niemann, 1998, p. 449).

Secondary cardiac arrest occurs in situations where the initial defect is in an organ other than the heart. The prime example of this is cardiac arrest secondary to respiratory failure (for example, drowning). When the lungs fail, there is decreased oxygen delivery to all the organs of the body, including the heart, which then ceases to function due to the loss of oxygen supply.

> *Young mum, Sarah Grey from Wells in Somerset, put her ELS [emergency life support] skills to use when an 18 month old child in her care got a plastic lid lodged in her throat. Sarah said; 'Ellie was frightened and I knew I had to act quickly. But thanks to my Heartstart training, I remained calm and confident and was able to stop her from choking.'*
>
> (British Heart Foundation, 2001)

Respiratory failure, although the most common, is not the only cause of secondary cardiac arrest. Trauma, head injury, shock (a drop in blood pressure below levels necessary to perfuse vital organs), poisons and metabolic derangements may all cause secondary cardiac arrest.

What unites both primary and secondary cardiac arrest is the endpoint, death. The loss of the vital functions of head, heart and lungs ends in death. Thus, the final stages of a number of different pathophysiological processes are similar enough so as to benefit from the application of the ABCDs of CPR.

The chain-of-survival

> The ECC [emergency cardiovascular care[11]] endeavor [has] been likened to links in a chain. If any link is weak or missing, the chance of survival is lessened, and the EMS system is condemned to poor results .... The most important link in the ECC system in the community is the layperson. Successful ECC depends on laypersons' understanding of the importance of early activation of the EMS system, their willingness and ability to initiate effective CPR promptly, and their training in and safe use of AEDs [automated external defibrillators].[12] Accordingly, providing lifesaving BLS at this level can be considered primarily a public, community responsibility.
>
> (American, 2000, p. I.1)

For CPR to be effective, it must be administered in an ordered and timely fashion. It is subject to what the AHA terms the 'chain-of-survival', which entails:

1. Early access: recognition of early warning signs, emergency telephone number, ambulance (EMS) dispatch.
2. Early CPR: bystander CPR.
3. Early defibrillation: short defibrillation response times, access to AEDs.
4. Early advanced care: ACLS response teams, short transport times, hospitals capable of reperfusion therapies (Cummins et al., 1991a, p. 1832).[13]

The chain-of-survival is presented as a relay race – a set of acts performed by different individuals cooperating in a temporal series. The patient is the baton and life the prize. The cardiac arrest patient, progressing from street to ambulance to ER to ICU, is passed from lay rescuer to paramedic to emergency medicine specialist to cardiologist, ideally undergoing BLS then ACLS then reperfusion therapy. This progress – from street to institution, from layperson to professional, from lifesaving protocol to definitive care, from death to life – is presented by medicine, accepted by the general public and represented in popular culture as an example of modern medical science triumphant.[14]

58-year-old Charles Slaven was recently saved by staff at his local gym when he collapsed with a cardiac arrest. He says; 'I am only alive today because onlookers knew about ELS [emergency life support] and the part it plays in the 'chain of survival'. If there had been just one 'weak link' then I probably wouldn't be here to tell the tale so I'm urging people to ask themselves, 'Would I know what to do?'

(British Heart Foundation, 2001)

A short history of CPR[15]

The 'birth' of CPR is usually dated at 16 September 1960, when Peter Safar, William Kouwenhoven and James Jude presented to a meeting of the Maryland Medical Society in Ocean City recommendations for combining mouth-to-mouth ventilation with chest compressions (Benson, 1961, p. 398; Safar et al., 1963, p. 34; American, 1966, p. 373).[16] Later that year, Safar, Brown and Holtey added the triple airway manoeuvre to mouth-to-mouth ventilation, external cardiac compressions and electrical defibrillation to produce what is now recognized as the CPR protocol. This they published in the *Journal of the American Medical Association* under the title: 'Ventilation and Circulation with Closed-Chest Cardiac Compressions in Man' (1961, p. 574). In February 1962, the AHA's Ad Hoc Committee on Closed Chest Cardiac Resuscitation proposed the term cardiopulmonary resuscitation and the acronym CPR. In September 1963, The AHA formed the Committee on Cardiopulmonary Resuscitation. The protocol they recommended received formal backing from the National Academy of Sciences-National Research Council. The recommendations of the National Research Council's Ad Hoc Conference on Cardiopulmonary Resuscitation were published in the October 1966 issue of the *Journal of the American Medical Association*, becoming, in essence, the first CPR manual (American, 1966, p. 373).

Initially, the technique was restricted to trained medical personnel. The AHA and American Red Cross were hesitant to sanction its teaching to the lay public for fear of inappropriate application and complications due to incorrect technique. In 1964, a grassroots lay organization, Resuscitators of America, began to teach CPR to the lay public. It was not given recognition by the AHA and fizzled out in 1968. In Seattle in 1972, Leonard Cobb began the first AHA-sanctioned CPR training programmes for laypersons. In 1973, the Second National Conference on Standards for CPR and Emergency Cardiac

Care (ECC) launched an extensive campaign to train the lay public in CPR (American, 1974, p. 833). The responsibility for research, training, dissemination and maintenance of the protocol was taken up by the AHA and became an integral component of its institutional structure. Their goal was to train the public, starting with schoolchildren in the eighth grade. The AHA convened subsequent conferences on CPR in 1973, 1980, 1986, 1992 and 1999 to review the current state of knowledge, update resuscitative procedures and publish those results in the form of new editions of BLS and ACLS manuals.

The promotion of CPR training constitutes one of the largest public health campaigns ever conducted in the US. Between 1973 and 2000 more than 70 million Americans learned CPR (American, 2000, pp. I.22–I.59). 'Many public health experts consider CPR training to be the most successful public health initiative of modern times. Millions of people have been willing to prepare themselves to take action to save the life of a fellow human being' (Cummins, 2001, pp. 41–2).

> *Barbara Miller, from Ayrshire, administered life-saving CPR when a man collapsed in front of her on a busy street. Barbara, who learnt ELS through the Heartstart initiative, kept the gentleman alive until the ambulance arrived. She adds: 'I was shocked and distressed that I was the only person at the scene who knew what to do.'*
>
> (British Heart Foundation, 2001)

Life-saving courses run by organizations such as the Royal Life Saving Society and the American Red Cross were gradually pre-empted, co-opted by or themselves adopted the AHA's CPR protocol. CPR was 'snatching life from the jaws of premature death' (Eisenberg, 1997, p. xi). This bold declaration appeared to be borne out, with survival rates as high as 49 per cent in early studies (Jude, Kouwenhoven and Knickerbocker, 1961, p. 1063; Eisenberg, 1979, p. 1905; Cobb et al., 1980, p. 453; Cummins et al., 1985, p. 114).

> Resuscitation ... may truly be called a miracle. Death, the eternal and dreamless sleep, was not permanent. Life was restored – a feat consigned to the gods or fantasy in previous generations. True, it wasn't the ultimate miracle of immortality itself – death is, after all, still inevitable. But its premature visitation, though allowed to cross the threshold of mortality, could now unceremoniously be ushered back. Sudden and untimely death was reversed. (Eisenberg, 1997, p. 30)

'The myth of CPR' (?)[17]

There were numerous attempts to duplicate the results of the early studies. Most were disappointing. Long-term survival rates[18] in the largest cities in the US throughout the 1980s and 1990s were in the range of 1.3–5 per cent, though some mid-sized urban areas with excellent emergency medical systems achieved survival rates of 15–35 per cent (Cobb, Werner and Trobaugh, 1980, p. 31; Eisenberg et al., 1980, p. 812; Eisenberg et al., 1990, p. 179; Becker et al., 1991, p. 355; Becker, Smith and Rhodes, 1993, p. 86; Lombardi et al., 1994, p. 678; Gallagher, Lombardi and Gennis, 1995, p. 1922; Sweeney et al., 1998, p. 234). Since the revision of the protocol in *Guidelines 2000* to include first-responder and bystander defibrillation with AEDs, there has been improvement in survival rates in the special case of: witnessed arrest, initial rhythm ventricular fibrillation, bystander CPR within four minutes and defibrillation within six minutes. In these special cases, long-term survival rates have been reported as high as 34–58 per cent, though most centres report survivals in the 12–20 per cent range, and some even lower (Beck and Leihnenger, 1962, p. 357; Karch et al., 1998, p. 249; Valenzuela et al., 1998, 414; Nichol et al., 1999, p. 517; Stiell, 1999, p. 44; Stiell et al., 1999, p. 1175; De Maio et al., 2000, p. 142; Bunch, 2003, p. 2626; Culley et al., 2004, p. S1525).[19] Though the whole thing must be ringed by qualifications and caveats, it is probable that for out-of-hospital cardiac arrest, long-term survival rates of 10–20 per cent for all rhythm groups and 40–50 per cent for witnessed ventricular fibrillation with very early defibrillation are not unreasonable expectations in the present system with the current technology (Nichol et al., 1999, p. 517; De Maio et al., 2000, p. 139, Valenzuela et al., 2000, p. 1206).[20] Since 2000, defibrillation has gradually taken increased precedence over mouth-to-mouth and external chest compressions in BLS, and complicated drug regimens in ACLS. These changes in the protocol over the last few years will be discussed in the chapters that follow.

This is a controversial topic in contemporary medicine. The assessment of resuscitative protocols is extremely complex. Definitions of what constitutes 'success' vary. The sudden and serious nature of cardiac arrest makes the mounting of random control trials, the 'gold standard' for the assessment of therapeutics, difficult. There are problems of informed consent in the unconscious patient. Despite 40 years of research, there is no comprehensive database devoted to CPR collecting, collating and interpreting data to track the success or failure of resuscitative attempts (such as the cancer and cystic fibrosis registries). There is a lack of standardization of data, though this has been addressed to some extent by the introduction of the Utstein criteria in 1991 (Cummins et al., 1991b, p. 960; Gallagher, Lombardi and Gennis, 1995, p. 1922; Nichol et al., 1999, p. 517; Timmermans, 1999, pp. 68–73). Meta-analysis, which uses statistical methods to combine the results of multiple studies, is proving helpful in clarifying some of the conflicting results between studies. Large, prospective, multi-centre cohort studies, such as the OPALS (Ontario pre-hospital advanced life support) study, are underway and are beginning to produce significant results (Stiell, 1999, p. 44; Stiell et al., 1999, p. 1175).

Factors that have the largest effects on survival rates include the following.

1. *Presenting rhythm*: If the presenting rhythm is ventricular fibrillation or ventricular tachycardia (VF/VT) as opposed to PEA or asystole, success rates are higher. In ideal circumstances where the arrest is witnessed by EMS personnel and defibrillation is timely, there can be survival rates as high as 34–58 per cent for VF/VT as opposed to only 2.4 per cent for PEA/Asystole (Beck and Leihnenger, 1962, p. 357; De Maio et al., 2000, p. 142; Bunch, 2003, p. 2626; Culley, 2004, p. S1525) and essentially 0 per cent for asystole (Bonnin et al., 1993, p. 1460). Van Walraven showed that unless a patient met one of three criteria –

- arrest was witnessed,
- initial rhythm was VF/VT,
- the patient regained a pulse within the first ten minutes of resuscitation,

their chance of discharge from hospital were 0.09 per cent, and return to pre-arrest function, 0 per cent (2001, p. 1602). However, VF/VT is the initial rhythm in only 20–39 per cent of cases of cardiac arrest (though it may be as high as 70 per cent in selected populations) and asystole in up to 41 per cent (Bonnin et al., 1993, p. 1460; Saklayan, Liss and Markert, 1995, p. 163; Valenzuela et al., 2000, p. 1206). The presenting rhythm is not something that either the protocol or the rescuer has much control over, though the earlier the intervention, the more likely that the rhythm will be VF/VT, and the more likely it will be to respond to treatment.

2. *Early defibrillation*: A short time to defibrillation is probably the most significant factor in improving survival rates of VF/VT (Cummins

et al., 1985, p. 114). The chance of survival decreases 7–10 per cent for every minute that passes without defibrillation. A number of studies claim that defibrillation at less than six minutes can double survival rates (Eisenberg, Copass and Hallstrom, 1980, p. 1379; Stults et al., 1984, p. 219; Olson et al., 1989, p. 806; Vukov et al., 1988, p. 318; Mosesso et al., 1998, p. 200; White, Hankins and Bugliosi, 1998, p. 145; Davis, McCrorry and Mosesso, 1999, p. 60; Hurlitz et al., 1999, p. 121; Culley et al., 2004, p. S1525). Between 6 and 11 minutes there is still an increase in survival with every minute that is saved (van Walraven et al., 1998, p. 544; Nichol et al., 1999, p. 517). Anything after 11 minutes is usually too late, with survival rates for VF/VT of only 2–5 per cent (Blouin and Moore, 1999, p. 517; Niemann et al., 1999, p. S4; American, 2000, pp. I.22–I.59). Defibrillation is good for what it is good for – witnessed VF/VT (see chapter 4).

3. *Early bystander CPR*: There are improved survival rates with early bystander CPR (Lombardi et al., 1994, p. 678; Gallagher, Lombardi and Gennis, 1995, p. 1922; Nichol et al., 1999, p. 517; Stiell, 1999, p. 44). Four minutes is considered as being the upper limit of the 'golden period' in which the commencement of CPR is most useful. The rate of bystander CPR varies greatly between different communities, and in most places is in the range of 10–30 per cent; even Seattle, with its comprehensive education programmes, has a rate of only 50 per cent (Becker, 1999, p. 353; Stiell et al., 2003, p. 1939).

4. *Secondary arrest*: Cardiac arrests secondary to hypoxia (respiratory arrest) have better survival rates than those due to primary cardiac failure (van Walraven et al., 2001, p. 548).

The presently accepted normothermic arrest time (that is, cardiac arrest with no CPR and thus no blood flow to the brain in a patient who is not hypothermic), which is reversible without brain damage, is five minutes. It should be noted that CPR commenced later than five minutes after arrest coupled with defibrillation administered later than ten minutes after arrest has, in general, a 0 per cent survival rate (Cummins et al., 1985, p. 114). The average ACLS ambulance response is ten minutes (Safar, 1996, p. 8S). This time gap is also the period in which defibrillation shows the greatest improvement in success rates. It is becoming increasingly apparent that the most important factor in improving survival rates is decreasing time to defibrillation, ideally to less than three minutes after collapse. The crucial question is whether CPR can maintain a circulation adequate to the metabolic needs of the two most vital organs, the heart and the brain, until definitive treatment (that is, defibrillation), is available.[21] Some say 'Yes'; some say 'No'. The marginal ability of CPR to maintain circulation is the major reason why the use of AEDs is now being pushed so strongly, in the hope that by putting defibrillation in the hands of the layman, it can be administered within the 'golden period' of less than six (or even three) minutes, and thus obviate the need for prolonged circulatory support.

The point of this short review of survival following CPR is not to come up with definitive survival rates or a definitive answer about the effectiveness of CPR. Rather, my point is to highlight some of the controversies and to demonstrate that, though CPR is effective, it is much less effective than is generally thought. And, that though survival rates are improving, they are doing so on the basis of changes in the protocol that are making it quite other than what it initially was.[22]

This is an area in which it is difficult to sort the wheat from the chaff, and I have come to my own conclusions. CPR is a protocol of proven but limited clinical efficacy. It is effective – but much less so than is generally thought.[23] Its disappointing results are due, largely, to the nature of the conditions it sets out to correct. The protocol is not called on except *in extremis* – when the chances of reversing the dying process are already very slim. CPR *is* better than no CPR. Effective CPR *is* better than ineffective CPR. Early CPR *is* better than late CPR. Its techniques *are* effective for what they are effective for, that is, defibrillation for witnessed cardiac arrest due to VF/VT and mouth-to-mouth ventilation for respiratory arrest. Survival rates, though well below public expectation, are still significant, especially if you are one of the survivors. Nevertheless, CPR has not proven to be the panacea for sudden death that was hoped for in the early 1960s; overall average rates for long-term survival for all cases of out-of-hospital cardiac arrest continue to hover around the 5–6 per cent range. What can be stated with some certainty is that expectations of the protocol continue to outstrip its capabilities. CPR *has* failed to live up to its early promise, the hopes of the public and its heroic image on television and cinema screens (see chapter 7).

Disappointment with the protocol has resulted in increased criticism from both outside and within medicine. Based on its poor survival statistics, the sociologist Stefan Timmermans, in *Sudden Death and the Myth of CPR*, points out that the dehumanizing violence of resuscitative protocols simply does not appear justified by their empirical success or, rather, lack thereof. He ascribes this illogical behaviour to society's denial of death, medicine's enthralment by technology and the politics of the healthcare system. He points to the powerful coalition of acute care medicine, certificatory and educational bodies such as the AHA, the government, courts and insurers, which all have a vested interest in the perpetuation of the protocol. Individual physicians are condemned for allowing themselves to be blinded by the technological imperative of a positivist worldview – if it *can* be done, it *should* be done – and the general public is reproached for colluding with medicine in the denial of death, for allowing itself to be co-opted into a fantasy of immortality (1999, pp. 56–89). All these accusations must be taken seriously.

Such a critique of the 'medicalization' of death is part of a well-established tradition, which sees physicians so blinded by science or enamoured of power that their duty to their patients becomes distorted or displaced (Gorer, 1965; Illich, 1976; Ariès, 1981; Elias, 1985; Baumann, 1992; Baudrillard, 1993). And there is no question that the above factors do operate and do, at least in part, explain the apparent folly of CPR. There is no doubt that the medical system as a whole and individual physicians within it have very real stakes, personally, professionally and institutionally, in the success of resuscitative protocols. The politics of medicine as a powerful late-modern institution and the limitations of a society that denies death *do* conspire in the promotion of the protocol. However, though these may be necessary, they are not sufficient cause.

The structure of protocol

CPR is a medical protocol. In general, a therapeutic protocol gives instructions for the performance of a specific series of acts aimed at a return to normal function. This series of acts (for example, CPR) is dictated, ideally, by physiological theory and empirical evidence, and it is formulated, or at least approved, by an authoritative body (for example, the AHA). Protocols are called into play in the face of doubt – where choices are not clear and judgment is suspect, where there is a significant lack of predictability in the results of the actions taken. Protocols guide us through the hinterlands of empiricism where cause and effect are insecurely wed.

The survival of a protocol depends not only upon the empirical success of its component techniques but, just as crucially, upon a logically consistent theory binding those techniques into a coherent whole greater than the sum of its parts. Protocol is not merely a random grouping of techniques but has a highly organized structure enacted according to a specific logic. In its practice, a protocol is a rigidly defined, algorithmically structured, decision tree validated by an underlying theory of function. Psychologically, a protocol allows us to put our faith in a higher authority, the expertise embodied by the certifying institution, rather than rely on our own knowledge and judgement. Symbolically, a protocol is an expression of universality, conformity and the exercise of power.

Universality

> The development of modern cardiopulmonary-cerebral resuscitation has given every person the ability to challenge death anywhere.
>
> (Safar, 1996, p. 3S)

Like many other examples of deathbed therapeutics, the CPR protocol was formulated in the hope that it might prove to be a panacea – a uniform, unified and universal response to a comprehensive set of terminal conditions causing sudden death.

> The ILCOR [International Liaison Committee on Resuscitation] Universal Algorithm and the Comprehensive ECC Algorithm are the only teaching/learning displays rescuers will need because they treat everyone in cardiac arrest this way. (American, 2000, pp. I.136–I.165)

CPR was developed to deal primarily with cardiac arrest as the result of ventricular fibrillation caused by coronary artery disease. However, it has always aspired to application to all forms of sudden death. In *Guidelines 2000*, we see BLS expanded to cover burns, electrocution, lightning injury, poisoning, near-drowning, haemorrhage, head trauma and seizures. ACLS manuals now have sections on stroke, asthma, anaphylaxis, drug overdoses, toxins, hypothermia, trauma and electrolyte abnormalities (American, 2000, pp. I.165–I.229).

The protocol aspires to universality in more than just its indications; it also works towards universality in terms of who applies it: 'Everyone can learn [CPR] and everyone should' (American, 2000, pp. I.77–I.85).

> Whether we think of ourselves as AHA delegates or European Resuscitation Council delegates matters nothing. We are now the World's Resuscitation Council; we hold a sobering responsibility to

rise above national pride and self-interest and work together to achieve our simple goal – to reduce morbidity and mortality from cardiovascular and cardiopulmonary disease .... Throughout the process of writing the International Guidelines 2000, the Senior Science Editors and the Editorial Board have attempted to create a work that is geopolitically neutral .... Research is needed to identify the best content, process, and structure of the curricula. Such a program will ensure widespread dissemination of CPR and other BLS skills to citizens around the world. (American, 2000, pp. I.1–I.11)

The universality of the protocol operates on a number of levels. It is universal in its technique (the unity of the algorithm), in its practice (anywhere, anytime), in its application (by anyone to anyone) and in its function (the reversal of all forms of cardiac arrest). Most importantly, it is motivated by a universal value – life.

Despite its aspirations, the CPR protocol is, in fact, no panacea. Its universality is both a strength and a weakness. The CPR protocol, in generalizing technique, provides an easily remembered and comprehensive response to sudden death, but in so doing it sacrifices specificity and, though it claims not to, restricts the exercise of judgement in the particular instance. It is a statistical gamble that does not always pay off. Not all of its actions are appropriate to all its applications. It has been argued that the universalizing ambitions of the CPR protocol are the consequence of the medicine's inability to admit that not all deaths can be reversed and hi-tech, critical-care medicine's protection of its technical expertise (Timmermans, 1999, pp. 57, 97). There is no doubt that both these factors are key in the protocol's universalizing tendency and its rapid growth. However, important as the denial of death and the power politics of modern medicine are, the drive towards universality is a force inherent in the very structure of protocol, all protocol.

Modern medical protocols answer the call to universality through the use of algorithms. An algorithm is a logically branching decision-making progression represented by a mnemonic image somewhere between table and diagram, text and image, instruction and narrative, to produce something akin to a map of action. If something happens, these are your choices; you choose one of them; do it, something happens as a result, which leads you on to further choices, and so on and on, until you reach a predetermined end-point.

The algorithm provides a programme that, at its onset, aims to be as inclusive as possible, moving on to increasing levels of specificity as it

40 The Contemporary Deathbed

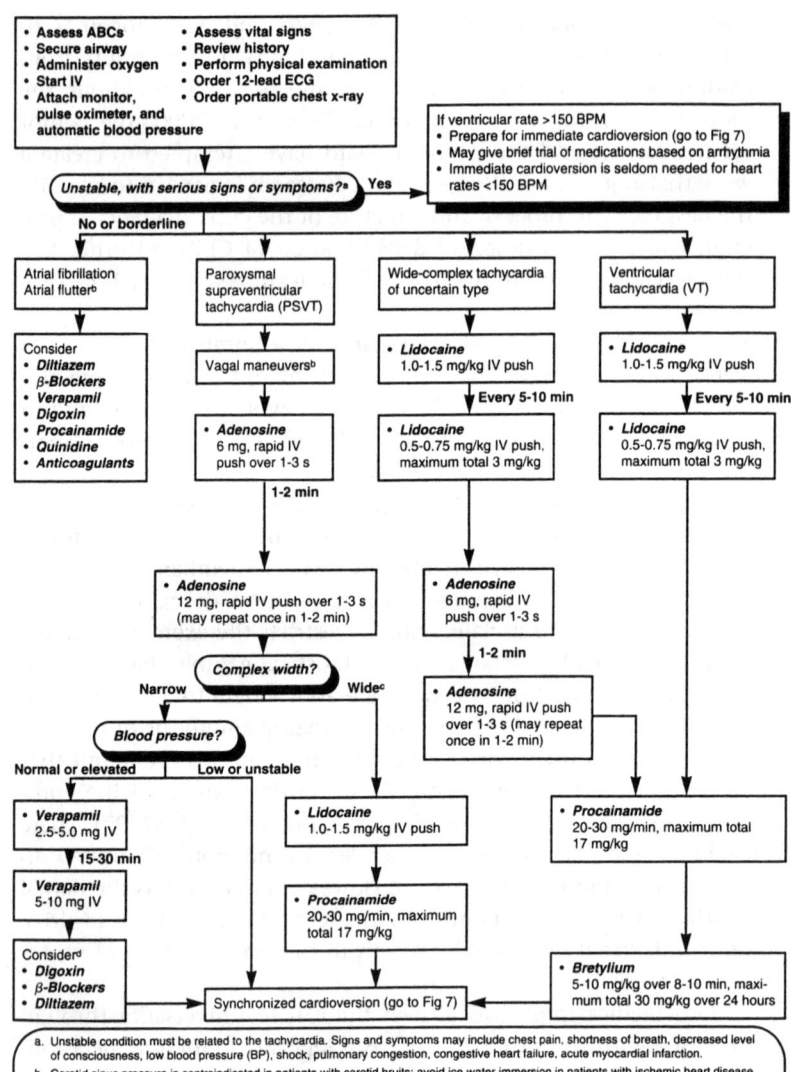

Figure 2.1 Tachycardia Algorithm[24]
Reproduced with permission
Advanced Cardiac Life Support
© 1997, Copyright American Heart Association

progresses towards a common desired outcome. Although its application is not necessarily identical in each case, it provides a comprehensive set of possibilities for action, leading to a desired outcome. In medical protocols, the algorithm is a means of taking a number of symptomatic presentations, reducing them to a common causal factor, then formulating a set of actions leading back to normal physiological function, while taking into account the particularities of each case. That is, its aspiration is to be a universal and unified response to a multiplicity of causes, ultimately effecting a single result. All in all, a rather tall order.

The creators of algorithms usually present them as mnemonic devices, to be used as aids to the practitioner's skills and judgement. This mnemonic function is especially important in the treatment of situations requiring complex action under conditions of high stress with crucial temporal limits. However, the need for a mnemonic device is, I would maintain, frequently due less to the complexity of the procedure and the ability of our little grey cells to remember it (though it does serve that function), than to the unpredictability of the condition being treated and the need to impose structure upon it.

A mnemonic device is not just an aid to memory, but is also an imposed structuring of both memory and the phenomenon represented by the mnemonic. Protocols, with their algorithmic structures, have their greatest utility in complicated pathophysiologies that are poorly understood where the therapeutic results are unpredictable. Algorithms help make sense of a confusing world, in fact, one might say, they help construct that world in a comprehensible fashion – both symbolically, via the structure of the algorithm and in fact, by directing the protocol's therapeutic techniques, which actually do change the portion of the world upon which they are practised. The algorithm is an architecture of response. It is a unified space in which the occult realities of the physical world and our subjective perception of them meet, and are made to 'fit'. All protocols seek to create a comprehensive response to an incomprehensible world, and, in so doing, organize that world into a comprehendible order. Protocol is as much about communication as it is about memory, as much about symbolic structure as it is about practical action.

In bringing together mouth-to-mouth, external cardiac compression and defibrillation into a unified and universal protocol, CPR attempts to correct the proximate physical causes of cardiac arrest – hypoxia, shock and arrhythmias. The symptoms – apnoea, unconsciousness and pulselessness – that identify the above physical processes are also the symptom complex that identifies clinical death. As a result, it becomes difficult to prevent practical responses (mouth-to-mouth, external cardiac compression and defibrillation) to specific physical derangements (hypoxia, shock and arrhythmias) from sliding into a symbolic dialogue (revival) with a universal ontological state (death).

Conformity

> An algorithm presents a way to treat a broad range of patients. By their very nature, however, algorithms over-simplify. The effective ACLS provider follows algorithms wisely, not blindly. Some patients may require extra care not specified in algorithms. The AHA accepts and encourages flexibility when clinically appropriate. Algorithms do not replace clinical understanding, nor should they be considered endorsements, requirements, or 'standards of care' in a legal sense. You will not find everything you need to know in the algorithms, but they are good memory aids. The algorithms list many interventions and actions as 'considerations' to help providers think. Although the algorithms provide a good 'cookbook', the patient always requires a 'thinking cook'.
>
> (Cummins, 2001, p. 5)

That's unarguably good advice. The experienced physician does try to operate as a 'thinking cook', relying on his or her judgement, using the algorithm as a guide. But the fact that it is deemed necessary to insert this caveat into *Guidelines 2000* is proof that the opposite is frequently the case.

CPR *is* performed slavishly. CPR was (and to a large extent still is) taught with an almost religious obsession in the precise application of the algorithm and the physical performance of the techniques it prescribes. Anyone who has taken one of these courses will be familiar with how unforgiving of variation they can be. One begins to suspect that perfection in performance is demanded less because it makes a huge difference to outcome than because perfection in performance is a possibility in a situation (the deathbed) where predictable effect is not. Despite attempts in *Guidelines 2000* to temper the obsessive character of the teaching and application of the protocol, algorithms continue to be treated as 'gospel'.

Resuscitative protocols were designed less for the cardiologist than for non-specialist medical staff and the layperson. The specialist, with his store of knowledge, is theoretically 'above' protocol, relying instead on judgement and experience. However, now that the protocol has become instantiated in ERs and ICUs, now that its practice is dictated by hospital policy and fear of litigation, it frequently precludes professional judgement. All practitioners, regardless of the level of their expertise, are held to its standard. Adherence to set resuscitative protocols has become the 'standard of care' in court judgments of physicians' performance.[25]

CPR has attained an unusually protected status within the law. CPR was the spur to the passing of 'Good Samaritan' legislation in many states of the USA. This legislation gives rescuers immunity from prosecution for damages done in an attempt to provide help in an emergent situation. No matter how inappropriate their actions or incorrect their technique, as long as the intent is to help and their actions do not exceed those of a prudent person, they will not be held liable. In the US, one of the most litigation-minded cultures in the world, there have been only a handful of suits against rescuers performing CPR since its inception in the early 1960s. None of them has been successful (Eisenberg, 1997, p. 133). The US courts have given resuscitative protocols not just protection but preference within the law. This is exemplified by the attempt to legislate AEDs into the workplace, airplanes, bowling alleys, and so on (see chapter 4).

> To the present [2001], there have been no reports of legal actions against anyone using an AED. On the other hand, lawsuits have been filed against facilities for failing to provide AEDs and train employees in CPR. (Cummins, 2001, p. 45)

Thus CPR's position under the law is not merely permissive, in that it gives one leave to practise the protocol, but has become, if not in fact then at least in practice, prescriptive. Not only is one safe from prosecution for doing it, appropriately or not, but one is liable for prosecution (in situations where a duty of care is established) if one fails to do it, appropriately or not.

Despite the practical wisdom of approaching protocol as a 'thinking cook', the above developments in medicine and law indicate that protocol, once established, commands disciplined adherence to a prescribed structure. This does not rule out reason, judgement and variation absolutely, but it does construct an internal tension that, on the one hand, results in an obsessive concern with following the rules and, on the other, requires caveats such as the above to legitimize appropriate deviation.

Power

The great strength of protocol is that it can be practised 'in the dark'. When facts are scarce and judgement difficult, we resort to protocol. Protocol is a set-piece behaviour that can be called on in a crisis, where the usual processes of judgement are suspended because of the need to act in the face of a lack of skill, information or time.

Though based on and supported by theory, protocol does not require knowledge of theory for its practice. One does not need to know the oxyhaemoglobin dissociation curve to give mouth-to-mouth, or normal cerebral perfusion pressures to do external cardiac compression or the physiology of ventricular fibrillation to operate an AED. All one needs to know is *how* to do them. Though theory is essential to the construction of the protocol, understanding of it is superfluous to its day-to-day practice; if not, it would not be protocol, but an exercise of judgement. Rescuers on the street require no knowledge of why they do what they do; all they require is the knowledge of how to do it. This is the enormous strength of protocol – it gives access to power in the absence of knowledge, and, perhaps even more importantly, in the absence of wisdom; that is, it removes much of the responsibility for judgment. All it requires is the ability to recall and follow rules. Despite praise of the 'thinking cook', protocol, in its purest form, relieves us of the necessity to think and of responsibility for judgement; the only knowledge necessary is that needed to perform the protocol, our only responsibility being to perform it correctly.

Strict adherence to protocol *is* important, because protocol is a means of exercising and distributing power. Protocols extend the power of an elite group to the wider population, in the case of CPR, that of physicians to lay rescuers. It is not just a way of the former exercising power over the latter, though it is that, but it is also a means of sharing of power. It allows the professional to use the hands of the man-in-the-street as tools in his crusade to save life, and it gives the man-in-the-street power over life and death. Control of the protocol does remain with the professional, but the necessities for its enactment are placed in the hands of the layperson.

> The most important part of the system [are] people like June Colven, who either know CPR themselves or can follow a 911 dispatcher's instructions – and do it well enough the first time to bring the person back from the dead. (Eisenberg, 1997, p. 11)

The protocol allows the professional, the institution and society to delegate power to the layperson without losing control over him or her.

Thus, the protocol becomes a means of social control, or, more charitably, a mode of negotiation between the larger social group and the individual. It is one means by which a community – in this case a community defined by its specialist knowledge and technical expertise – not only imposes its will upon, but also shares its power with, the individual man or woman in the street.

In the operation of protocol, power comes from a transcendent source: the institutional body that gives the protocol its imprimatur. It is transmitted through the institutionally determined structure of the protocol to the representative of that authority, in this case, the individual functioning in the role of rescuer. Distinct individual subjectivity is traded for a role determined by the structure of the protocol. The responsibility of the incumbent of that role is determined less by the success or failure of their actions than by their fidelity to their role, that is, their adherence to the formula of the protocol. In this instance, 'We did all we could' can be translated as 'Don't blame me, I did it correctly'. Culpability is transferred from the head to the hands. Blame, if it is placed, is less for poor judgement than for inaccuracies in application. Protocol allows for the replacement of incumbent by role and judgement by technique, and in so doing shifts responsibility for the act from the judgement of the person acting to their application of technique and, ultimately, onto the act itself – a sly but nevertheless useful manoeuvre, especially at the deathbed.

Though the role-playing imposed by protocol transfers blame for failure from the judgement of individual to the application of the protocol, there is a further transference, whereby the prescribed logical structure of the algorithm relieves its individual components (techniques) of responsibility for failure by also blaming deficiencies in application. This is exemplified in the AHA's emphasis on breaks in the chain-of-survival.

> It is a cliché to state that a chain is only as good as its weakest link, but in resuscitation the cliché is valid. If each link or step occurs rapidly, there is a good chance for successful resuscitation. Any delay in a step, however, means death is inevitable, regardless of how efficiently the other steps occur .... Each link summarizes a series of small but vital actions, which must flow flawlessly. Again, any delay in action can destroy the integrity of the entire chain. (Eisenberg, 1997, p. 255)

The disappointing survival statistics of CPR are (almost) always blamed not on the inherent shortcomings of the protocol's techniques, but on breaks in the chain-of-survival, that is, a breakdown in the ordered response of bystanders, EMS and hospital (Cummins et al., 1999a, p. 1832). 'If any link in the chain is inadequate, survival rates will be poor' (American, 2000, p. 1358). Mickey Eisenberg, one of the great proponents of CPR (and a member of the Seattle-King County researcher group) states:

> Cardiac arrest in Seattle is no different from arrest in New York or Chicago, and yet the likelihood of survival is 10 times higher in Seattle. The explanation: Seattle can deliver CPR, defibrillation and advanced care quickly. There are no mysteries or secrets; any community can do the same. (1997, p. 259)

However, this claim is disputed. Other communities have achieved high rates of bystander CPR and yet still failed to achieve high survival rates. Even in-hospital CPR, where there is less likelihood of a break in the chain-of-survival, has long-term survival rates as low as 15 per cent (Schneider, Nelson and Brown, 1993, p. 91; Gallagher, Lombardi and Gennis, 1995, p. 1922; Saklayan, Liss and Markert 1995, p. 163; De Maio et al., 2000, p. 139).

The chain-of-survival is a valid concept, and its breakdown is a real danger. No matter how effective the constituent parts of a protocol are, a breakdown in the delivery system will damage overall results. Failures in the chain-of-survival do have a profound effect on the chances for success and these failures are potentially correctable. However, true as this is, any protocol can only be as effective as its component parts even when applied efficiently. And, as we shall later see, there are persistent problems with each of these techniques that appear to be ignored in favour of blaming 'breaks in the chain'. In the end, the responsibility for a particular unsuccessful result can always be shifted from the individual to the protocol ('I did all I could') and blame for the generally poor performance of the protocol transferred onto the lack of organization of the community exercising it (failure of the chain-of-survival).

Success thus becomes defined, less by the practical effect of the protocol – its survival statistics – than by the construction of a functioning community around an intact chain-of-survival. The CPR protocol, though validating itself through scientific fact, becomes suspiciously like the Catholic Mass – faith and faithful performance lead to salvation, not just of the individual but also of the community structured by that performance. Indeed, both protocol and ritual are means of incorporating the individual into the larger social structure and negotiating a power-sharing agreement between them. Both CPR and the Mass are means of insuring an intact chain-of-survival: the one in this life, the other in the next. The relations between protocol and ritual will be explored further in the following chapters (see chapter 6).

Influence

Resuscitative protocols operate in the larger context of a changing (some would say, failing) healthcare system. At present, there is a somewhat desperate search for alternatives to the kindly old family doctor dealing out pills and platitudes from his neighbourhood surgery – a paradigm of healthcare delivery that has become outmoded for any number of economic, social and political reasons. I am not going to get into whose fault this is, why it has happened, or whether it is a good or bad thing. What I wish to point out is that the chain-of-survival, increasingly, has become one paradigm for the restructuring of modern healthcare delivery. As I have implied, protocol is a form of social structure, so it should not be surprising that it should generate social structure. It is no secret that, though not the exclusive origin of critical care medicine, the requirements of CPR and the chain-of-survival were essential to the development of pre-hospital EMS systems, ERs and ICUs (Pantridge and Geddes, 1967, p. 271; Eisenberg, 1997, pp. 203–18; Gibbs and Ross, 1997, p. 70). The ABCD mnemonic of CPR translated into the chain-of-survival is enacted in the journey of the individual patient from street to ambulance to ER to ICU, from lay rescuer to paramedic to ER doc to intensivist. This is not to deny alternative modes of access to healthcare and other structures of healthcare delivery. Rather, it is to point out that the critical care paradigm, symbolically represented and constructed by the chain-of-survival, has come to dominate certain institutional modes of healthcare.

CPR, not only its resuscitative content, but more importantly its organizational structure, that is, the chain-of-survival, has become the model upon which not just critical care medicine but, increasingly, primary care is being patterned. The growing importance of the ER (and its off-shoot, the walk-in clinic) as a critical node in the distribution of healthcare and a dispenser of 'MacDonald's medicine' (to the disgust of many) is not unrelated to its crucial position in the chain-of-survival. The chain-of-survival has become a structural formula for facilitating the interdependence of changing modern bureaucratic institutions. For better or worse, the chain-of-survival is writ large on the structure of late twentieth-century healthcare. The import of resuscitative protocols is as much in their covert organization of increasingly large areas of healthcare as in their more overt function of 'snatching life from the jaws of death'. Newly emerging patterns of healthcare are realized in institutional structures that are physical reiterations of the concept of 'life' as imagined by the chain-of-survival. The chain-of-survival is not merely a device for ordering the protocol of revival, but is a heuristic project, generating a concept of being that constructs the social structures responsible for survival, both the protocol's own and ours.

Furthermore, CPR is a tool for integrating the individual into that structure of being. As the patient is passed from the hands of rescuer to paramedic to physician, from street to ambulance to ER, he or she traverses the chain-of-survival, moving not only towards a concept of life defined by the protocol, but just as surely towards a death constructed by that same chain. As the following chapters hope to demonstrate, CPR has as much to do with identifying the dead as with restoring life, as much to do with constructing a concept of 'life' as with battling death, and as much to do with representation as with reality. I hope to show that CPR's integration of both the living and the dead into the medical systems it has helped construct is less a conspiracy against the past and against the dead, as it is often portrayed, than a necessary response to the exigencies of the modern and life in it.

3
The Royal Humane Society: The Method

Many and indubitable are the instances of the possibility of restoring to life persons apparently struck with sudden death.

(Humane, 1774, p. 2)

Henley, June 9, 1776...
Sir,
I take the earliest opportunity to transmit the particulars of my success in the recovery of a child, apparently dead by drowning, which happened in the afternoon yesterday, about four o'clock .... Thomas Mellet's son of this place, a child between four and five years old, was bathing yesterday in the river Thames, (which runs close by the side of the town). The child accidentally fell down in the river, and was under water above a quarter of an hour. He was taken up, at a considerable distance, to all appearance dead. The extremities and the body were cold, the jaws fallen, and no pulse to be discovered. The person that took him up, suspended him by the legs for some time, then he was immediately taken home, to a house at a small distance, and was laid on the bed between the blankets, when I was called upon for assistance. I diligently pursued the usual methods of strong frictions by warm flannels, stimulants to the nose, and blowing with great force into the mouth down the throat: In about a quarter of an hour there appeared symptoms of life by small gaspings, and as soon as the child was able to swallow, I got down a small quantity of brandy and water, and in an hour the child was perfectly recovered....

I am, Sir, Your most obedient humble servant,
Wm. Clowes

(Humane, 1777, pp. 14–15)

The Royal Humane Society

Though the 'birth' of CPR is usually dated at 1960 and is looked on as being a product of late twentieth-century medicine, its constituent techniques and the concept of the resuscitative protocol have earlier origins. In the latter half of the eighteenth century, in both Europe and America, a number of philanthropic societies were founded 'for Affording Relief to Persons Apparently Dead from Drowning' (Hawes, 1774, p. 1). The first of these appeared in Amsterdam in 1767. Institutions with similar goals sprang up in Milan and Venice in 1768, Hamburg 1769, Paris 1771, St. Petersburg, London and Norwich 1774, Cork 1775, Liverpool 1775, Philadelphia 1780 and Boston 1786. The list continues until, by 1800, there were over 30 such societies in Great Britain, with the London Society being in correspondence with an equal number overseas.

'The Institution for Affording Relief to Persons Apparently Dead from Drowning' was inaugurated at a meeting on 18 April 1774 in the Chapter Coffee House, St. Paul's Churchyard, London by Drs William Hawes, Thomas Cogan, John Coakley Lettsom and some 13 other physicians, surgeons, apothecaries and surgeon-apothecaries practising between Westminster Bridge and London Bridge. The name 'Humane Society' was adopted later that year. In 1787, it became the 'Royal Humane Society' on receiving a royal charter from George III.[1] Its founding document, *The Plan of an Institution for Affording Relief to Persons apparently dead, from Drowning. And Also For diffusing a general Knowledge of the manner of treating Persons in a similar critical State, from various other Causes; Such As Strangulation by the Cord, Suffocation by noxious Vapours, &c. &c.*, outlined its goals and methods (Hawes, 1774, p. 1). Its aim was the 'restoration of life'; its methods were experiment, instruction and reward. To this end, it took upon itself the tasks of raising funds, rewarding rescuers, instructing and educating the medical and lay public through pamphlets and lectures, publishing its resuscitative protocol (*Methods of Treatment for the Recovery of Persons Apparently Dead from Drowning*[2]), providing personnel and equipment to enact that protocol, refining the protocol through the collection and scrutiny of case reports and encouraging scientific progress through experimentation.

The Method of the Humane Society initially included mouth-to-mouth ventilation, various forms of physical stimulation, re-warming, embrocations, purgatives and tobacco smoke enemas. The Method was first published by the Society as an appendix to its founding document of 1774, but had its origin in earlier works. The Method was, for the most part, a translation by Thomas Cogan of a Dutch protocol of 1763 (Johnson, 1773, p. 119). The earliest protocol mentioned in the eighteenth-century literature, though an exact date is not given, appears to be that of Dethardingius, a Swedish physician, who developed a system that included re-warming, tracheotomy, friction and abdominal compressions (Physician, 1746, p. 39). In 1740, René-Antoine Ferchault de Réamur of Montpelier published *Avis pour donner du secours a ceus l'on croit noyez* (*Notice in Order to Give Help to Those Believed to Be Drowned*). In this, besides recommendations for agitation and stimulants, were instructions on the importance of re-warming, the use of bellows to introduce air into the mouth and, as a last resort, 'bronchotomy', that is the surgical opening of the trachea so that 'air will then freely enter the lungs'. Réamur's recommendations later found their way not only into the drowning protocols of Humane Societies throughout Europe, but were published in their entirety in Jean-Jacques Bruhier's 1742 edition of his sensationalist *Dissertations sur l'incertitude des signes de la mort* (*Dissertation of the Uncertainty of the Signs of Death*), which is often credited as triggering late eighteenth-century fears over premature burial (Bondeson, 2001, p. 81). In 1744, John Fothergill published the first English-language report of the use of a resuscitative protocol in 1732 to revive a miner overcome by noxious vapours (1782, pp. 110–19). The recommendations Fothergill makes in this report are almost identical to those later made in the Dutch protocol and then in the London Humane Society's Method.

It is worth noting that a number of the techniques, such as mouth-to-mouth and purgatives, were already in use in certain medical circles long before the Humane Society's publication of The Method. However, it was the Humane Society that gathered these techniques into a formal protocol, specifically for the purpose of communicating it to the public. Furthermore, it was the Humane Society that instituted the necessary financial, political and institutional structures to accomplish this. However, before we move on to The Method and its specific therapeutic techniques, it may be useful to examine the condition it was primarily designed to treat: drowning.

Drowning: the floating grave

Sudden death in the eighteenth century, excluding epidemic years, was most likely to be the result of accident, childbirth or war. One common form of accident was drowning. Oceans and rivers were a risk to the traveller, an occupational hazard for the transport worker and a temptation to the suicide and child. It is therefore not surprising that the problem of the resuscitation of the drowned should surface in the ports and centres of ocean-going empires, such as London and Amsterdam. In the years 1781–2, the number of lives reported in English publications as being lost to drowning amounted to 'upwards of 10,000' (Macpherson, 1783, pp. 121–2).

Until the seventeenth century, knowledge of the pathophysiology of drowning was still based on the writings of Galen. Galen had postulated that water entered the orifices of the body causing the internal organs to swell and burst. In the sixteenth century, with the rebirth of anatomy, new structuralist perspectives resulted in the refutation of much of Galen's anatomy and physiology. Post-mortems of drowning victims in the mid-1700s showed that, unless the victim had been long dead in the water, their lungs were not, as had previously been thought, filled with water:

> By dissection after drowning, the quantity of water found in the lungs is very inconsiderable, and totally insufficient to produce the changes which take place. From this we may infer that the exclusion of the atmospheric air from the lungs, is the cause to which we must attribute every effect arising from submersion. (Bartlett, 1792, p. 9)

Asphyxia was thus correctly ascribed to the exclusion of the air from the lungs caused by small amounts of inhaled water triggering laryngospasm.[3]

Today, asphyxia is used as a synonym for suffocation, that is, exclusion of air from the lungs causing hypoxia. Throughout most of the eighteenth century, asphyxia (ασφυξια) still carried its literal meaning: pulselessness. Any cause of pulselessness – suffocation, primary cardiac arrest, hypothermia, blood loss – was subsumed under the term asphyxia. It was roughly equivalent to the term 'cardiac arrest', that is, a clinical state characterized by loss of respirations, pulse and consciousness leading to sudden death. By the late eighteenth century, there were two competing theories as to how exclusion of atmospheric air from the lungs might cause asphyxia: the mechanical and the vitalist. These corresponded, respectively, to the pathophysiological processes of apoplexy and suffocation.

The Humane Society's Fothergillian Essay competition of 1788 nicely sets out both sides of this debate. Charles Kite, the Silver Medal winner, presented the iatromechanical argument, positing apoplexy as the proximate cause of death (1788). Iatromechanists, like Kite, influenced by William Harvey's explanation of the circulation of blood, saw the human body as a hydraulic system – made up of pipes and conduits, valves and locks. Apoplexy was thought to be a disorder of neurological function due to increased pressure on the brain caused by congestion with excess quantities of blood. In this theory of drowning, the lungs were seen not as organs of gas exchange but as pumps assisting the movement of blood through the pulmonary circuit from the right to the left side of the heart. Exclusion of air from the lungs was thought to result in the collapse of the small blood vessels in the lungs, thus obstructing the blood's pulmonary transit. This had two effects: first, the left side of the heart, no longer stimulated by the inflow of blood from the lungs, would not be excited to contract and propel blood through the arteries. Second, blood backing up in the venous system would cause congestion in the brain leading to increased intracranial pressure and the cessation of vital functions, that is, apoplexy. Based on the apoplectic theory, Kite observed that therapeutic bloodletting from the external jugular veins might be beneficial because of their direct connection to the cerebral circulation, but he concluded that artificial ventilation in the form of mouth-to-mouth or bellows ventilation was the most efficient means of relieving cerebral congestion by its opening up of the pulmonary circuit.

Edmund Goodwyn, the Gold Medal winner in that same year, presented a more vitalistic point of view (1788, pp. 1–98). He maintained that there was some quality of, or substance in, atmospheric air that entered the blood stream and was responsible for the 'irritability' of the organs, that is, for their ability to react to stimuli. In this formulation, suffocation prevented this vital quality or substance from entering the lungs. Through a series of elegant experiments Goodwyn demonstrated the relation between suffocation and asphyxia. He showed how water entering the hypopharynx induced laryngospasm, resulting in atmospheric air being excluded from the lungs. This exclusion resulted in dark venous blood no longer acquiring the florid colour of arterial blood as it traversed the pulmonary circuit. When this occurred, the animal lost consciousness, respiratory movement ceased, the heart stopped beating and death ensued. These effects could all be reversed through the prompt reintroduction of air into the lungs by artificial ventilation.[4]

Drowning was the paradigmatic condition that the Humane Society's Method was designed to treat, just as ventricular fibrillation is the paradigmatic lesion upon which CPR is based. But, like CPR, The Method was expanded to cover what were seen as closely related and analogous conditions. To drowning were added suffocation, strangulation, asphyxia due to fire damp and choke damp,[5] and deaths from lightning, opium, syncope, freezing, convulsions, cardiac fits, hysterical passion, alcoholism and stillbirth (A. Hawes, 1774, p. 8; Fothergill, 1795, p. 167; Curry, 1815, p. ix). In fact, as with CPR, The Method came to be called on in many cases of sudden, unexpected death of varying aetiology.

Death: absolute and apparent

> About nine o'clock in the evening the 2nd of November last [1787], the *Ann and Elizabeth*, was driven on a rock near Margate; the sea ran high ... bursting through the cabin windows .... At ten the cabin was full of water, and the waves washed over the deck; the crew, consisting of five men and a cabin boy, about 15 years of age, in hopes of saving themselves ... were compelled to quit their retreat and seek refuge in the shrouds, climbing the mast and lashing themselves to the cross-trees; about three in the morning Roger Mares [the cabin boy] appeared totally exhausted with cold and fatigue ... and at about six they supposed him dead .... The horror of the night had even on those who were on shore, awakened the most serious apprehensions for the many distresses which the next morning might bring to light, and as soon as the day appeared, the sloop Anne and Elizabeth was discovered in the utmost distress, all the people on board being seen hanging from the shrouds .... As soon as the ebbing of the tide would allow ... a boat went off to them .... It was with great difficulty the sloop could be boarded, and the mariners rescued, who had suffered most sensibly from the wet and cold of so dreadful a night, and the menaces of surrounding death .... All the crew were safe landed; but the boy, supposed to be dead, remaining lashed to the shrouds. Among the spectators on shore who was waiting with anxiety the return of the boat, was Nicholas Styleman, Esq.; of Norwich, who was on a visit at Margate, and perceiving that, though they had brought away the people, there still remained a lad tied in the shrouds, he expressed his wonder that the boy was left behind; the answer of all the people who came on shore, was that the boy had been dead several hours. Mr. Styleman

earnestly entreated the boatmen to go back and fetch the boy; this they objected to ... as the vessel could not be boarded without great danger ... but being allured by the reward of Five Guineas, which this gentleman offered to them, to bring the body, whether dead or alive, they returned, and brought the body from the vessel. It was landed under every appearance of confirmed death, perfectly cold, limbs stiff, the eyes fixed, and the jaws locked. Mr. Styleman had him put into warm blankets.... The usual endeavours of restoring heat and mobility by warm flannels and friction being found very ineffectual, he was carried to a warm bath in the neighbourhood .... In about an hour laborious and convulsive reparation returned, sometimes at very long intervals; the heart commenced its action, and a slight pulsation was soon afterwards perceptible ... he then lifted up his eyelids, but the eyes appeared motionless and the pupils widely dilated .... At about nine in the evening he swallowed some broth with difficulty, but with much avidity.... He was full of gratitude to his deliverer, but knew nothing of what had happened; he remembered the vessel going on the rocks, and the sea bursting into the cabin, but here his recollection closed; all that after occurred was lost in oblivion, so that he may be said to have undergone death without knowing it ... On the boy being happily restored to life, [Mr. Styleman's] kindness was again conspicuous, as he purchased clothes for him, and likewise took him repeatedly to church, in order to return thanks for the great mercies received.... A great number of genteel families enjoyed infinite satisfaction from the recovery of the boy, and contributed to fitting him out in the most comfortable manner for the naval service.

(Royal, 1790, pp. 109–12)

The diagnosis of death has never been entirely unproblematic.

Many, various, and even opposite appearances, have been supposed to indicate the total extinction of life. Formerly, a stoppage of the pulse and respiration were thought to be unequivocal signs of death: particular attention in examining the state of the heart and larger arteries; the flame of a taper, a lock of wool, or a mirror applied to the mouth or nostrils, or a cup of water to the *scrobiculus cordis* [pit of the stomach]; were conceived sufficient to ascertain these points: and great has been the number of those who have fallen untimely victims to this erroneous opinion. Of late, some have formed their prognostic from the livid, black, cadaverous countenance: others from the heavy, dull, fixed or flaccid state of the eyes; from the dilated pupil, the foaming at the mouth and nostrils, the rigid and inflexible state of the body, jaws, or extremities; the intense and universal cold, &c .... it is evident, that these signs will not afford certain and unexceptionable criteria, by which we may distinguish between life and death. (Kite, 1788, pp. 92–5)

As Kite, and other physicians of the eighteenth century, point out, none of the clinical signs of death is absolute – loss of breath, cessation of pulse, unconsciousness, lack of movement, dilated, unreactive pupils, cold flesh, pallor, stiffness – none is a sure indication of death.

To draw the line, that separates life and death; and to mark the precise limits of either, we need here hardly remind our readers, who are in the least conversant with the subject, that the *celebriori nomina* of the medical art have owned, this most important, and if solved, decisive question in Physic, is wrapped in shades of almost impenetrable darkness. (Medical, 1791, p. 6)

It is no easy thing, even today, to identify the dead. The so-called 'vital signs' – consciousness, pulse and breath – are signs of the functioning of the vital triad of brain, heart and lungs. They are important signs of life, but their absence, at least in certain cases, does not always indicate death. In some circumstances, it is difficult to distinguish the appearance of death from the reality of death – difficult to distinguish 'apparent death' from 'absolute death'.

In such drowning accidents ... a stoppage of the vital functions, as breathing and the circulation of blood, often produces a state of apparent death – Even the suppressed pulse of the arteries, imperceptible respiration, the coldness and rigidity of the limbs, the want of contractibility in the pupil of the eye, the involuntary loss of excrementitious substances – all these symptoms of approaching dissolution should not discourage us from trying the proper means of recovering the patient's life. In children and young persons, in particular, we must not too hastily decide, whether they be absolutely dead or not .... And here the excellent rules published by the Royal Humane Society of London, for the recovery of persons apparently dead, cannot be recommended in too strong terms. (Willich, 1809, p. 100)

The Humane Society's protocol became a useful means of distinguishing between absolute and apparent death, and avoiding a particular threat:

> Thousands have been hurried to the grave without the confirmation of death; and no doubt, amidst such numbers, many have revived to feel all the horrors of a second, and more dismal dissolution. (Royal, 1789, p. 64)

As previously mentioned, Bruhier's book *Dissertations sur l'incertitude des signes de la mort* (*Dissertation of the Uncertainty of the Signs of Death*), which contained Réamur's drowning protocol, is often credited with triggering anxieties over premature burial (Bondeson, 2001, p. 80). The preface to the English translation of this book claimed that the successes of Réamur's drowning protocol were a proof of the unreliability of the traditional signs of death. However, the propensity of the drowned corpse to return spontaneously to life had long had an honourable place in folklore. The authors of the Humane Society's *Reports* enjoyed quoting instances of prolonged submersion followed by miraculous recovery: the more improbable, the better. Professor Johann Nicholas Pechlin of Sweden reported a gentlemen submerged for eight days, his feet being stuck in a river's muddy bed. He was particularly troubled by fish, which made attacks on his eyes, and by the deafening noise of people filling their water-buckets in the river (Physician, 1746, p. 14). Kite, in his essay on the revival of the drowned, points out the dangers of too hasty a diagnosis of death:

> A lady in Hampshire was buried three or four days after her supposed death, the next day, a noise being heard in the vault, it was opened, and she was found just expiring. Maximilian Misson tells us of Francis de Civille, of Rouen in Normandy, who is recorded to have been three times dead, three times buried, and as many times raised from the dead. Upwards of half a dozen stories are related of persons who, being buried, were roused from their trance by the attempts which were made to rob them of valuable rings which they had on their fingers; and a greater number of instances were said to have happened, where persons being prematurely confined

to their coffins, have not only devoured their shrouds, but have been reduced to the necessity of eating part of their own flesh. Many more similar cases might be given; but, in all probability, what has been said will be thought fully sufficient. (1788, pp. 189–220)

Quite. Legislation was passed in Germany, Austria, England and France requiring some delay – as much as three days – before burial, so that putrefaction might be allowed to commence (Bondeson, 2001, p. 19). The first public mortuary constructed for this purpose was opened in Weimar in 1792. But why should the dead awaken so inopportunely?

Hypothermia: cold and dead

The revival of the drowned, at least in northern Europe, is complicated by the fact that victims are not only wet but also cold. At its extremes, cold kills, but up to certain temporal and pathophysiological points, it saves. Importantly, the form this defence takes mimics death. Hypothermia produces a state of suspended animation from which 'absolute' death must be differentiated. It was the hypothermia related to cold water drowning that allowed the Humane Society's distinction between absolute and apparent death. It also allowed for the drama of reanimation and promoted the fear of premature burial.

In many, probably most, instances, victims were not so much dead as cold. Like the hedgehogs studied in their winter torpor by eighteenth-century naturalists, the heart slows, breathing becomes imperceptible and consciousness fades: apparently dead, still you live. One can chart

Table 3.1 Signs and Symptoms of Hypothermia

Core Temp. in °C	Signs and Symptoms
37.6	Normal core body temperature. Pulse = 60
35	Shivering maximal
34	Amnesia. Speech difficulties
33	Incoordination
32	Stupor
31	Cardiac output drops. Pulse = 40
30	Risk of cardiac arrhythmias
29	Coma. Pupils dilate
28	Respirations drop
27	Loss of reflexes
24	Blood pressure drops
23	Loss of corneal reflexes
20	Pulse = 20
19	Electrical silence on electroencephalogram
18	Asystole – the heart stops

the ebbing of life against core body temperature. As temperature drops the signs of life wane consecutively, until, at some imperceptible point, long after the appearance of death has marked the body, the line is crossed and death itself, finally, truly arrives.

Hypothermia may usefully, albeit artificially, be broken down into a triple relation with death:

1. Cold as the *cause* of death: The body's physiological processes function within a very narrow temperature band. When ambient temperature decreases, it triggers a number of automatic and behavioural changes designed to maintain internal core temperature. When these compensatory mechanisms are exhausted or overcome, the body begins to lose heat and its temperature sinks below levels critical for metabolic function. If the core body temperature sinks low enough, respiration and circulation cease, and death ensues from the combined effects of hypoxia and ventricular fibrillation brought on by the drop in core temperature.
2. The cold body as a *result* of death: Body heat is the product of the metabolic process of energy production. When an animal dies, for any reason, and cellular metabolism ceases, heat production ceases and the body becomes poikliothermic. Like a cup of coffee cooling on the desk, the body's temperature drops to ambient temperature.
3. Cold as a *defence* against death. The physiological changes produced by hypothermia can act to protect the living animal against further damage. It may seem paradoxical that the loss of heat, which threatens life, also acts to preserve it, but such is the case. Hypothermia acts as a defence against hypoxia. As temperature decreases, metabolic processes slow down, decreasing the cells' requirements for oxygen, glucose and other substrates. Respiration and heartbeat are slowed to the point of being imperceptible, but because of the decreased metabolic requirements, they remain adequate to the task of providing metabolic substrate.[6] This is particularly important in the heart and the brain, the two organs most sensitive to hypoxia, and the two organ systems from which the major signs of death are derived. Even in the eighteenth century, there were inklings of cold's defensive value:

> Some however, affirm, that a Principle of Life may in the deplorable State of Submersion, be retain'd for a long Time, because the Coldness of the Water renders the Circulation slower, and suppresses the Transpiration of the vital Air contain'd in the Blood. (Physician, 1746, p. 17)

Because of the difficulties involved in diagnosing death in the hypothermic patient, 'No one is dead, until they are warm and dead'. This ambivalent relationship between cold and death is, at least at the phenomenal level, a trigger for fear of the 'living dead'. Hypothermia is, *par excellence*, the living death from which absolute death must be differentiated. As importantly, the recovery from hypothermic near-death is one of the most awe-inspiring physiological phenomena that one might ever witness.

It is more than probable that those awakening in the tomb were not so much dead as cold. And it is certain that the drowned, resuscitated by the Humane Society in the eighteenth century, were more cold than wet. Careful review of the detailed case reports presented in the Humane Society's publications between 1774 and 1784 indicates that somewhere in the region of 90 per cent of *successful* resuscitations from drowning were resuscitations not from hypoxia, but from hypothermia. With hindsight, it is apparent that those who were pulled dead from the water and stayed dead, died, for the most part, from the combined effects of hypothermia and asphyxia; but those who responded to resuscitation were almost exclusively hypothermic, and the successful response to The Method was, in the vast majority of cases, more a response to re-warming than to any of the other manoeuvres in the protocol.

In the nineteenth century, expectations of revival, from all forms of sudden death, came to be based on the special case of near-death due to hypothermia. The restoration of the apparently dead by the Humane Society's Method gave proof of science's ability to triumph over death. Not entirely serendipitously, the identification and treatment of this particular mode of death coincided with the birth of the modern. The secularization of the world, necessary for the modern project, required that man be given at least some control over life and death. And the restoration of the drowned, via the dramatic though unappreciated effectiveness of revival from hypothermia, gave proof of that power. The fact that drowning was complicated by the obscurely recognized causal factor of hypothermia was to haunt both the comforting image of revival and the more disturbing image of premature burial throughout the nineteenth century, feeding not only people's wonder at science's power, but also their fear of nature's duplicity.

The importance of the conjunction, at the end of the eighteenth century, between occult hypothermia, fears of premature burial, the doctrine of vitalism and The Method will be explored further in the chapters that follow. The unacknowledged vision of the hypothermic patient awakening from the dead is a secular fantasy that continues to haunt our expectations of death 300 years later. The portrayals of resuscitation in TV shows, such as *ER* and *Casualty*, though they may be resuscitations from heart attacks, trauma, drug overdoses and so on, remain, in their unduly optimistic statistics and dramatic re-awakenings, more rooted in the occult fantasy of hypothermic death, than the reality of the emergency room (See chapter 7). Our hopes of revival still aspire to a script where the victim, with 'every appearance of confirmed death, perfectly cold, limbs stiff, the eyes fixed, and the jaws locked .... [is] happily restored to life .... full of gratitude to his deliverer .... returning thanks .... [to our] infinite satisfaction'.

The Method

> *The METHOD For The RESTORATION of the APPARENTLY DEAD*
> CAUTIONS
> 1. When in the stream, by accident, is found,
> The pallid body of the recent drown'd;
> When every sign of active life is fled,
> And all are ready to pronounce it dead,
> With nimble speed the clay-cold body lay
> In flannel warming, and with care convey
> To some kind home, or nearest friendly hut,
> There gently slop'd–a little rais'd the head –
> The lifeless corpse lay on a couch or bed.
> If chilling cold or damps extend their gloom,
> Let moderate fires attemper soft the room:
> But if the sun in potent strength is seen,
> Expose the body to the solar beam.
>
> FRICTION
> 2. Then, when with tepid cloths it is well dried,
> Let friction soft, with flannel, be applied:
> Sprinkle the flannel, ere you do begin,
> With rum or brandy, mustard, or with gin.
> Or heated bricks, or tiles, should next be got:
> These, wrapp'd in flannel with precaution meet,
> Should be applied to both hands and feet.
>
> INFLATION
> 3. And if you'd see, what you so much desire,
> The object of your care again respire,
> Let one the mouth and either nostril close,
> While th' inflating bellows up the other blows.

The air with well-adjusted force convey,
To put the flaccid lungs again in play.
Should bellows not be found, or found too late,
Let some kind soul with willing mouth inflate.
Then lightly squeeze–awhile compress the chest,
That the excluded air may be exprest.

TOBACCO FUMES
4. Yet, should not these, with every care succeed,
With vigour still to other means proceed:
Tobacco-smoke has often proved, indeed,
Of wond'rous use, in cases of such need,
Try ev'ry means, not even this neglect,
With this herb's fumes, the bowels to inject.
Thrice administer the same within the hour;
and, if it proves inadequate in power,
To clysters of this pungent herb apply,
Or other juice of equal potence high.

AGITATION
5. Nor yet th'important doubtful task forego,
Nor quit the scene of misery and woe:
Try other means, nor yield the glorious strife,
Till gain'd the prize of slow-returning life.
Oft agitation proves a wond'rous aid,
And to suspended life a friend is made,
Let some assistant hands, with sinews strong,
The undulating force a while prolong.

COMMUNICATING OF HEAT
6. When all these means an hour have been pursu'd,
And no faint gleams of cheering hope are view'd,
If brewhouse, bakehouse, or a glasshouse nigh,
Quick for assistance to the nearest fly:
The remedy with speed should be embrac'd,
And in the grains, or lees, or ashes plac'd,
Th'envelop'd body there should gently meet
The latent blessing of attemper'd heat.
The temp'rature but little should exceed
What is standard of good health agreed.
Much good from hot-baths, if with ease obtain'd,
With early means applied, is often gain'd.

ELECTRICITY
7. Likewise, th' electric fluid, when death doth reign,
And stagnant life is cold in every vein,
(Drawn from the choice—the best of Nature's fires)
A kindly warmth, a gentle heart inspires;
Breathes thro' the whole a vivifying strife,
And wakes the torpid powers to sudden life.
Yet more: the shock of life is oft the test,
When all who're present are of doubt possest:
Let fly the sudden shock: if life remain,
Contractions, spasms, instantly are plain.
No longer doubt, no more the case debate,
The body's in recoverable state.
If these are seen, or other signs appear,
Being well assured the returning life is near,
Into the mouth some luke-warm water pour;
And if to swallow is returned the power,
A little wine or brandy tepid give,
Or what is nearest, or he can receive.

PERSEVERANCE
8. Three or four hours with ardour persevere,
Ere you resign your subject to despair.–
A fatal error it too oft has been,
When latent life has not been quickly seen,
Their courage fail'd–they thought they could not save,
And doom the body to untimely grave.

LIFE RESTORED
9. Thus, when the patient, snatched from instant death,
Has been restored to draw his vital breath,
Convey him quickly, with a friendly arm,
T' enjoy the comforts of a bed that's warm.
There cease from noise–his half-shut eye-lid shows
He wants the blessings of a sweet repose.
When he from slumbering shall again awake,
Of health and vigour he'll once more partake.
Restor'd to kindred and society,
He'll live to bless your kind humanity

(Hawes, 1797, pp. 8–10)

Though the form is amusing, the content is a reasonably accurate reflection of the instructions issued in the Society's *Methods of Treatment* between the years 1774 and 1811.

Ventilation: the breath of life

> In every case of apparent death, the instituting an artificial breathing, by assiduously inflating the lungs with fresh air, is one of the first and most necessary measures to be taken for recovery.
>
> (Curry, 1815, p. 39)

The form of artificial ventilation recommended in The Method was mouth-to-mouth or bellows ventilation. The Humane Society found that mouth-to-mouth was easily taught, easily performed and the equipment – the rescuer's mouth and lungs – was always at hand. It appeared to be safe and was occasionally effective:

> The operation of inflating the lungs completely, demands considerable address; and as it constitutes the most important part of the process, it were to be wished, that not only medical pupils of all denominations, but also some other intelligent persons, in every parish, were fully instructed how to perform it with dexterity – A circumstance of no small consequence, especially in country-places remote from medical aid. The operation may be tolerably performed by the common people. (A. Fothergill, 1795, p. 117)

As Anthony Fothergill pointed out, it was a universal response that might be applied to very many cases of accidental death by all people at all times in all locations.

Kite gives instruction on bellows ventilation:

> The medical director, standing at the right side of his charge, must keep the mouth perfectly closed with his left hand, while with his right, making a suitable pressure on the prominent part of the windpipe, he prevents the air passing into the stomach, till, finding the lungs are properly distended, he is to press strongly on the chest, removing, at the same time, the hand from the mouth, so as to let the air pass out: when, by these means, the lungs are compressed, the same process is immediately to be repeated, that, as far as can be, the manner of natural respiration may be imitated ... it is

one persons business to work the bellows ... another must be employed in making the occasional pressure on the breast .... (1788, p. 145)

I need hardly point out, though the theoretical justifications differ, the similarities to the ABCs of CPR. However, both mouth-to-mouth and bellows ventilation were soon to fall under suspicion and, for reasons which will be examined in greater detail in chapter 5, both were dropped from The Method in the 1830s.

Circulation: the pulse of life

Though theories regarding the relation of respiration to circulation were in a state of flux at the time of the first publication of The Method in 1774, Harvey's mechanistic description of the circulation of the blood was well accepted. It was accepted that the heart was a vital organ, that its function was central to life and that the circulatory system was essential to the functioning of the other systems labelled as vital: the respiratory and the nervous. The majority of the vigorous therapeutic manoeuvres recommended in The Method – concussion, agitation, friction, and electricity – were aimed at physically stimulating the circulation of the blood and strengthening the heart's pumping action:

> Successive concussions ... communicated to the heart and internal organs, tend to put the stagnant blood in motion; to renew oscillations of the moving fibres; and to incite the hidden springs of life into action. (A. Fothergill, 1795, p. 143)

It was believed that the vital organs (the brain, heart and lungs) were in 'sympathy' with each other and with the external environment as mediated through the sensory organs of the skin, stomach and bowels. Stimulation, eliciting irritability in one organ, might rouse the dormant powers in another, restoring its functioning.

In the seventeenth and early eighteenth centuries, many of the folk therapies employed in the resuscitation of the drowning victim involved the use of considerable physical force. Victims were hung by the heals and beaten with sticks, rolled back and forth over a barrel, jogged up and down on the back of a horse and subjected to other robust physical manoeuvres in attempts to rid the lungs of water and to excite the fading life-force back into action (Physician, 1746, p. 6). One of the primary goals of the Humane Society, stated explicitly in

The Method, was to mitigate the more violent of these 'pernicious' practices (Hawes, 1774, p. 2). However, the idea that a short, sharp shock was somehow beneficial kept creeping back into The Method. In the *Annual Report* of 1783/4, contrary to earlier recommendations of the need for gentle treatment of the body, the Humane Society recommended, 'that the body should be well shaken every ten minutes .... In a variety of instances agitation, in conjunction with the methods laid down, has forwarded the recovery of boys who had been drowned' (Humane, 1785, p. 168). The use of chest and abdominal compression as forms of stimulation will be examined further in chapter 6.

Electricity: the spark of life

> Let the heart be excited by a gentle electrical shock, passed obliquely from the right side of the chest through the left, in the direct course of the heart.
>
> (A. Fothergill, 1795, p. 127)

In 1767, Joseph Priestley summarized what was then known about electricity in his book *The History and Present State of Electricity, with Original Experiments* (1772). In 1773, one year prior to the Humane Society's first published protocol, John Walsh discovered the electrical nature of the discharge from the torpedo fish and John Hunter found evidence of electrical phenomena in other aquatic species. Animal electricity manifest in the nervous system through its 'irritability' became a contender for the title of *vis vitae* – the life-force. Underlying most of The Method's therapeutic techniques was the vitalist concept of the 'life-force' which, like the dying torch engraved on the Society's medals, might be fanned back into full flame by the application of the correct techniques.[7]

Electricity was useful in the resuscitative situation on two counts. The first was that it acted as a kind of gauge measuring the strength of the vital force:

> Electrical shock is to be admitted as the test, or discriminating character of any remains of animal life; and so long as that produces contractions, may the person be said to be in a recoverable state; but when that effect has ceased, there can be no doubt remain of the party being absolutely and positively dead. (Kite, 1788, p. 125)

If an electrical shock was applied to a body and there was muscular contraction, then some quantity of the vital force must still be present.

The complete lack of any response was a taken as a sign of the loss of viability. Electricity could thus be used to diagnose death, an issue that was becoming increasingly important towards the end of the century as fears of premature burial grew.

Electricity's second use was as a stimulant, to rouse the ebbing vital force to action:

> Much having lately been done in the recovery of persons apparently dead, by drowning, by the Societies very laudably instituted for that purpose; it hath frequently occurred to me that there is, in nature, a power, which may probably upon trial, prove a more speedy and effectual remedy, than anyone hitherto employed for that purpose. The power I allude to is ELECTRICITY:[8] and from careful observation of its effects on the human body, I am strongly of opinion that (together with warmth and friction) a few electrical shocks, from a jar containing one hundred or two hundred square inches of coated surface, fully charged (from which not danger, I think, need be apprehended) and passed in different directions through the body, but particularly through the heart and lungs, might produce the desired effect, in a very short time; when perhaps all other applications after a long and unremitted perseverance, may have proved wholly ineffectual. Those who have considered the rapidity and violence with which a charge of electricity passes through the human body, and the *internal concussion*, (procurable by no other means) which is given to those parts that are brought immediately into the circuit will, I imagine, be instantly convinced of the probability of its success, in the case of those unfortunate persons, for whose benefit I now wish to recommend it.... Why not have recourse to the most potent stimulus in nature, which can instantly pervade the inmost recesses of the animal frame? Why not immediately (if a machine can be procured) apply electrical shocks to the brain and heart, the *primum vivens* & *ultimum moriens* of the animal machine? (*Reports*, 1775, p. 77)

Animal experiments had shown that the heart could be stopped by electrical shocks and started again by the same:

> The effects of electricity were, sometime ago, finely illustrated by the ingenious Abdilgard, in many curious experiments on apparently dead animals; wherein by dextrous management of its power, he is said to be capable of alternately suspending and restoring animation at pleasure .... From the above phenomena, which appear

to be no less singular than interesting, it seems reasonable to conclude, that electricity ought to be principally directed to the thoracic viscera in form of gentle shocks: That these should be so accurately adjusted to the tone of the moving fibres, as may renew the perfect unison of action, which is natural to the system. (A. Fothergill, 1795, p. 127)

Fothergill demonstrates in the above an inkling of the true nature of fibrillation and role of defibrillation. He realizes that it is not merely stimulation, but the coordination of muscular contraction that is important. He goes on to point out that electricity and artificial respiration may have an additive effect:

[Electricity] may be used, with perfect safety, during any part of the process. That artificial respiration, however, may contribute not a little to its success, can scarcely be doubted. Therefore to make them co-operate, their forces must be combined, or employed in succession. (pp. 127–9)

Though a number of means were used to generate electrical shocks, a device designed by Charles Kite specifically for the Society bears the closest resemblance to today's defibrillators (1788, p. 193).

Heat: the fire of life

It is evident that the first step to be taken for the recovery [of the drowned] is, to restore the heat of the body .... For this purpose, the body as soon as possible, is to be stripped of its wet cloths, to be well dried and to be wrapped in a dry, and, if possible, warm coverings.

(Cullen, 1776, p. 8)

As discussed above, hypothermia is an inextricable part of drowning in the waters of the temperate and polar zones. Re-warming was accomplished by stripping off wet clothes and getting the victim into a warm environment: in front of a fire, into the sun, into a warm bath, placing him or her in bed between two volunteers, applications of warm foments, hot bricks, bags or socks filled with warm sand, friction with warm flannels, and so on. Again, as already discussed, it is evident from examination of case reports that, in hindsight, the most successful therapeutic act of The Method was re-warming. Though the importance of re-warming was recognized, the somewhat complex cause-and-effect relationship of decreased body temperature to symptoms remained unclear. Because of the difficulties in linking causes (apoplexy, asphyxia, loss of animal heat) to symptomatic effects (pulselessness, apnoea, decreased body temperature), other therapeutic techniques (agitation, chest and abdominal compressions, friction, bleeding, ventilation, tobacco smoke enemas, electrical shocks) were often given credit for the successful effect that the removal of wet clothing and placement near a fire had silently accomplished.

Drugs: elixirs of life

Most of the drugs used in The Method could be classed as 'stimulants', whether they were embrocations, inhalants, emetics, purgatives or the rather special case of tobacco. Gin, rum, brandy, vinegar, sal ammonia, spirits of hartshorn, tincture of benzoin, rosewater, lavender and various other compounds were rubbed on the skin, waved under the nose or applied to the temples and wrists (Cullen, 1776, p. 12). The hope was that the excitation of the cutaneous, olfactory or visceral nerves by embrocations, volatiles, emetics and purgatives would communicate itself to the muscles of respiration and the heart. Emetic tartar (tartaric acid and antimony), ipecacuana in wine, heavily salted water or tickling the back of the throat with an oiled feather were all variously recommended by the Society (Cullen, 1776, p. 24). However, the Society was never very enthusiastic about the use of drugs, other than tobacco, and by 1810, most had fallen out of favour (Curry, 1815, p. 57).

An unusually popular method of stimulating the bowel, which was thought to retain the vital principle of irritability to the greatest degree, was the *enema fumosum*, that is, tobacco smoke fumigations of the rectum (*Reports*, 1775, p. 78). Such was the enthusiasm for the *enema fumosum* that special fumigators were manufactured for inclusion in the Humane Society's resuscitation kits and, for many years, it was considered the piece of equipment most essential to revival (Humane, 1785, p. 24). However, in case of emergency, other mechanisms might suffice:

> Whilst some of the Spectators of this melancholy Accident were advising to hang her by the Heels, and others ordering different Measures to be taken, a Soldier with his Pipe in his Mouth, came to ask the Reason of such a Concourse of People; upon being informed of the Accident, he desir'd the disconsolate Husband to give over

weeping, because his Wife would return to Life very soon. Then giving his Pipe to the Husband, he bid him introduce the small End of it into the Anus, put a Piece of Paper perforated with a Large Number of Holes upon its Mouth, and thro' that blow the Smoke of the Tobacco into her Intestines, as strongly as he possibly could. (Physician, 1746, p. 45)

The woman is reported to have returned to life, grateful for the canniness of the soldier and the devotion of her husband.

As early as 1776, Cullen, though recommending the *enema fumosum*, thought its effectiveness due more to its heat rather than to the medicinal effect of the smoke (1776, p. 16). In 1788, Kite questioned the whole theory of sympathetic irritability and whether the stimulation of the intestines was communicated to the heart (1788, p. 184). In 1791, Coleman declared that the use of tobacco smoke 'is quackery in the highest degree' (1791, p. 236). The Humane Society ceased recommending the use of fumigations after 1811, when Sir Benjamin Brodie demonstrated that he could kill dogs with tobacco (Curry, 1815, p. 128).

The Lancet: blood and life

> Nature, in this, as in other critical situations, sometimes happily triumphs over the *remedy*, as well as the *disease*.
>
> (A. Fothergill, 1795, p. 102)

Those familiar with eighteenth-century medical therapeutics may be surprised to find bloodletting omitted from The Method. Throughout the eighteenth century and into the nineteenth, bleeding was, as it had been for centuries, one of the chief weapons in the medical armamentarium. In the Galenic humoral theory of disease, blood was one of the four humours; its excess or deficit thought to be the cause of illness. Galen taught that surplus humours, if allowed to accumulate in some body part, resulted in putrefaction, excess heat and fever. The humoral balance could be restored by removing such superfluities through bloodletting. As the humoral theory gave way to iatromechanism, the technique, bloodletting, persisted, but it acquired a new justification. Instead of a humoral imbalance, disease became the result of blockage and 'congestion' in the great hydraulic machine that was the body (re: the apoplectic theory of drowning). Bleeding was thought to relieve pathological congestion, thus returning normal function to the system and restoring life.

However, the Humane Society was never very keen on bleeding. In early versions of The Method, bleeding was mentioned, but cautioned against, other than in very unusual circumstances:

> Opening a vein in the arm or neck may prove beneficial, but the quantity of blood taken away should not be large; nor should an artery ever be opened, as profuse bleeding has appeared prejudicial, and even destructive to the small remains of life. (Hawes, 1774, p. 9)

In the earliest series of case reports, there were two deaths that the editors of the *Annual Reports* believed might have been hastened by the inappropriate use of bleeding (*Reports*, 1775, p. 77).[9] As early as 1744, John Fothergill stated his opposition to the lancet, pointing out that, regardless of what appeared reasonable in the light of the then dominant apoplectic theory of drowning, bleeding simply did not appear to work (1782, pp. 110–19). Later, the leading lights of the Society (Hawes, Lettsom and Hunter), as committed vitalists, saw blood as a prime candidate for the *vis vitae* (if not the thing itself, then at least the vehicle for it). Loss of it could only mean loss of life-force.

> Bleeding deprives us of the most important point which it is our object to promote, viz. irritability; and when symptoms of recovery are apparent, if we diminish this power it will always prove injurious and sometimes fatal. (Bartlett, 1792, p. 9)

The triumph of the hypoxic theory of asphyxia over the apoplectic should have put paid to bleeding by pulling any theoretical justification out from under it. Nevertheless, it took a long time dying. Though the Society condemned bleeding outright in 1795, this condemnation was persistently ignored by physicians in correspondence with the Society. Medical practitioners continued to sing the praises of bloodletting in the Society's *Case Reports* well into the nineteenth century. It was not until 1835 that the lancet was finally prised from their fingers by Pierre Louis. Using his *méthode numérique*, he famously proved in *Recherches sur les effets de la saignée* (1835) that bloodletting had no discernible effect on the outcome of patients with pneumonia (R. Porter, 1999, pp. 312–13).

However, bloodletting's persistence as a last-ditch therapeutic manoeuvre exemplifies three important points that have more general application. The first is the phenomenon of the persistence of a practice or a therapeutic technique through a series of conflicting theoretical justifications. This is touched on by Bynum in reference to the use of both bleeding and cathartics. Bloodletting, he points out, had worked its way through several theoretical justifications before being proved both empirically ineffective and logically invalid, and finally being dropped from medical therapeutics. Bynum states that: 'There is a great deal of historical continuity in therapeutics, much more so than in theories of disease' (1994, p. 18). Technique persists; theory changes. Techniques are not always abandoned in the face of changing ideology; rather ideology is often bent to accommodate technique. Indeed, the therapeutic act persists not merely in the face of changing theory, but because of it. Therapeutic technique, when under threat, is often salvaged by a sudden and radical transformation in the explanation of both the therapeutic effect of the act and the pathophysiology of the underlying disease, in what amounts to a sort of ideological conversion. Why an empirically ineffective technique should persist when theory changes, or even because theory changes, requires some explanation.

Habit and the external influences of culture, politics, economics and suchlike all have their role to play in the persistence of technique, but in the rather special case of therapeutic acts at the deathbed there is more to it than mere inertia or secondary gain. This brings us to the second important point exemplified by the use of bloodletting *in extremis*. Alongside bleeding's therapeutic use, there was a diagnostic purpose. In the moribund patient, the absence of a brisk bleed on opening a vessel and a dark colour to the blood were indications of the patient's failed respiratory and circulatory systems.[10] Folk custom in some locales and even occasionally written wills required the opening of a vein prior to consigning the corpse to the grave. This was not merely to make certain that the diagnosis of death was correct, but should that diagnosis be wrong, the opened vein itself would insure that, in due time, it would be made right. If the victim was not dead, he or she soon would be and thus be spared the horror of awaking to find him or herself mistakenly interred. This last form of insurance is the third important function of a deathbed therapy. Terminal therapeutics is subject to a terminal paradox: What does not cure kills.

The Method

> It was thought impossible, after a complete suspension of the vital functions had once taken place, that a restoration could be effected; had it been attempted, it would have excited a

sneer, and been considered as a proof of folly. This happy and enlightened age claims the honour of giving birth to humane societies. By their establishment the polished world became possessed of an invaluable gem ...

(Bartlett, 1792, p. 6)

Though physicians had long treated the moribund, prior to the eighteenth century their participation in deathbed activities was limited. Once they had bled, forced vomiting or induced diarrhoea, there was little more help (or damage) they could give, and so the physician usually made a strategic exit making room for the priest (R. Porter, 1999, p. 302). As religious ritual became increasingly attenuated in the sixteenth and seventeenth centuries, the position of the physician at the deathbed was increasingly strengthened. By the end of the eighteenth century, religion, by its continence of the use of opium in ameliorating the suffering of the body, had given implicit permission for the doctor to do something in the face of death (though the actual administration of drugs was usually left in the hands of family members) (Ariès, 1981, p. 409).

It began to be accepted that human intervention might be exercised to restore life. Science might actually have something to offer at the deathbed. Something *could* be done in the face of death. What developed was 'an obvious contest ... between the skilful practitioner and the overwhelmed powers of nature: [where] attention and care was necessary on his part in order to insure victory' (Hawes, 1774, p. 14). *Could* quickly became *should*. The imperative to save life, to do something, became couched in the language of empire and war (a trope that medicine continues to exploit, as many have pointed out). A battlefield immanent within the body replaced the outward journey of the soul towards the transcendent. The deathbed had always been a site of struggle, in that the forces of good and evil were locked in a battle over the soul of the victim, but with increasing secularization the nature of this struggle changed. The adversary was no longer a transcendent force – the devil – and the reward transcendent bliss – heaven. The adversary now became the process of transcendence itself – death – and the reward was now a postponement of that transcendental journey – a return to life.

The Method of the Humane Society gave the physician something 'to do' at the deathbed. The sudden appearance of death, far from discouraging hope, became a call to action. The Method enabled and encouraged heroic intervention in the process of sudden death. The protocols for the drowned were a secular intervention at the deathbed, organized, perhaps not as broadly and comprehensively as religious deathbed ritual, but organized, none the less, along similar lines. Like religious ritual with its liturgy, these medical protocols required a carefully specified mode of performance, a supporting institutional structure, participation by professionals and laity, an underlying theoretical doctrine and a certain amount of faith.

The *Annual Report*: 'The correspondence of the learned and ingenious ...'

> There is every reason to hope, that a generous spirit of trying these salutary experiments, with vigour and perseverance, will be diffused over the whole kingdom; productive of the most happy consequences to the multitude.
>
> (Hawes, 1774, p. 9)

The Humane Society, as was the case of many nineteenth-century philanthropic societies, practised a form of secular evangelism. It had good news, that of revival, and it needed to spread it. The Society used a number of means: pamphlets, posters, public demonstrations, lectures and sermons. Its main propaganda organ was its *Annual Report*. Initially, each *Annual Report* was a slim volume, but subsequent editions grew larger and larger, often to over 500 pages. Editions from the mid-1780s on contained the latest recension of The Method, a financial statement, scientific papers, diagrams for instruments, editorial comment, letters from individual practitioners, communications from other Humane Societies, extracts from sermons, poetry and, on one occasion, a play. However, the bulk of each *Annual Report* was taken up with case reports. These were meant to provide an empirical fund of clinical experience that might be applied towards the perfection of the protocol:

> The advantages resulting from the reception and publication of Communications are many and indisputable. Science, in general, is advanced by the correspondence of the learned and ingenious. Errors are thereby discovered and just principles attained. Even an acquaintance with the unsuccessful attempts of others, joined into an examination of the causes of their failure, often leads to a happier practice. (Humane, 1781, p. v)

Especially in the early years, 1774–90, considerable effort was expended in detailing attempted revivals. A representative of the Humane Society would interview the victim (if the revival was successful), the rescuers and as many witnesses as possible. These case reports recorded not just the facts surrounding the accident itself and the techniques used in reanimation, but details of both the victims' and rescuers' social situation, family, physiognomy and personality.

The tone of the case report was often more that of a 'Boy's Own Adventure' than our modern idea of a clinical file. Certainly, much of that impression is due to an anachronistic reading of (what we see as) the rather purple prose of the period; but beyond that, the *Reports* were self-confessedly more than merely archival. Initially no more than a manual of technique, with appended empirical justification in the form of case studies, the *Reports* became much like an evening's programming on BBC2 television – some news, some information, a little art, a bit of religion and lashings of drama. The *Reports* came to include research, instruction, propaganda and entertainment.

In 1787, the demands of propaganda and entertainment led the Humane Society to revise its criteria for the inclusion of case reports. Before 1787, reports of all cases, successful and unsuccessful, were published. After 1787, unsuccessful cases were no longer reported:

> But as so dismal a catalogue can answer no valuable purpose in the subsequent years, the particulars will be omitted, and the numbers only of the premature deaths stated. It must be more pleasing to our readers, as well as to ourselves, to dwell upon the preservations which have occurred ... and other interesting subjects connected with animation. (Royal, 1789, p. 71)

Of course, on a crude psychological level, no one likes to broadcast their mistakes, but there was much more at stake than a threat to the physicians' esteem. The case studies had become dramatic adventures evoking the dangers of the commonplace. They celebrated the victory of life over death and sent out a call for a new kind of hero saving a new kind of victim – the 'common' man.

Victims: 'Taken from a watery grave ...'

> The design for which [the Society] was established can hardly be opposed, when it is remarked, that it was formed to protect the industrious from the fatal effects of unavoidable accidents; the young and inexperienced from being sacrificed

to their recreations and the unhappy victim of desponding melancholy and deliberate suicide from the miserable consequences of a disgraceful death .... Of what value is life to the community, or how it is estimated by individuals, is hardly requisite to state; in the strength and number of the people, consist the true opulence and security of the nation; and next to the hopes of blissful futurity, LONGEVITY is deemed the greatest blessing conferred upon the human race – Individuals prize it on the score of their relative and social connections. How painful is it to be torn suddenly from an indulgent parent, a dutiful child, a beloved wife, or an affectionate husband. Judge then, when hope itself is nearly fled, how great the joy to be unexpectedly restored to all these near and tender attachments. Nor will even religion be silent on this occasion; she will rejoice that the triumphs of her enemy are diminished, and that those whom the wisdom of providence thinks fit to afflict, though they become desponding from distress, are prevented from being criminal by self-murder.

(Humane, 1781, pp. x–xi)

On reading the Society's tracts, there is little doubt that the men and women supporting it were genuinely concerned with alleviating the suffering attendant upon unnecessary and sudden death. However, the Humane Society was not merely involved in the relief of personal suffering. It was an institution labouring in the great Enlightenment project of the rational construction of a 'good society'. As such, it saw itself in service to the institutional pillars of society – industry, religion and the family. The Society chose its victims (so to speak) on the basis of the needs of those important social institutions. The ideal victim was young, healthy, industrious and open to salvation.

> We have seen the child unexpectedly restored to the arms of its fond parents; the father, and support of a family, to his wife and children; the suicide has been snatched from the guilt of becoming his own destroyer. (*Reports*, 1775, p. vi)

The three most common situations in which the protocols were employed were work-related accidents involving men employed on the water, suicide attempts by young women and the accidental drowning of children.

The workman

> The industrious *Poor* ... from working upon the water, and in mines, &c. are necessarily exposed to the disasters mentioned above; and have they not a kind of demand upon us, to interpose, and avert, if possible, the fatal consequences to which they are rendered liable by serving the community with their labours, and gaining honest livelihood? Nay, is it not our *interest*, as well as duty, to replace them, if possible, in their sphere of usefulness, that they may again work for their wives and families; whereby these may be snatched from immediate misery and want, and the community be relieved from an expensive burden?
>
> (Hawes, 1774, p. 45)

The most efficient means of transporting goods and people in the swiftly industrializing eighteenth century was on the water. The vast majority of adult male drowning victims were employed in the water trades: sailors, watermen, bargemen, stevedores and drunks (the last category is perhaps not strictly occupational). Miners, kiln stokers and brewery workers were also exposed to death by asphyxia. The Society pointed out that the loss of a good workman was felt by his family, his employer and society as a whole. The literature of the Society spoke the utilitarian logic of its Nonconformist founders:

> Every person in society must be esteemed worth a certain sum to the community; what the average value may be estimated at I am unable to determine, calculators being much divided in their opinions; but I presume, that the mean proportion of the inhabitants of Great Britain cannot be rated at a less value than ONE HUNDRED GUINEAS each. Upon this calculation the HUMANE SOCIETY has, under the Divine Providence, saved our country A HUNDRED AND TWO THOUSAND, ONE HUNDRED AND FIFTY SIX POUNDS, within eight years. (Royal, 1789, p. 165)

The relationship between the health and wealth of nations was prominent in political and economic thought of the eighteenth century. As the modern state, characterized by centralized government, began to emerge, so ideas of the value of the nation's health began to appear (D. Porter, 1999, p. 49). As the individual was the source of that wealth, so society had a vested interest in the individual:

> Let us for a moment ... survey the Inhabitants of such a kingdom swarming over the aqueous element – extending its limits, and increasing its already wide dominion! Let us behold the most valuable and industrious members of the community ploughing the dangerous bosom of the ocean, that thence a more plenteous harvest of wealth may be reaped by the state, than even the fruitful fields could afford! Let us consider the vastness of the numbers thus employed; fairly appreciate their value, and their importance to their country – to their families! – Let us estimate the dangers to which they are constantly exposed in their struggles to provide for those Families, and to aggrandize the power and opulence of that Country! (Royal, 1789, pp. x–ix)

The 'power and opulence' of the nation depended upon the strength, number and health of its people. The Society, in preserving the 'industrious poor', preserved the wealth of the nation.

The suicide

> We have learned, that this unhappy creature is of good character; that she had thrown herself into the water, having been stripped of all her clothes, and turned out of doors by her inhuman step-mother.
>
> (Humane, 1777, p. 51)
>
> The unfortunate creature was only thirteen years of age; she had embezzled some money to the amount of 15 or 16 shillings, and afterwards fearing detection, and its consequent punishment, she was tempted to commit the horrid crime of suicide.
>
> (Humane, 1777, p. 32)
>
> The distressed unfortunate gave me the following account: That she was a native of Stratford upon Avon, was married, and had four children, and was pregnant with the fifth; that her husband became idle and disorderly, and that her friends had taken to the children; that her husband prevailed on her

to accompany him in search of work (being by trade a linen weaver) that she went with him to Manchester, Stockport, and many other places, and last to Wolverhampton, where he left her; that she followed him towards Kidderminster, but despaired overtaking him; that having neither money nor friends, and being deserted by her husband, she determined to put an end to her life.

(Royal, 1789, p. 210)

Suicides comprised up to 29 per cent of the annual cases of attempted revival in the years prior to 1780. Between 1774 and 1776, out of 78 adult cases of successful reanimation 24 were female, and of these 13 (54 per cent) were suicide attempts. For males, the incidence of suicide as a cause was 9 per cent. In most cases, there is mention made of straitened financial circumstances, inability to get work or homelessness. 'Unhappy', 'unfortunate', 'distressed' – emphasis is placed on the social conditions occasioning the fatal decision. On the other hand, the suicide was 'stained with the guilt of murder' – the perpetrator of a 'horrid' and 'horrible crime':

> With respect to the latter class, although it is *misery* in one shape or another that drives anyone to commit the horrible crime of suicide, yet every serious and considerate mind must earnestly wish to snatch them from such a destruction; so that their souls may not rush into the presence of their Creator, *stained with the guilt of murder*, and that their relations may also be rescued from the *shame* as well as *loss* to which such rashness exposes them .... [One] must feel an additional pleasure in recalling a miserable creature from the very brink of eternity, into which he was precipitating himself by his own guilt; which guilt has this alleviation – it was occasioned by *wretchedness*. (Hawes, 1774, p. 45)

The popularity of suicide by drowning may have initially drawn the Society into this line of work, but once involved, it began to respond to suicides of all types. Hanging had always been common and overdoses with opium were becoming more so. These conditions whose proximate cause of death is, like drowning, respiratory failure, proved satisfyingly amenable to The Method.

The saving of suicides was a double salvation. Not only was life snatched from death, thus fulfilling the 'humane' remit of the Society, but these unfortunates were saved 'that their souls may not rush into the presence of their Creator, stained with the guilt of murder'. Though organized religion had, by and large, conceded to medicine the right to interfere in death's advance, the Society's interference with Providence did not go entirely unquestioned. It was important that the Society have a Christian validation for its actions, for, in raising the dead, it trod on sacred ground. However, this interference might be excused if it could be interpreted as doing the Lord's work. The case of the suicide, where redemption depended on revival, provided a neat justification for The Method's place in God's plan. Saved from death. Saved from crime. Saved from sin. The Society was thus able to justify its reanimative activities on a number of fronts. Its revival of the common man served humanity; its preservation of the industrious poor Mammon, and its rescue of the suicide God.

The child

> And how many a parent is hourly subject to the danger of seeing a sprightly and adventurous son brought home to him a breathless corpse! What would they not give at that instant for the most distant hopes of recovery!
>
> (Hawes, 1774, p. 6)

The third group of victims were children. Approximately 40 per cent of cases between 1774 and 1800 were children under the age of 15 years. Drowning was, and remains, a particular danger to small children who walk before they can swim, and to older children who leap before they look. The small child's combination of curiosity, poor motor skills and unfamiliarity with water puts him or her at great risk around rivers, ponds and wells. The peaks of incidence in the paediatric age group in eighteenth century were the same as they are today: toddlers of both sexes and 12–15-year-old boys.

Children were ideal victims. Their potential for the future made them particularly worthy of revival. Furthermore, the innocent child embodied the Enlightenment ideal of innate virtue, upon which the future of both the man of reason and the good society might be built. Man might be made good because as a child (like the noble savage, the child of history) he was born good. Childhood and the child were becoming central to a concept of the family as the incubator of social progress. Childhood innocence became a precious commodity to be protected and nurtured by the good society so that such innocence might survive into adulthood and blossom as virtue.

The child was not only the spotless lamb, ideal (paradoxically) as both sacrificial victim and candidate for rescue, but the paediatric body is an ideal physiological substrate for the techniques of revival. Contrary to popular belief, children are not the delicate buds they appear. They are in many ways, like the bud, hardier than the full-blown flower, at least when frost is in the air. Children, though particularly prone to hypothermia, are also unusually resistant to its deleterious effects and especially well served by its protective ones. The revival of the hypothermic child is, and remains, particularly gratifying.

'The humble and the illustrious'

Though there were alcoholic ne'er do wells, ungrateful suicides and infants smothered in their cots, by far the majority of cases were portrayed as examples of one of the three ideal models of victim. Each of these may be taken as embodying an important component of eighteenth-century social structure. The economic system represented by the industrious workman as the support of the family and the state; religion by the penitent Magdalene saved from both the grave and hell; and the family embodied in the beloved child, the centre of the family unit and the future of society. The Society not only saved the individual victim, but also was portrayed as saving society itself. How then could society not support it?

> On what can the liberality of a rich and powerful nation be better bestowed, than on an institution which stretches forth its preserving hand alike to the humble and the illustrious, to the favoured child of affluence and grandeur, and to the unhappy vassal of poverty and misfortune; nay, to the heedless votary of treacherous pleasure, and to the desperate victim of blasphemous despair? (Royal, 1789, p. vii)

Benefactors: 'The service of the community ...'

> Non fasces, non purpureum, non divitias, non ingenium, sed animum communi utlitati inservientem, dignitas sequitur.
>
> (Royal, 1789, p. 4)[11]

Those who laboured to achieve the Society's goals were a diverse group. They varied in the form of their attachment to the Society, their mode of participation and their social, professional and economic status. One became a director in the Society by contributing one guinea per annum. Membership provided a subscription to the Society's *Annual Report* and the opportunity to attend its annual banquet. Initially the Society was a middle-class mix, with heavy representation from medicine and the Church. Among the 104 directors listed in the *Reports* of 1774, there were five physicians, 19 surgeons, 14 apothecaries, 17 surgeon-apothecaries, six clergymen, a plumber, printseller, printer, builder, jeweller and the Comptroller General of His Majesties Customs in America. The first president, an honorary position, was the Lord Mayor of London, Frederick Bull. The list of directors grew from 104 in 1774 to close to 500 in 1776. By then it included a few titled names, women, government and institutional donors (Worshipful Company of Fishmongers, Company of Coalfactors and Lightermen, Worshipful Company of Drapers, and so on). Early celebrity members included the playwright and physician Oliver Goldsmith, the actor David Garrick, the surgeon John Hunter and the physician William Heberden. In 1783, George III became patron of the Society, and thereafter the Humane Society was the Royal Humane Society. As the years went on, the Society became a popular recipient of bequests – or sometimes not:

> The amiable old gentleman, it seemed, had intended to leave the whole to the Royal Humane Society, and had indeed executed a will to that effect; but the Institution, having been unfortunate enough, a few months before, to save the life of a poor relation to whom he paid a weekly allowance of three shillings and sixpence, he had, in a fit of very natural exasperation, revoked the bequest in a codicil, and left it all to Mr. Godfrey Nickleby; with a special mention of his indignation, not only against the society for saving the poor relation's life, but against the poor relation also, for allowing himself to be saved. (Charles Dickens, *Nicholas Nickleby* [1839], 1990, p. 2)

The clergy too were prominent among the subscribing members of the Society and were especially valued as apologists for its activities. Though fears of accusations of impiety were sometimes expressed in the Society's literature, there is little evidence of objections to reanimation from organized religion. Many sermons were given propounding God's approval of medicine's presumption:

> 'The Son of Man is not come to destroy men's lives, but to save them' [Luke 9: 56]. The words of our Lord ... naturally lead us to consider the value of human life, and the duty of preserving it by every method in our power .... He at once gave demonstration of

the power which he had received from his Father in Heaven, and of the value which he sat on human life .... when he raised *Lazarus* from the grave, after he had been buried for four days.... There is no evil which we so generally dread, as the loss of life: 'All that a man hath he will give for his life.' Every conceivable enjoyment on this side of Heaven depends on the continuance of life. Crowns and sceptres lose their value as their owners draw near the grave. In that dark abode, the slave and the sovereign are equally impotent: In the grave there is no knowledge – no mental enjoyment .... As all sensation depends on the organs of life, so when those organs are destroyed, we have reason to fear all mental exercises must cease, until he who first gave us existence shall restore us from the ruins of nature, and bring us forward to resume the task, and complete the work which we left unfinished .... Institutions have been formed in various parts of the world, for the recovery of persons, after they had tasted death, and sunk into a state of insensibility, from which, if left without assistance, they could not have awoke, 'till the morning of the resurrection. A proposal for a society, for the purpose now mentioned, in former days of ignorance and superstition, would no doubt have been treated as impious and absurd: But the success which has attended the exertions of societies formed for the recovery of the dead, particularly such as were drowned, has far exceeded expectation. (Lathrop, 1787, pp. 6–15)

This, like most sermons preached on behalf of the Humane Society, presents a line of reasoning that saw medicine and science as manifestations of God's grace, part of the Creator's gift to man and meant to be used in service to man's salvation.[12]

Rescuers: 'Persons of every description ...'

It was recognized that the most important factor leading to the 'recovery of the apparently dead, is the length of time that elapses before the proper remedies can be applied' (Kite, 1788, p. S2). In sudden death, whether it from cardiac arrest in the twentieth century or drowning in the eighteenth, there is a temporal imperative that necessitates drawing the layperson into the protocol. This temporal imperative was, and is, the justification used for the universal dissemination of both The Method and CPR:

> But although Medical Men are, from the nature of their studies and profession, particularly qualified for being useful on such occasions, it by no means follows that they are exclusively so; on the contrary,

repeated experience has shewn, that intelligent persons of every description may readily acquire sufficient information upon the subject, to render them the happy instruments of recovery. (Curry, 1815, p. iv)

The Method required and the Society hoped for participation by waterman and physician, natural philosopher and clergyman, peasant and prince. The Society sought to encourage participation by these diverse social groups by providing rewards suitable to the status of each.

Reward was as central to the Humane Society's goals as promulgation of The Method. Even before the Society had been officially founded, its main mover, William Hawes, offered out of his own pocket rewards to the Thames watermen for bringing to him the bodies of the drowned. When the Society was established, rescuers were rewarded for pulling the victim from the water and for applying The Method to the victim. The necessity of monetary reward was coloured by the Society's opinion of the lower classes:

> It is now universally acknowledged, that an immense number of lives have been preserved by the instantaneous efforts and immediate exertions of watermen and others, on the alarm of accidents by drowning, &c. It is too well known that such characters are only to be stimulated by the certainty of pecuniary encouragement; which are regularly ordered to be paid by the Managers of your valuable Society; therefore the gratuities allowed and expended on such interesting occasions, as rescuing the human race from the jaws of death, are highly laudable in an institution established for the security and preservation of life. (Royal, 1789, p. 64)

The humanitarian concern of 'such characters' was thus encouraged by four guineas for every life saved, two for an unsuccessful attempt and one to the publican who allowed his premises to be used for the exercise of The Method. The reward could be refused and often was, even by 'the lower class of people',' who frequently requested that the money be given to the victims' families.

The medical profession was expected to, and did, provide its services *gratis*. The medical practitioner attended the scene of the accident as a skilled technician, a reliable scientific observer and a sort of medical police officer:

> We embrace with pleasure this opportunity of observing, that the grand advantage of our Institution over that of other nations, seems

to be derived from this voluntary Service of Gentlemen of the Faculty. As they are in a public capacity, the places of their abode are readily found, and the *best* assistance is immediately afforded. For although the modes of treatment are such that they may be applied by those unacquainted with the Medical art; yet it is natural to imagine that these Gentlemen will be more expert in the use of them than others; that they will be more cautious not to employ the pernicious and justly-exploded methods of suspending the body with the head downwards, rolling it upon the ground, or on a barrel, &c. A man of skill in his profession will also have opportunities of making such observations and improvements as may be productive of still greater success. The early presence of a gentleman of character is moreover a security against imposition. The reward given to the first messenger that applies to a Medical Gentleman, effectually prevents any neglect in that article; and when he is present, he is in a situation to make such enquiry, and collect such intelligence from the numbers around him, as leave no room for deceit and collusion; so that of the numerous cases which have already fallen under our inspection, we have not, had the least reason to suspect any intended fraud. (Humane, 1777, p. 100)

As the above quote implies, the idealized Enlightenment physician was to be a champion of reason against superstition, free inquiry against dogmatism and truth against fraud. The clinician/scientist was to be a hero leading the fight against death, suffering, want and fear – or at least that was the hope. Contributors to the *Reports* portrayed each other as a combination of scientist and saint: 'The happy instrument of Heaven, in turning the sorrows of multitudes into joy, and their lamentations into exclamations of gratitude' (*Reports*, 1775, p. vi).

In lieu of money, medals were awarded to those medical men who provided their time and services free of charge. Many rescues involved considerable danger to the rescuer, and those who put themselves in danger were also awarded medals. The Society's original medal, designed in 1774 by Dr Watkinson and engraved by Thomas Pingo of the Royal Mint, was silver, two inches in diameter and portrayed a young boy blowing on the 'torch of life'. It was inscribed *LATEAT SCINTILLA FORSAN*: 'Perhaps a Spark May Yet Remain.' The obverse was engraved with the civic crown, the reward given in ancient Rome to those who saved the life of a fellow citizen. Surrounding this was the inscription *HOC PRETIVM CIVE SERVATO TVLIT*: 'He Has Obtained This Prize for Having Saved the Life of a Citizen'.

The Society's highest award was the Gold Medal, reserved for acts of exceptional bravery in a dangerous rescue, or, as in the following case, a modicum of sagacity in an exceptional rescuer:

> On The Second Alexander, Emperor of All the Russias, Restoring a poor Man to Life who had been drowned by The Rev. James Plumtree, M.A.
>
> By widows' tears and hapless orphans' moans,
> By nations' cries, and by a whole world's groans,
> From Macedonia Alexander rose,
> And built his fame upon his subjects' woes;
> Then wept, unable to extend his state,
> And all succeeding times agree to call him Great.
> On Wilna's stream, as Russia's Monarch stray'd,
> A peasant's body on the bank was laid,
> Of seeming life bereft; a friendly band,
> Forth from the flood, had brought it to the land,
> And gather'd round with unavailing zeal,
> If signs of life they haply might reveal:
> But all in vain. Yet with paternal love,
> The Prince himself would every means approve;
> With unremited energy applied,
> Till thrice the hour revolv'd; then, lo! The tide
> Of life again renew'd, and sighing breath
> Gave token he'd repass'd the gate of death.
> With eyes up-rais'd the Father Monarch stood,
> 'The brightest day is this of all my life, good God!!!'
> Tears from his eyes the pious words attend,
> And Alexander lives the poor man's friend.
> You, who the story hear, the hearts elate,
> Say, is not Russia's Emperor THE GREAT?
>
> (Royal, 1814, pp. 12–13)

The Tsar's actions consisted of little more than ordering that the man's wet clothes be removed and chafing his wrists. However, to give the Tsar credit, when the imperial physician rode up and told him that he was wasting his time, Alexander insisted on continuing the rewarming process and the peasant eventually regained consciousness. It all ends happily with the Tsar 'giving the poor man some money' and eventually being rewarded himself with the Royal Humane Society's Gold Medal and this 'splendid' poem (Royal, 1814, p. 13).

Spectators: 'Behold them alive from the jaws of death!'

Resuscitative protocols, then and now, are designed to be universal in their practice – anywhere, anytime, by anyone. The Society worked towards this ideal universality by disseminating The Method as widely as possible, one means being the exercise of The Method in public. Restorations tended, as most accident do, to gather crowds:

> She was to all appearances quite dead .... There were upwards of one hundred spectators who had the satisfaction of seeing the proper means employed, which fortunately restored the young woman alive to her disconsolate friends. (Humane, 1785, p. 90)

The activities of the Society came to be something of a spectator sport. Many restorations were carried out in the drinking houses that lined the Thames. The Society provided monetary compensation to publicans who allowed their establishments to be used and when the Society began to set up 'general receiving houses' where reanimative equipment might be stored, pubs were frequently chosen.[13] Whether out of a sense of duty, monetary reward or the fact that restoration was thirsty work in front of a thirsty audience, publicans appeared willing to allow their premises to be used.

However, spectators, like the ambulance chasers of today, could hinder rescue efforts. By 1783, the large numbers of spectators that gathered had become a significant problem and The Method began to warn of problems occasioned by attracting crowds. Nevertheless, spectatorship at these events continued to be high, and the Society, somewhat ambivalently, continued to play to the crowd in demonstrations of its 'revivals'.

By 1783, the Society had instituted a public Annual Festival, at which rescuers were presented with their medals and the 'saved' were paraded around a hall in solemn procession (Humane, 1785, p. 5). Surviving victims were presented with, 'a Bible, a Common Prayer, and another religious book, *The Great Importance of a Religious Life,* with a view of rendering them thoroughly sensible of the great mercies received, and of preparing them for future happiness' (Hawes, 1797, p. viii). Speeches were made and sermons given extolling the virtues of The Method and the Society:

> Of all the means, which divine or human exertions can employ, to lift the admiration, or win the love of a beholding world, none can ensure these more completely than calling back into life those who are dear to us .... There some of them, who are monuments of the

blessings of this HUMANE SOCIETY, now stand before you. Behold them alive from the jaws of death! They were buried by the overwhelming deep, or they felt the strangling hand of death in other ways. They were consigned to the state of darkness, which you never seriously reflect on but with trembling. They actually entered that land of the enemy, compared with whose captivity, every bondage, every evil upon earth is welcome to your minds; and even to retard whose approach, you count all the wealth of the world cheaply laid out, in the hour when he threatens you with his grasp .... Had you seen them in the tumultuous moment, when every little remnant sense was struggling for rescue from the cruel element, which strove to extinguish it; what, that the hand or purse could have spared, in the impatient endeavour to save a sinking brother? ... Even now perhaps, while we speak, a beloved child, a father, or a mother just taken from a watery grave, or gathered up from the suffocating stroke, are bedewed with the tears of surrounding and inconsolable relations, whilst the motionless eyes cannot repay with one single glance the bursting sobs, which fain would wake them into life: – They run, they cry aloud for the blest hand, for the dear, humane, divine art, that shall give salvation. (Bromley, 1782, pp. 9–27)

The Society had reasons other than self-aggrandizement for staging such formal displays and encouraging the practice of The Method in public. Most obviously, these were effective ways of spreading the enthusiasm, knowledge and skills necessary to help the individual victim. But as importantly, the Society, as a support to the state, a friend to industry, a guardian of the family, a saviour to the sinner and a rewarder of virtue had not only to do all these things, but had also to be *seen* to do them. Justification for both the Society and The Method was not merely in the life saved, but in the 'Virtue' engendered in both the individual and society as a whole. Good must not only be done, but be seen to be done. The Society exercised its laudatory aims not just as ends in themselves, but as the means towards encouraging, through example:

Gentlemen, I cannot resist calling your attention to the establishment of a *Humane Society* under our auspices at ALGIERS. – I repeat Algiers; for, it is surprising, and almost incredible, though indeed we know it as a fact, that in that barbarous soil *a spark of humanity* is at length kindled. – May it expand, illumine, and soften, the heart equally dark and callous! – What a grateful contrast does this present of the CHRISTIAN SYSTEM to the barbarity of infidels. – In that land, where a Muley Ishmael immolated with his own hands eighty of his relatives – the *amities of the gospel* have led to an establishment that saves the life of even a stranger! ... We have witnessed enough to encourage zealous perseverance in its promotion. – *The little cloud, not a hand's breadth, has expanded even beyond our horizon.* – May it be diffused and expanded to the extreme limits of the universe! (Lettsom, quoted in A. Fothergill, 1795, pp. iv–v)

Humanity and the Humane Society

OCCIDIT, QUI NON SERVAT.

(Hawes, 1797, p. 8)[14]

The Humane Society saw drowning as a particularly democratic form of death as 'no person from the Prince to the Peasant can at all times be secure from those dreadful disasters, which suddenly suspend vital action' (A. Fothergill, 1795, p. 189). All men were equal in the face of such a death and it behove all men to rise against it. The system of revival instituted by the Society thus strove to involve all strata of society from peasant to prince. It provided a structure in which public, profession, church, state and commerce all had roles. It sought to produce a universal and universalizing protocol that could be applied to all forms of sudden death, at all times, in all places, by all people.

> These establishments [Humane Societies] intend a general benefit. They provide a possibility of restoration, which may affect individuals in any sphere of life, either in their own persons and connections. There is scarcely any one but what is exposed to accidents by water, where business or pleasure may call them. (Hawes, 1774, p. 6)

The application of The Method functioned not merely to revive the individual victim, but to redeem society itself.

> It is probable that the moral benefits resulting to the community from these Institutions, may rival the advantages conferred upon the numbers who have been saved from destruction. (Bath, 1806, p. 41)

The Society encouraged the rescuer through the good act to become the good man helping to build the good society. The Humane Society, as its name baldly states, was as much about constructing 'Humanity' as about rescuing the drowned:

> Tis thine, when vital breath seems fled,
> To see the awful confines of the dead;
> Drag the pale victim from the whelming wave,
> And snatch the body from the floating grave;
> To breathe in the life re-animating fire,
> Till warm'd to second life the drown'd respire.
> Hark! As those lips once more begin to move,
> What sounds ascend of gratitude and love!
> Now with the GREAT REDEEMER'S praise they glow,
> They bless the agent of His pow'r below;
> New sprung to life, the renovated band,
> Joyful before their second Saviour's stand;
> And oh, far sweeter than the breathing spring'
> Fairer than Paradise, the wreaths they bring!
> The blissful homage rescued friends impart;
> Th'enraptured incense of a parent's heart;
> O'eraw'd and wond'ring at themselves they see
> And feel the pow'r of soft HUMANITY!

(Pratt, in Royal, *1789*, p. 61)[15]

In Pratt's poem, the conflation of the divine 'Great Redeemer' and the mortal 'second Saviour', through the latter being the former's 'agent of His pow'r below', shifts the authority and responsibility for nature (and the life it quickens) from a transcendent power – God – to a corporate force – humanity. It expresses the hope of a better world through man's mastery over nature. Human society might develop through its own efforts and the individual was capable of a similar self-directed development. Civilization was a progressive, human process. The Enlightenment imposed a new narrative on culture – one that, though recognizing the hand of Providence, was primarily secular. It valued the universal, the novel and the rational over the local, the traditional and the superstitious. A human-centred and progressive society was possible through the active manipulation of social institutions in such a way that they might encourage the humanity of man and his commitment to a humane society.

The dream of the united brotherhood of man moved to common action by a universal threat was one that was shared by other philanthropic organizations of that period, as well as by revolutionary movements in both Europe and America. This was outlined in a letter from Thomas Russell, the President of the Massachusetts Humane Society, to Grenot Vaublanc, the President of the revolutionary French National Assembly:

> Civil liberty takes its root in philanthropy, and will always produce institutions favorable to humanity, and to all the social virtues. From the progress of that freedom, which the revolution effected in your country, is calculated to produce the most useful institutions …. Indeed the world is convinced, that a nation, which has made the happiness of the whole human race, the basis of its civil constitution, cannot fail to exert all its powers in the completion of the glorious plan …. We behold, with rapture, the French and American nations, inspired with the same ardour for human happiness – and feeling the most intimate alliance with Frenchmen, we will only try to emulate them, in the glorious work of restoring the whole world to the situation one great family, dwelling in peace, liberty, and safety …. Impelled by the most exalted feelings of liberty and gratitude, the Americans have embraced the French as their brothers; and as both nations breathe the same spirit of patriotism and humanity, the cement of their affections can never yield to any adverse occurrence, or even to time itself. (Bartlett, 1792, p. 9)

The blossoming of philanthropic societies in the nineteenth century owes much to an evangelical fervour to improve society and the individuals in it through example, education and participation. The Humane Society was well situated to play its own small role in the much larger enterprise of constructing (implicitly, if not explicitly) a humanity free from superstition and the errors of the past. It possessed, in The Method, a practical means of linking all elements of society together in the revival of the drowned and the redemption of the rescuer. 'Humanity' was not merely an abstract concept necessary to the Enlightenment's gradual secularization of the world; but, as a reification of corporate power, it became a practical instrument in the hands of modernity. Humanity was struggling to become something one could lay one's hands on, and, in the restoration of the drowned, one quite literally did.

On a practical level, the application of The Method saved the victim's life and was the essential act upon which the institution of the Humane Society was built and through which its goals were achieved. However, the goal of any technique is seldom absolutely identical with that of the institution that supports the technique. The goal of The Method was revival: the return of life to the victim. The goal of the Society was the redemption of the rescuer, and through redemption of the individual, redemption of society. Salvation depended not on the worship of a transcendent deity, but on a commitment to one's fellow human beings. Ultimately, the revival of the victim and the redemption of the rescuer were in service to the construction of the good society. Something that advocates of CPR are not shy of expressing even today:

> There is another answer to the question of whether resuscitation is worth it. It is true that only a few will be resuscitated. But we must also acknowledge a greater truth: the effort of resuscitation is ennobling. It reveals much about our society's values.... Medicine imposes compassion, reason and decency on a random universe. (Eisenberg, 1997, p. 253)

Both The Method and CPR are thus seen not merely as medical therapeutics but as moral acts. Though the application of the protocol gives benefit to the individual victim, and is the essential objective act upon which the institution is built and through which its goals are achieved, it is, more importantly, a form of social action. Enactment of the protocol not only mediates the relations between the victim and the rescuer, and between the individual and the collective, but helps construct those very entities of self and society.

The Method, used in this way, is a performative act. The mere performance of the humane act is its effect – the construction of humanity. The application of The Method, whether successful or not as a practical act, has already at the moment of its enactment, accomplished the symbolic act of binding the individual participants together in a common humanity. In the performance of the act, a common 'we' is born of an individual 'I'. This ontological shift from the individual to the corporate is less the result of an objective argument than a conversion experience for the subject. Protocol, if it is to achieve the aim of its supporting institution, joins the psychological to the social. It unites the individual psyche to a consciousness of community through shared subjective affect. In what was becoming an increasingly secular universe, to *be* good, one must *do* good; but in being good, one need also *feel* good. To be part of humanity, one need feel human: 'It is a new species of feeling that is awakened, when we shew the dead restored to life' (Bromley, 1782, p. ix). In demonstrating 'the dead restored to life', the Humane Society sought to foster a humane society based on a universal humanity identified by its access to a 'new species of feeling' – the 'humane'. This new species of feeling sought not only to unite all men in the subjective experience of humanity, but the humane feeling was itself that very experience of unity it sought to engender. In a happy tautology, it might give birth to itself, the means not becoming, but being always already the end. This shared affect of the humane would be found in 'the breasts of those of its members who have rescued the prisoners of death, [who] have experienced sensations, the very idea of which the powers of description are too feeble to convey' (Bartlett, 1792, p. 6). A more specific discussion of these 'sensations' must wait on the discussion of the fate of the techniques of the resuscitative protocol given in the following chapters (pp. 173–6).

The future

Grasping religion with one hand and science with the other, the Humane Society seemed set to march into the nineteenth century confident in its task of conquering death and despair:

> It gives us unspeakable pleasure, that we are now able to unite our evidence with that of other nations, in confirmation of a fact equally interesting as it is curious and surprising, *viz.* that persons may, either by immersion in water, or by other species of strangulation, have every faculty totally suspended, so that they shall, to all appearance, be dead for a considerable length of time, and yet it may be in the power of art to recover them ... *we have succeeded;* and we congratulate our countrymen upon having demonstrated a fact, which we hope will, in the process of time, wipe tears from the eyes of thousands: we congratulate ourselves in being the instruments of so much happiness. These were our motives; these our rewards; and we desire no other. (Hawes, 1774, p. 11)

By 1800, we have, if not in exact detail, at least roughly, a resuscitative protocol that is recognizable as such to us today. The theory may have been tentative, but it came to the correct conclusions – if you maintain brain, heart and lung function, you maintain life. The technology may have been crude, but it was sound – re-warming, mouth-to-mouth ventilation and attempts to stimulate cardiac function through electricity and drugs. The delivery system may have been limited, but

The Method was based on the same premise as the chain-of-survival – utilize the lay public and motivate them through education, propaganda and reward. The Society succeeded in building an institutional structure that provided funding, professional personnel, communication, transport, equipment, physical facilities and liaison with the political and economic powers of the day.

However, something happened. Within 60 years, The Method was abandoned. Interest waned in reanimation techniques. Mouth-to-mouth, electrical shocks and most of The Method's other therapeutic manoeuvres fell by the wayside. The focus of the Humane Society narrowed to awarding medals to the brave and the provision of life-saving equipment. Ultimately, even that latter duty was given up and what remains of the Humane Society today is the awarding of medals and citations for bravery. The Method, woven of threads gathered from folklore, established medical practice and the new experimental science, unravelled during the nineteenth century, to be knit again as CPR in the twentieth. How this came about will be explored in the next three chapters.

Part Two
The Techniques

Part Two

The Techniques

4
Defibrillation: *Scintilla Vitalis*

Defibrillation now transcends both ACLS and BLS care.

(American, *Guidelines* I.90)

When after a winter flurry, the sun climbs into the cold blue sky, snow, new fallen on the prairie evens out the irregularities of the ground beneath, hiding grass and weeds, tin cans and dead cats. Spring's green shoots, summer's insects, the slow corruption of autumn lie stilled beneath. When it is very cold, below twenty below, the snowflakes fall small and dry, and the drifts they form are light as down. When you throw yourself backwards into one, it catches you with soft arms. Powdery clouds of white rise to settle back onto your face. Lying in a quiet snowdrift on a bright February day I shut my eyes not to darkness, but to the red warmth of the sun shining through my lids. The snow is warm. How delicious it would be to steal a nap in this clean, soft bed.

22:55 hrs. Crackling over the ambulance-ER radio,
'Teenager, male. Found down in snowdrift on golf course. Naked. Time down unknown. Cold and unresponsive. Pupils fixed and dilated. No respiratory movement. No palpable pulse. CPR's commenced. C-collar applied. V-fib on monitor. Defibrillated × 3. No response. Intubated and bagged. ETA ten minutes.'
23:10. Paramedics roll into the trauma bay, one straddling the stretcher pumping on the boy's chest, one at the head of the bed bagging, the third carrying the IV's and monitor. A quick look at the monitor shows V-fib. A quick look at him shows hard, white Parian marble. Cold and unresponsive. Rectal temp, 26 degrees.

Pupils fixed and dilated. No respiratory movement. No palpable pulse. 'Run D5-normal saline at 42 degrees. Set up for a peritoneal lavage. Get a catheter in. An n/g tube down. Get respiratory to set up ventilator with heated neb. Start a second line. Call County and tell them to send the chopper. We have a hypothermic in V-fib, 26 degrees, will need rewarming by bypass ...'
23:20. 'Doctor, County's bypass unit's in use. Will be for four hours.' 'Damn !... Give me a 14 blade, I'm going to crack his chest.' Start an incision just to the left of the sternum in the fourth intercostal space curving down below the left nipple to the posterior axillary line. Almost no bleeding, but what there is bright red as it runs down his pale flank. 'Large curved Metz.' Cut through the intercostal muscles with the heavy, curved scissors, from the sternum to where his flank meets the table. 'Rib spreaders, please.' Difficult to get them through the incision between the ribs. Hard to crank them apart; chest is so stiff from the cold. Get hand in chest and hold the lung out of the way. Incise the pericardium. Heart cradled in hands. Cold and still. Begin internal massage.
23:30. 'Just pour the warm saline straight into the chest, over my hands.... Keep pouring .... More .... Keep pouring ...'
24:00. Hands are finally warm, so is the heart. Maybe there's a flicker of activity. 'Let's defibrillate. Set to 15 joules. Stand clear' Zap! Heart remains still. 'What does the monitor show? ' 'Fine fib or flat line, I can't tell.' 'Set to 30. Stand clear' Zap! ... 'Again' ... Zap! ... 'Again' ... Zap!
00:15. 'There's a QRS,[16] *there's another, look.' His heart beats, once, pause, again, again, again. It assumes a slow but regular rhythm. 'He's in sinus. Slow. 40. But I can feel a pulse.' 'Keep pouring the warm saline in. Call ICU. Let's get a hold of cardiology and cardiovascular. Jesus! Look, he's beginning to pink up.'*

Defibrillation

A brief history

> Let me tell you, my friend, that there are things done today in electrical science which would have been deemed unholy by the very men who discovered electricity, who would themselves not so long before been burned as wizards. There are always mysteries in life.
>
> (Bram Stoker, *Dracula*, 1993, p. 246)

The ancient Greeks were familiar with electrical phenomena. Thales of Miletus describes how rubbing amber (ηλεκτρον, *elektron*) would cause it to attract light objects, such as feathers. However, it was not until the seventeenth century that various natural curiosities were brought together into a system that allowed them to be labelled 'electric'. By the end of that century a great deal was known about electricity and its effect on the animal body. Inevitably, this mysterious electrical fluid began to be touted for its therapeutic proper-ties. Electricity penetrated to the very core of the body to 'rouse the dormant powers of life' (A. Fothergill, 1795, p. 127). By the beginning of the nineteenth century, electricity had become, quite literally, the 'spark of life'.[17] As we observed in the preceding chapter, the Humane Society used electrical shock to re-excite the fading life-force into action, and failing that happy outcome, used it to insure that the mysterious life-force had actually fled, thus avoiding the horror of premature burial.

For the first half of the nineteenth century, electricity was, in many ways, a cure in search of a disease. 'Electro-quackery' was rife.[18] In 1850, the German researchers Karl Ludwig and Moritz Hoffa focused attention on the connection, which had been sporadically observed since the early 1700s, between cardiac arrhythmias and electricity. They succeeded in inducing ventricular fibrillation in a dog's heart by the application of electrical current (Schecter, 1983, p. 68). Between 1887 and 1889, in a series of dog experiments, John McWilliam proved that sudden cardiac death was due to ventricular fibrillation rather than, as had been previously believed, asystole (1889a, p. 6; 1889b, p. 348). McWilliam speculated that sudden death under chloroform anaesthesia might also be due to ventricular fibrillation. In 1911, Alfred Goodman Levy and Thomas Lewis conclusively demonstrated the connections between chloroform, ventricular fibrillation, cardiac arrest and sudden death (1911, p. 99).

As Europe and the United States went electric in the 1880s, there were an increasing number of deaths from electrocution. In 1899, Jean Louis Prevost and Frederic Battelli (and, independently, R. H. Cunningham) reported that a current passed through the heart would cause it to go into fibrillation, and that a second stronger shock was capable of reversing the fibrillation (Cunningham, 1899, p. 622; Prevost and Battelli, 1899, p. 1267). In 1926, the Consolidated Electrical Company of New York and the Rockefeller Institute funded further research into fatal electrical accidents. It was found that more than 50 per cent of fatalities in electrical accidents were caused by ventricular fibrillation. In the 1930s, Edison commissioned William

Kouwenhoven, an engineer at Johns Hopkins University, to develop a portable defibrillator that could be used in the field. His group at Johns Hopkins demonstrated that an electrical shock applied externally to the chest would induce ventricular fibrillation and that a second shock, also applied externally, would correct it. In experiments on dogs, Kouwenhoven achieved survival rates of 99 per cent when the heart was in fibrillation for 30 seconds, 90 per cent at one minute, 27 per cent at two minutes and 0 per cent at four minutes (Kouwenhoven and Hooker, 1933, p. 475).

Claude Beck, professor of surgery at Case Western Reserve University in Cleveland, has been credited with the first successful human defibrillation (1947) in the case of a 14-year-old boy who developed ventricular fibrillation while under anaesthesia (Beck, Pritchard and Feil, 1947, p. 985; Beck et al., 1960, p. 133). Using openchest massage and internal defibrillation with alternating current, he converted the boy's fibrillating heart to a normal sinus rhythm.[19] Throughout the 1940s he championed the use of internal cardiac defibrillation and later introduced the concept of 'hearts to good to die'.

In the mid-1950s, Kouwenhoven and Zoll working independently developed external cardiac defibrillators and reported successful resuscitations of patients with ventricular fibrillation using external defibrillation (Zoll et al., 1956, p. 727; Kouwenhoven et al., 1957, p. 550).[20] This move from internal to external defibrillation was important for it meant that it was no longer necessary to split the chest open to administer the electrical shock. The procedure was thus no longer limited to the operating room (or, infrequently, the hospital ward). It became applicable to any area in the hospital to which the then quite bulky machinery could be trundled. It also widened the circle of rescuers who might be capable of administering a therapeutic shock. Not only surgeons but also physicians without surgical skills, cardiologists, residents, junior doctors and nursing staff could all perform the procedure.

The next move in broadening defibrillation's field of application came with the development of portable defibrillators. In 1962, Bernard Lown invented a defibrillator that used direct rather than alternating current. As a result, defibrillators, which had been large machines of over 100 pounds, could be carried by hand. This decreased response times and meant that the defibrillator was no longer confined to the hospital; it might be taken out into the community (1964, p. 863). Ambulances were provided with portable external defibrillators in the early 1960s, first in Prague, then Moscow, Seattle and Belfast (Pantridge and Geddes, 1967, p. 271). We thus arrive at the point where our discussion of defibrillation within the modern CPR protocol commenced in chapter 2.

Machines: AEDs

Defibrillation introduced sophisticated instrumentation into modern resuscitative protocols. The use of the defibrillator necessitated a level of technical expertise that, in the early 1960s, though possible within the hospital, was beyond the reach of the layperson. Much in the fashion of tobacco fumigators in the eighteenth century, defibrillation marked a threshold within the protocol. Anything less than defibrillation – basic airway manoeuvres, mouth-to-mouth ventilation and external cardiac compressions – was in the remit of the layperson and was labelled BLS. Defibrillation and anything more technically sophisticated – intubation,[21] IVs and drugs – were the responsibility of the professional and became ACLS. Defibrillation and the defibrillator marked this boundary.

The sophistication, of both equipment and skills, necessary to accomplish ACLS contributed to the increased medicalization of the dying process. In order to practise the full protocol – defibrillation, sophisticated airway techniques, IVs and drugs – trained personnel within adequately equipped institutions became necessary. On the street, a system of paramedics, equipment depots and transport was necessary. Though the development of EMS (emergency medical services) systems arose primarily out of military triage and pre-existing fire and rescue services, the presence of a technology that required sophisticated equipment and specialized skills was a major factor in the accelerated evolution of pre-hospital care systems. Increasingly sophisticated technological innovations were also having an effect within the hospital by moving resuscitation and post-resuscitative care out of the hospital ward and into specialized critical care areas, such as the ER and the ICU. Thus, the CPR protocol, in its ACLS mode, contributed to the institutional sequestration of death behind an increasing number of closed doors.

On the other hand, CPR in its BLS format was moving the response to sudden death out into the community. As mentioned in chapter 2, Claude Beck, using the AHA's recommendations for mouth-to-mouth ventilation and closed-chest cardiac compression, established the Resuscitators of America in 1961, an organization whose aim was to teach these techniques to the lay public. At that time, the AHA remained reluctant to instruct the laity in the protocol and the Resuscitators of America faded into obscurity. In 1972, public instruction, this time sanctioned by the AHA, was introduced in King County, Washington and the laity was brought back into the picture. In 1984, King County became the first EMS system to institute the use of AEDs (automatic external defibrillators) in ambulances (Eisenberg, 1997, p. 188). Since then the development and use of AEDs has pushed forward, decreasing the time between cardiac arrest and defibrillation by putting the necessary technology into the hands of the lay rescuer.

CPR, despite its ACLS mode promoting an exclusionary professionalization of resuscitation, is, in its BLS mode, a means by which the community, represented by the individual rescuer, is drawn towards the deathbed. This bi-directional movement, which pulls death behind the doors of the ICU and pushes CPR out onto the street, creates a permanent tension within the resuscitative protocol that both brings us into proximity and distances us from death.

> Several experts have observed that great amounts of time and money are spent on the development of new defibrillation waveforms, novel antiarrhythmics, innovative vasopressors, and fresh approaches to ventilation and oxygenation. The total combined effect on survival of these interventions is equivalent to nothing more than cutting the interval from collapse to defibrillatory shock by 2 minutes. (American, *Guidelines* I.136–I.165)

Among the most significant changes in *Guidelines 2000* is the increased emphasis on immediate defibrillation enabled by the introduction of AEDs (American, *Guidelines*; Cummins, 2001). At its inception in 1960, CPR was presented as no more than a temporizing measure until definitive treatment, that is electrical defibrillation, could be accomplished (Kouwenhoven, Jude and Knickerbocker, 1960, p. 1064).

> Never delay defibrillation! Airway and ventilation are secondary to prompt defibrillation if defibrillation can be performed in the first minutes after arrest. (Cummins, 2001, pp. 65–6)

AEDs make this possible. One of the most important consequences of the introduction of AEDs is defibrillation's move from ACLS (where it is in the hands of professionals) into BLS (where it becomes a task for the layperson).

Public access defibrillation (PAD) is a healthcare initiative to make AEDs available throughout the community for use by trained laypersons. PAD holds promise to be the single greatest advance in the treatment of VF arrest since the development of CPR. (American, *Guidelines* I.22)

In adult cardiac arrest (certain exceptions aside), current recommendations are that resuscitation should begin by activation of the EMS system. Then, if an AED is present, shocks are immediately given × 3. Only then, if those shocks are unsuccessful, the ABCs of airway-manoeuvre, rescue breathing and external cardiac compressions are begun. 'The use of defibrillation now transcends both ACLS and BLS care' (American, *Guidelines* I.90). If no AED is present, the ABCs are commenced until an AED arrives (American, *Guidelines* I.22–I.59).[22]

AEDs are touted as becoming as ubiquitous as fire extinguishers (Mercier, 2001). They have shrunk to the size and weight of a small laptop computer, costing about $3,000 (£1,650). The American Heart Association, the American College of Emergency Physicians and the European Resuscitation Council have all advocated the widespread dissemination of AEDs. The US Cardiac Arrest Survival Act of spring 2000, directs government regulators and the Federal Aviation Administration to install AEDs in federal buildings and airplanes. On 12 October 2000 the Rural Access to Emergency Devices Act was passed. This provides $25 million over three years to facilitate placement of AEDs in small communities and rural areas. There has been heavy investment by many communities in supplying AEDs to police and fire personnel, and positioning them in public venues such as shopping malls, theatres, sports stadiums, transportation terminals, and so on.

At present, training in the use of AEDs is recommended for individuals with a 'duty to care': police, firefighters, flight attendants, lifeguards, security personnel, ferryboat crews, sports marshals, ski patrollers, and so on. The use of AEDs is 'not discouraged' in what are called 'targeted responders' or 'citizen responders'. These are members of the general public who are given special responsibility by institutions, such as the companies in which they work. The same recommendation is made for family members of patients at risk. AEDs are now available for purchase on doctor's prescription by the general public for use in the home. It is projected that, ultimately, defibrillation with an AED will be taught to all CPR providers (American, *Guidelines* I.60–I.76). Defibrillation, like mouth-to-mouth and external cardiac compression, is envisaged as being administered by anyone, in any place, at any time.

Legislators have also been instructed to draw up a bill protecting Good Samaritans using AEDs from lawsuits. There have, to date, been no lawsuits over deaths following the use of AEDs, and, in fact, Richard Hamburg, spokesman for the AHA has pointed out that 'If there's any threat of litigation, it is more for not providing the device' (D. Brown, 1999, p. 33). Lawsuits have been filed against facilities for *failing* to provide AEDs and train employees in CPR (Cummins, 2001, p. 45).

Early defibrillation of ventricular fibrillation has, in some studies, improved survival from witnessed ventricular fibrillation to as high as 34–94 per cent (Eisenberg, Copass and Hallstrom, 1980, p. 1379; Stults et al., 1984, p. 219; Cummins et al., 1985, p. 114; Vukov et al., 1988, p. 318; Mosesso, 1993, p. 1311; Valenzuela et al., 1998, p. 414; Hazinski, Cummins and Field, 2000, p. 6; Caffrey et al., 2002, p. 1242; Culley, 2004, p. S1525). Some studies, though showing increased success in reversing ventricular fibrillation, have long-term survival rates of only 11–13 per cent (Olson et al., 1989, p. 806; Haynes et al., 1991, p. 545). Other studies demonstrate little increase, for example 2.1–2.9 per cent (Brison et al., 1992, p. 191), or no increase in survival after the introduction of AEDs (Kellerman, Hackman and Somes, 1993, p. 1433; Pepe et al., 1994, p. 1037; Sweeney et al., 1998, p. 234). However, in all studies, it is apparent that the shorter the time between collapse and defibrillation, the better the survival rates. In a 1985 study by Cummins of witnessed out-of-hospital cardiac arrest, if CPR was commenced at less than five minutes after collapse and defibrillation accomplished at less than ten minutes, survival was 37 per cent. If CPR was commenced at more than five minutes after collapse and defibrillation accomplished at more than ten minutes, survival was 0 per cent (Cummins et al., 1985, p. 114). Though both time to CPR and time to defibrillation are significant, time to defibrillation is much more so. For AEDs to be maximally effective, they should be used within six minutes of arrest, and preferably within three minutes. Every minute after that decreases the chances of survival dramatically. There is a claim made for a doubling of survival rates with early defibrillation when compared to mouth-to-mouth and chest compressions alone (Pell et al., 2001, p. 1385).

Most authors agree that immediate defibrillation of witnessed arrest is an effective therapeutic intervention. However, there is controversy over its cost-effectiveness. A University of Glasgow study assessed the cost utility of AEDs in airports, railways stations, and other public settings and calculated the cost per quality-adjusted life-year (QALY) gained at $68,924 (£40,000) (Walker, 2003, p. 1312). This figure exceeds the commonly accepted cut-off level for funding of $50,000 (£27,500) per QALY gained:

> The American Heart Association and the Department of Health in England are both strong advocates of public place defibrillators .... However, decisions to expand provision of public place defibrillators have been taken in advance of adequate information on their clinical and cost effectiveness .... Without information on the value for money of such a strategy, it is impossible to determine whether greater improvements in survival and quality of life could be achieved by investing the same amount of money in alternative strategies such as reduced emergency medical service response times or the provision of defibrillators to other first responders. The decision on whether or not to provide public place defibrillators should be based on objective evidence and not political expediency .... public place defibrillators are a 'good news story'. They are novel, highly visible, and empower the public and, therefore, attract positive media coverage. These factors in isolation are not sufficient to justify their funding from public monies. They need to be supported by clinical and economic evidence. (Pell, 2003, p. 1376)

Other studies have shown costs as low as $13,000 per QALY gained, depending on the likelihood of cardiac arrest occurring at a particular site – the higher the incidence the cheaper the cost (Nichol et al., 1998, p. 1315; Cram et al., 2003, p. 745; Nichol et al., 2003, p. 697).[23] However, in all such studies, the assumptions upon which estimates are made are often controversial (Kirchheimer, 2004).

On reviewing the literature, there is no question that early defibrillation does indeed increase long-term survival, but again not to the extent that the profession hopes or the public believes, and that the costs involved need to be carefully considered. The emerging consensus appears to be that while the use of AEDs by first-responders (for example, police and fire services and other personnel in 'high probability' locations, such as airports and casinos) may be justified, the 'fire-extinguisher' model of public access defibrillation is unlikely to prevent many deaths. Timmermans raises the question of whether 'the infinitely optimistic emergency community [has] ... chosen to ignore signs that the effectiveness of automatic defibrillating may be limited [and] ... indiscriminate defibrillation ... promoted as a way to achieve immortality' (1999, p. 77). I suspect that both medicine's optimism and Timmermans' caveat are valid.

Living and life

> Defibrillation is the spark of life.
>
> (Eisenberg, 1997, p. 178)

Electrical shock, as part of the CPR protocol, not only attempts to reverse death by correcting ventricular fibrillation, but, failing that, it retains its eighteenth-century diagnostic function 'as the test, or discriminating character of any remains of animal life' (Kite, 1788, p. 125). If the heart fails to respond to defibrillation, then the patient is dead – another example of the terminal paradox, where what is therapeutic is also diagnostic.

The phenomena of electricity are, and have been since the eighteenth century, important visualizations of the fantasy of life. At the beginning of the twenty-first century, life and death as enacted on the street and portrayed on the television screen are made manifest in the image electric. The convulsed spasm elicited by defibrillation, the glowing QRS complex on the cardiac monitor, the jagged pattern of brainwaves on the electroencephalogram retain vitalist connotations of electricity as 'the spark of life'.

That the living and the dead are different would seem self-evident. How they are so is less obvious. One way of comprehending this phenomenon is to postulate some *thing* called 'life'. We denominate 'life', in the sense of both naming it and assigning it value. By so doing, we bestow upon that accumulation of physical, chemical and physiological processes a kind of being. It was at about the same time as the institution of the Humane Society, in the late eighteenth century, that two conflicting physiological doctrines, 'mechanism' and 'vitalism', were squaring up to battle over the designation 'life'.

Mechanism

In the seventeenth century, natural philosophers, such as Pierre Gassendi and Robert Boyle, resurrected Democritus's pre-Socratic doctrine of atomism. Mechanism was based on the concept of particulate matter in motion. The cosmos, from the smallest particle to the stars in the heavens, obeyed mechanical laws and was mathematically measurable. Following mechanism's success in explaining many of the workings of the physical world, iatromechanism[24] attempted something similar with the animate world, that is, it sought to explain the workings of the living body through the same laws of physics that were being used to explain inanimate nature. The doctrine of mechanism was most famously enunciated by René Descartes, who asserted that the body (*res extensa*) was no more than a machine, under the governance of an immaterial, immortal and rational soul (*res cogitans*). Cartesian dualism, by separating the mind/soul from the body, gave iatromechanism space in which to develop free from the interference of God and other transcendent forces. At the end of the seventeenth century and into the eighteenth, iatromechanists, such as Giovanni Borelli, Giorgio Baglivi and Julien Offray de La Mettrie, argued that animal functions were ultimately the result of mechanical causes. God worked through geometry (King, 1978, pp. vi–34). La Mettrie (*L'homme machine*, 1749) even sought to do away with God, reducing all living beings, including man, to machines.

Iatromechanism allowed Enlightenment physicians an alternative to animist notions of malign astral influence, religious doctrines of demonic possession and recently discounted Aristotelian qualities. Iatromechanism gave physicians the ability to explain health and disease on the basis of the structure of the body and the functional relations between its parts. It allowed for Harvey's discovery of the circulation of the blood, Descartes' description of the reflex arc and the Oxford Group's[25] delineation of respiratory function.

However, mechanism, though capable of explaining certain basic phenomena of the living body, did not seem quite up to an explanation of life as a whole. In 1747, John Stevenson complained:

> Not content with the ingenious and useful Application of Levers, Ropes and Pulleys; to the Bones, Muscles and Tendons, and other valuable *mechanical* and *hydrostatical* Pursuits: Not content with these, I say, Millstones were brought into the Stomach, Flint and Steel into the Blood-vessels, Hammer and Vice into the Lungs, & etc. But all to no good Purpose; there being certain Bounds beyond which mechanical Principles and Demonstrations do not reach. (*Cause of Animal Heat*, 1747, quoted in Mendelsohn, 1964, p. 97)

The rigid application of mechanical philosophy threatened to reduce the world to lifeless formulae. The resurgence of vitalist thought in the late eighteenth century is said to have been a reaction to this overly aggressive mechanism (Wear, 1995, p. 344). Surely, man was more than a machine, and life more than clockwork.

By the mid-eighteenth century, there were three major alternative explanations of life. La Mettrie's atheistic materialism attracted many natural philosophers, but troubled them as Christians. George Ernst Stahl, professor at Halle, attempted to translate the Christian soul into the realm of nature through the concept of the *anima*. This was a spirit, an immortal spark, implanted by God into the living body, giving both life and consciousness. Stahlian animism has been accused of being little more than concealed theology. Hermann Boerhaave proposed a dualism similar to that of Descartes. The body was a hydraulic machine, regulated by the flow of essential fluids through a system of conduits and reservoirs, but man also possessed an immaterial soul, supplying consciousness and governing will (R. Porter, 1999, p. 247).

Vitalism

Vitalism also sought to leave behind superstition and magical thought, but, unlike mechanism, hoped to preserve the unique and exalted status of the living being. 'Vitalism' is an omnibus term and has been used to cover such diverse doctrines as primitive animism, the Greek concept of *psyche* (ψυχή), Galenic *pneuma* (πνεῦμα), the Christian soul, animal heat, animal magnetism, animal electricity and organicism. Vitalist doctrine has been divided helpfully, if somewhat artificially, into three sub-types: transcendental vitalism is seen as little more than the animistic belief that soul or spirit, as the vehicle of life, is the gift of a transcendent power; substantival vitalism endows the quality of life present in animate matter with a real being, so as to make of it an immaterial substance, a fluid or essence somehow unlike the matter it animates; and critical vitalism (sometimes called organicism) maintains that the innate organization of the organism, and not some superadded transcendental principle, is responsible for the vital properties of living entities. This last form of vitalist thought merges with materialist structuralism to produce the modern functionalist approach to living organisms. Discussion of animism at the one extreme, and organicism at the other, is beyond the scope of this book. However, I should like to look briefly at the form of vitalism dominant at the time of the institution of the Society's Method – substantival vitalism.

> Apparent death consists in a total, tho' temporary cessation of all the powers of motion and sense; to be more particular, the lungs

cease to act; the heart and arteries to beat; and the brain and nerves to diffuse their energy. It, therefore, only differs from real death, in this, that the living principle is not extinct, but only lies dormant; which, sometimes spontaneously, but more frequently and certainly, when excited by proper means, again becomes active: In consequence of which, all the functions of life are restored. (*Governors*, 1789, p. 5)

The major difference between mechanism and vitalism lay in the interpretation of the word 'principle'. Is 'the living principle' a law or a force? In mechanism, the occult principle of life is a set of relations between objects – that is, it is a set of physiological laws. The ultimate implication of the mechanistic view is that the living organism is the result of a set of mechanical/chemical processes no different in kind from those that govern the inert physical world. Life is thus a secondary effect of the matter and structure of the living organism. The living being is no more than the sum of its parts.

In substantival vitalism, the living body is more than the sum of its parts and this 'more', the inexplicable residuum that is the peculiar essence of life, is the 'living principle': a vital force – that is, an agent, substance or power – with its own real independent or transcendent being, driving the biological processes we identify as unique to living things (Rousseau, 1992, p. 63). 'Life' is thus a cause rather than an effect of the structure and function of the living organism. Life might be distinguished from inert nature not only by its extraordinary complexity, a quantitative criterion, but because it is some *thing* altogether qualitatively different. This 'living principle' or vital force is a substance different in kind from the matter it moves. In a quest extending from the seventeenth to the twentieth centuries, vitalists actively sought this 'living principle'. Like the dying torch engraved on the Humane Society's medals, the life-force was as real an entity as the torch's fire; and the purpose of The Method was to fan it back to full flame.

Cartesian dualism gave the vitalists, as well as the mechanists, leave to set aside the *res cogitans*, the soul as mind, as an essentially unfathomable entity originating with God, the concern of theologians. This manoeuvre allowed vitalism to re-establish, the pre-Christian division of the 'soul' into *thymos* (θυμος for the Greeks and *animus* for the later Romans), and *psyche* (ψυχή and *anima*). *Thymos* roughly corresponds to the rational, voluntary processes of the mind, a consciousness-soul, which might then remain as an attribute of the divine soul.

Psyche drove the involuntary processes that kept the living body ticking over: a life-soul (Onians, 1951, p. 187; Snell, 1953, p. 15; Guthrie, 1981, p. 27). 'The *animus* is that with which we think, the *anima* that by which we live' (Nonius Marcellus, *De compendiosa doctrine*, p. 426). The problem that the vitalist philosopher faced was how to maintain the distinct status of the living being without relying upon religion and the miracle of a transcendental soul, on the one hand, and without falling back on tautological Aristotelian qualities, on the other.[26] Eighteenth-century vitalists hoped to solve this problem by proving the existence of an independent cause – a substantial 'life-force', the *vis vitae*. Natural philosophers, such as Paracelsus and Joan-Baptista van Helmont, hypothesized a force flowing into and through the bodies of living creatures, endowing them with motion and heat (Burwick and Douglass, 1992, p. 8). Even William Harvey, though his explanation of the circulation was mechanistic, believed that 'something more' powered and drove the human machine:

> Likewise in the Blood, there is a spirit of virtue, doth act above the power of the Elements (most conspicuous in the nutrition or preservation of each particular part) and also a nature, nay a soul in that spirit and the blood answerable in proportion to the elements of the Stars. (William Harvey, *De Generatione*, 1651, quoted in Wear, 1995, p. 336)

Substantival vitalism attempted to reify this life-force, that is, make it 'real', by clothing it in substance. The subtle substance of the life-force, though invisible, without weight or shape or colour, nevertheless had a real existence and was accessible to the senses, though in a way different from crude matter. In different eras, this substantial life-force became identified with different phenomena, the most significant of these being breath, animal heat and animal electricity – the imponderables.

The imponderables

The substantialization of the life force was not intended to be its materialization. Whatever the *stuff* of the life-force was, it was different in kind from the matter it animated. To maintain a status independent of the matter it moved and to prevent life from evaporating into a mere quality of matter, the life-force must manifest itself in a way different from that of mere matter. Mere matter, a lump of coal say, is visible, extensible (length, breadth and height) and ponderable (mass and weight). The life-force, as a force, is invisible and imponderable, that is, it lacks colour, shape and weight. However as a substantial force, though imponderable, it nevertheless can be felt. A whispered breath across the cheek becomes the movement of the divine *aether*. The heat of that cheek under a caressing hand discloses an animating fire. That hand convulsed by contact with a live wire feels power. Regardless of its form, the life-force, invisible and imponderable, is yet tangible, accessible to touch, felt as sensations like movement, heat or pain.[27] It is apprehended despite its strategic absences of visibility and extension. We know it as powerful because of its effects. We know it as real because we feel it. We know it is different because we cannot directly see or hold it.

The criterion of tangible imponderability limits somewhat the range of phenomena suitable for conceptualization as the immaterial substance of the life-force. Despite the multiplicity of names and forms these candidates for immaterial substance have taken, they are all (under normal circumstances) invisible and lack extension and mass (at least in the era before the discoveries of Boyle, Lavoisier and Maxwell). By far the most powerful, direct and comprehensive of vitalist images is that of concealed fire. All the imponderables – breath, animal heat and electricity – partake of fire. They manifest as the air that feeds the flame, the heat radiating from it and the energy stored within it. This image of an occult flame burning within the living body is a metaphor to which there is constant return.

The life-force, as embodied in the imponderables, gained a distinct and privileged status in the physical world as a *thing* felt but not seen. That these things can be felt means that they have substantial existence; that they cannot be seen denies them, at least in the imagination, material existence. The imponderables are all conceived of as substances in motion, as fluids. Air (later gas) and animal heat (later phlogiston and caloric) were conceived of as 'imponderable fluids'. These vital forces were made intelligible as currents flowing along gradients from areas in which they were in surplus to areas in which they were in deficit. Later, electricity and magnetism were also given the status of imponderable fluids. The hydraulic nomenclature of electrical current, magnetic flux and stream of electrons remains with us today. These imponderable fluids are sublime, as much in the alchemical as in the metaphysical sense, having shed physical qualities to the point of approaching pure movement (Tercier, 2002, p. 1). Substantival vitalism, while substantializing force or agency or change – moving it towards a material manifestation – at the same time, rather paradoxically, sublimates matter into motion. Experienced as immanent qualities, but conceptualized as distinct agents, these substantialized forces of vitalism formed a bridge between living flesh and dead meat.

Vitalism clothed life in substance, giving form to the occult, making the life-force comprehensible to the mind and apprehendable to the hand. The end-result was a reification of qualities: the transformation of a function into an entity. Living, an adjective qualifying a state-of-being, was made to obey an ontological imperative, becoming a substantive noun, a-*thing*-in-itself – life. Substantival vitalism, in privileging being over becoming and in explaining process by existence, worked to make an occult force, visible only to the mind's eye, responsive to the hand. It gave natural philosophy some *thing* it could manipulate. However, immaterial substance was an unstable compound: the 'substance' of it constantly in danger of precipitating into matter, and its 'immateriality' of sublimating into soul. Each of the candidates for *vis vitae* only reigned for so long.

Air and breath

It would be difficult for any culture to ignore the brute observation that the living breathe and the dead do not: 'Men and other animals live on *aer*, by breathing, and this is to them both soul and mind, as will be clearly demonstrated in this treatise; and if this leaves them they die and their mind fails' (Diogenes fr. 4). Breath has long been seen as the vehicle of life: 'And the Lord God formed man of the dust of the ground, and breathed into his nostrils the breath of life; and man became a living soul' (Genesis, 2:7). 'Air' comes from the Greek αηρ, via the Latin *aer*. What is to us a gas made up of nitrogen, oxygen and carbon dioxide was, to the ancients, one of the building blocks of the cosmos – earth, air, fire and water. The Greeks had no concept of a gas. *Aer* was conceived of as vapour, an exhalation rising from a liquid – like the mist over a field of dew-soaked grain or steam from newly spilt blood. *Aer* moved and was moving. It was the wind in the grass, invisible though manifest in its effect. Imponderable yet tangible, *aer* was the universal substance that pervaded and moved the cosmos. It was taken in by men and animals as *pneuma*, breath, and it animated the living body. *Pneuma* was the vehicle by which the divine instilled life in the mortal, animating the *psyche*, which was that which gave the body life. As the wind moved the dust of the earth and the waves of the seas, so *pneuma* empowered the *psyche*, moving invisibly within it, the cause of perception and motion.

The *psyche* survived as a shadow in Hades. Departing from the body at death, exhaled in the warrior's last gasp, the *psyche* rose like steam from the blood shed in sacrifice (Onians, 1951, pp. 93–123). As *aer* rose towards heaven, aspiring to the all-encompassing purity of *aether*, so man's *psyche*, made of *pneuma*, strove upward towards a similar unity with the divine. Macrocosm and microcosm were linked by *aer* (Rohde, 1925, p. 461). 'The *aer* within us is a small portion of the god' (Diogenes, quoted in Theophrastus, *De sensu*, pp. 39–45).

Aristotle, working with the Hippocratic doctrine of the four basic humours (blood, yellow bile, black bile, phlegm), articulations of the four primary opposites (hot, cold, dry, moist), in turn reflections of the four elements (earth, air, water, fire), fashioned a functional description of the soul. He declared that the soul, for which he used the term *psyche* and by which he meant life processes in general, existed in nutritive, animative and rational aspects. Following Empedocles and Plato, he located this soul in the heart. Blood produced in the heart was the vehicle of the nutritive-soul. *Aer*, analogous to *aether*, the active element which moved the stars, was breathed into the lungs, passed into the pulmonary blood vessels and thence was conducted to the heart, where it mixed with blood to form *pneuma*, the vital-spirit of the animative soul, which was discernible as *thermon* (θερμον) – innate heat. The heart was a cauldron in which the blood boiled, and it was the force of this ebullition that drove the blood through the body carrying heat and *pneuma* to all its parts where it acted as the principle of sensation (the perception of change) and motion (the ability to cause change) (Longrigg, 1993, pp. 52–3). Aristotle's choice of *pneuma* to link God through nature to man, and to link perception to response within the individual animal, was further refined and promoted by Praxagoras of Cos, Hierophilus of Chalcedon and Erasistratus of Ceos.

Galen of Pergamum took the Aristotelian hierarchy of souls and characterized them as being materially of the nature of *spiritus*, that is, breath. Nutritive-spirits were manufactured in the liver from chyle, produced by the digestive process and carried to the liver by the portal vein. This nutritive-spirit was then distributed in blood throughout the body by the venous system. Some of this blood reached the heart, where from the right ventricle a portion of it passed through invisible pores in the inter-ventricular septum into the left ventricle. In the crucible of the left ventricle, this blood, containing nutritive-spirit, was mixed with *pneuma*, brought from the lungs to the left ventricle by the pulmonary vein, to produce vital-spirit, which was then distributed, by the arterial system, throughout the body to vivify and warm it. Some of this blood imbued with vital-spirit reached the brain, where, in the *rete mirabile*,[28] it was further elaborated into the more ethereal animal- or psychic-spirit, which was then transmitted throughout the body by the nerves, producing sensation and motion (Temkin, 1973, p. 142).

Galen likened the vital heat produced in the heart to the flame of a lamp. The fat of the body was the oil that fed the internal fire; inhaled air, the wind that fanned it; and exhaled breath, its smoky waste. Galen brought lungs, heart and brain together in a tidy system using both breath and animal heat to explain living processes (Mendelsohn, 1964, p. 28). Despite its faults and inconsistencies, the Hippocratic-Aristotelian-Galenic axis is what we would recognize as a 'scientific' doctrine – discursively redeemable in that it seeks its answers from within, rather than from outside, its operating frame of reference, that is, it looked to nature rather than to a transcendent deity. The Galenic system was to dominate medicine well into the seventeenth century, by which time cracks had begun to appear.

Heat and combustion

> Death may usurp on Nature many Hours;
> And yet the Fire of Life kindle again
> The o'er-prest Spirits.
>
> (Shakespeare, *Pericles*, III.ii.82–6
> [Royal, 1789, frontispiece])

Andreas Vesalius could find no evidence of the Galenic *rete mirabile* in man. Ioannes Argenterius questioned Galen's assertion that the psychic-spirit was elaborated from arterial blood in the non-existent *rete mirabile*, and maintained, against what had by then become orthodox medical theory, that there were not three spirits, but only one, flowing from the heart and carrying heat, the instrument of life and motion. There were not three species of soul; rather, the different constitutions of brain, heart and lungs made the vital force operate differently in these centres as well as in the liver and other tissues. Bernardinus Telesius and Thomas Campanella taught that man had a God-given immortal soul that bestows reason, moral sentiment and religious feeling, but that he also shares with animals an animating soul, which in substance is spirit. This spirit, the *vis vitae*, 'vital force', is composed of heat and 'thin matter'. It dwells in the ventricles of the brain, and is desiring, comprehending and motive, flowing through spinal cord and nerves (Temkin, 1973, p. 142). Vital-spirit was immaterial, imponderable, invisible but powerful and tangible, felt as animal heat. For Paracelsus, life, the process of generation of animal heat, was like fire. On combustion of any material, mercury was that portion of it which is volatile like smoke; sulphur that which is hot and bright like flame; and salt that which is the solid residue like ash. Jean Fernel of Paris postulated a *spiritus*, which entered the body on the fortieth day of conception and imbued it with innate heat. This *spiritus* derived from the starry sphere and was the same as the *aether,* which gave heat to the sun. Harvey, like many others, believed that the innate heat found in the blood was a vital spirit of an 'aerial or aetherial nature', like to, but not actually, elemental fire. It was the purpose of the circulation to distribute this vital animal heat generated in the heart to the rest of the body. Descartes proposed a fire burning in the left ventricle. As blood entered that chamber it was vaporized, causing expansion of the heart and forcing the blood into the aorta and on through the arterial system. This hidden fire in the heart was held to be the mainspring and origin of all other bodily movements (Henry, 1997, p. 67).

On the other hand, the mechanist philosophers of the early eighteenth century saw animal heat not as a cause but as a consequence of vital activity, an epiphenomenon. Joan-Baptista van Helmont speculated that animal heat was not the cause of nutrition and growth, but rather the result. Furthermore, he rejected the premise that heat was essential for life – as fish were as alive as ferrets. Pitcairne, Hoffmann, Boerhaave, Hales, Douglas and von Haller all supported a mechanical model in which heat was generated by the motion of blood or particles within the blood – perhaps the friction of blood corpuscles on the vessel walls. These versions of the mechanical production of animal heat fitted very nicely with Newton's laws of thermodynamics. However, this mechanical theory of animal heat was in its turn displaced by theories of the 'caloric'. For Lavoisier, *oxygène* was a ponderable element containing within it the imponderable fluid, caloric. Caloric was present in all substances and was absorbed or emitted in chemical reactions. Near the end of the eighteenth century, this concept of a caloric fluid was challenged by Count Rumford who averred that heat was motion, not material substance. The experiments of Davy, Carnot, Kelvin, Joule, Helmholtz, Thomson, Maxwell and Mayer replaced the caloric theory with the kinetic theory of heat as work and motion.

The association of vital-spirit with air and heat was a spur to seventeenth- and eighteenth-century investigations of respiration and combustion. Lavoisier, Black, Priestley, Rutherford and Cavendish gradually sorted out the nature of atmospheric air as a compound substance made up of oxygen, carbon dioxide and nitrogen. Boyle, Hooke, Willis, Mayow, Lower, Crawford and Seguin made the step-wise connections between the exchange of air in the lungs and the production of heat and energy from the combined processes of respiration and digestion. These discoveries meant that it was possible to view the heat of the animal body as combustion's analogue in the biological world.[29] It was possible to envisage animal heat/combustion as a material bridge spanning the void that separated the realm of living processes from that of inert matter. Neither oxygen nor animal heat need be ascribed to some transcendent vital-force, but could be treated, in oxygen's case, as a substrate for a chemical reaction, and, in animal heat's case, as a result of a chemical reaction: matter acting on matter. Thus, both breath and animal heat, at slightly different times, but as part of the same phenomenon of respiration, crossed over the bridge from the metaphysical into the physical realm.

Electricity and irritability

In achieving material status, breath and animal heat were forced to abdicate their claims to the title of life-force. The quest for the life-force then shifted from the lungs and heart (the praecordium, ancient home of the *animus*) to the brain and nervous system (home to the *anima*), from respiration to motion, from the mechanical processes of life to the control of them. Attention focused on the actions of the nervous system, the property of irritability and the mysterious force of electricity.

It was via the concept of 'irritability' that electricity was to become the last imponderable. 'Irritability' was the term used to describe the ability of living matter to respond to external stimuli. On a local level, it was manifest by the ability of isolated muscle to contract in response to noxious stimuli. On a more general level, it was the ability of the living being to react to external stimuli with self-actuated movement. Though manifest by the living organism as a whole and in all its parts, irritability was seen to be under the control of the nervous system.

Newton, concludes the *Principia* (1687), thus:

> A certain most subtle spirit which pervades and lies hid in all gross bodies .... all sensation is excited, and the members of animal bodies move at the command of the will, namely, by the vibrations of this spirit, mutually propagated along the solid filaments of the nerves, from the outward organs of sense to the brain, and from the brain into the muscles.

This concept of stimulus and response – of awareness of change and an internal principle of motion in response to that change – was formalized by Descartes in the early seventeenth century as the reflex arc. Frances Glisson, in the 1670s, was the first to make 'irritability' the specific vital property of living tissue. For Glisson, this internal principle, which both sensed and caused movement, was the soul (Wear, 1995, p. 344). Albrecht von Haller, a century later, put irritability forward as the primary manifestation of life. However, Haller did not resort to animism to explain this activity, but insisted that irritability and sensitivity were properties inherent in muscle and nerve. He postulated that the 'nervous fluid' that activated this system might be the same as 'electrical matter' (R. Porter, 1999, p. 250).

The Montpelier vitalist Paul-Joseph Barthez gave vitalism its name. He coined the term *principe vital* for the irritable force, analogous to gravity, coordinating and directing bodily actions (Lesch, 1984, p. 25). Denis Diderot went further and posited a biological materialism, which did away entirely with both the soul and any form of life force, by investing matter itself with the property of irritability. Across the channel, Robert Whytt, William Cullen, John Brown and John Hunter sought to rescue irritability from the mechanically and atheistically inclined Gauls. John Hunter argued that life was the cause, not the consequence, of the organization of living beings. Whytt described a natural soul, operating through the nervous system, which was energetic, sentient at a non-conscious level and spatially extensive with the body. Cullen ascribed the source of nervous energy to an immaterial soul, which he identified as an aethereal fluid that was the basis of light, heat, magnetism and electricity (R. Porter, 1995, p. 376).

The leading lights of the early Humane Society, William Hawes, William Cullen and Anthony Fothergill, were committed vitalists. As will be recalled from chapter 3, at the time of the founding of the Humane Society in 1774, the apoplectic theory of drowning, essentially a mechanical theory, held sway. It was in part due to the vitalist orientation of the Society that the apoplectic theory was replaced by the asphyxial. The majority of The Method's therapeutic manoeuvres were based on the doctrine of irritability and the need to re-excite that waning life-force:

> We now know that the vital power, or in other words, the irritability of the system ... is not of so volatile or fugitive a nature, as to quit them on the immediate suspension of the action of the heart and lungs ... on the contrary, after it seems to have deserted the external parts, a remnant still tenaciously maintains its

residence in the principle vital organs a considerable time after motion and sensation have ceased .... the vital principle [remains], often in a dormant state, without betraying any sign of its presence, till it happens to be roused by the proper modes of excitation. (A. Fothergill, 1795, p. 11)

Most of the techniques in The Method – vigorous friction, agitations, chest compressions, tobacco enemas, smelling salts, the expansion of the lungs and re-warming – were aimed at rousing 'irritability' in the vital organs through the sympathetic action of physical force. It was to this class of manoeuvres that electricity belonged:

Electricity presents us with one of the most speedy and powerful stimulants hitherto discovered .... in the torpid sate of apparent death, it seems admirably calculated to rouse the dormant powers. (A. Fothergill, 1795, p. 127)

The vitalist equation of irritability with the life-force was easily electrified, as electricity was to some extent irritability described by cause rather than effect.

Electricity had been posited as a vital force as far back as the sixteenth century. In 1791, Luigi Galvani announced in *De Viribus Electricitatis in Motu Musculari Commentarius* (*Commentary on the Effect of Electricity on Muscular Motion*) that animal tissues contained an innate, vital force activating nerve and muscle, which he termed 'animal electricity'. Galvani's belief was that the brain was an organ secreting electrical fluid into the nerves, which then acted as channels for its distribution. As a result of the work of Galvani, Volta, Hales, Hunter and Priestley, by the end of the eighteenth century electricity had been introduced into medical practice as both a test of and a stimulus to life.[30]

The heart was considered most irritable, composed as it was of multiple layers of muscular fibres. It was in the heart that irritability clung on the longest. It was in the heart that the last flicker of life remained. It was towards the heart that the mysterious power of electricity should be directed. Animal experiments had shown that the heart could be stopped by electrical shocks and started again in the same way:

It has ... been ascertained by repeated experiments, that a moderate shock is peculiarly adapted to the recovery of animals whose vital functions have been suspended by very strong ones: and in this way animation may be alternately suspended and restored, a considerable number of times, as I have often experienced. (Kite, 1788, p. 242)

Throughout the late eighteenth century and into the nineteenth the relations between electricity and life remained a focus for experimenters. Wilhelm von Humboldt induced fibrillation in the hearts of carp. Giovanni Aldini recommended that galvanism be used in conjunction with mouth-to-mouth respiration in the revival of the near-dead. Xavier Bichat experimented on the effects of galvanism on the corpses of the guillotined (Schecter, 1971, p. 360). A series of similar investigations by others brings us back to the beginning of this chapter (p. 99) with Ludwig and Hoffa's induction of ventricular fibrillation in a dog's heart by the application of electrical current and the subsequent development of defibrillation as a therapeutic manoeuvre.

When air became gas, and heat caloric, then the life-force became electric. But almost at the moment that this new candidate for the life-force appeared, it was already being undermined by the investigative process that had brought it to prominence. The equation of electricity to life stimulated researches into the nature of other electrical phenomena, thus beginning electricity's quantification. On the biological side, through the work of Humboldt, Helmholtz, Nobili, Matteucci, Du Bois-Reymond and Mayer, electricity's relationship to cardiac and neural function was elucidated, and animal electricity shifted from being the movement of an imponderable fluid to becoming the self-propagating flux of ions across a cell membrane. On the physical side, the work of Coulomb, Faraday, Davy, Ohm, Orsted, Ampere, Kelvin and Joule eventually revealed the inter-convertibility of electricity, magnetism and mechanical work. Maxwell synthesized this knowledge of energy relations into his unified theory of electromagnetism. Thomson formulated the electron. Planck created quantum mechanics. Einstein described the special theory of relativity. It was thus revealed that matter was electric in nature. Energy and matter were interchangeable. When it became possible to quantify occult forces and render them visible in the form of formulae and equations, when everything felt by the hand could also be seen with the mind's eye, vitalism was forced to flee.

The flight of vitalism

Each imponderable was raised to the title of life-force only to be overthrown. Intended to be a defence against materialism, the bestowal of substance on agency began the progressive materialization of the occult – air became gas, heat the calorie and electricity the flux of electrons. The imponderables, on being made intelligible, became in a sense visible, and in so doing lost their sublimated status as substances made extraordinary by their deficiencies. Under the increased scrutiny of the scientific gaze, each was transformed from occult cause to revealed effect. As the gaze of science penetrated deeper and deeper into living matter, the life-force was forced to retreat before that gaze.

By the beginning of the nineteenth century, a radically different formulation of life was taking shape, based on the concept of organism and the power inherent in organization. Causal links between structure and function had long been being present in the work of those such as Vesalius, Harvey, Morgagni and the physiologists of the eighteenth century. Haller's concept of sensibility and irritability, as elaborated in Descartes' reflex arc, was seen as dependent upon the organization of the living body, leading vitalism away from the reification of life as an imponderable and towards the concept of life as self-organizing function. Functionalism stated that it was the unique arrangement of an organism's components that bestowed on it the vital characteristics of order, adaptation, evolution, growth and reproduction. Modern science denies the existence of 'life' as a distinct ontological entity and defines life is the functioning state of the living organism. In Bichat's famous words of 1800: 'Life consists in the sum of the functions, by which death is resisted' (1827, p. 10). It is a measure of the strength of positivism in modern science, in fact, of its identity with science, that such a tautology is no longer troublesome.

At the beginning of the twentieth century, vitalism made a last stand in the areas of embryology and evolution. The philosopher Henri Bergson, positing an *élan vital*, and the embryologist Hans Driesch, with *entelechy*, were the last serious proponents of vitalism within the realm of science (Bakhtin, 1992, p. 87; Rousseau, 1992, p. 63). Their critical vitalism continued to maintain that life was the cause of organization and not the result. In the end, with the help of molecular biology, critical vitalism was co-opted into positivist materialism, and vitalism, as a viable scientific doctrine, disappeared altogether. In the modern, 'life' is the sum of the relations which promote the survival and reproduction of the organized entity. The whole is not greater than its parts. The body has precipitated into matter, and 'life' sublimated into the laws governing that matter. Life has gone from being a divine gift to an occult force to a set of equations. Life became such fine stuff that it disappeared into thin air, which, however poetic, has left us very little to hang on to.

Though vitalism, as a scientific doctrine, might be a dead issue, vitalist modes of thinking survive. Life, like any tool long familiar to the hand, is not hastily cast aside. Hidden beneath our positivist approach to a material world is a nostalgia for a vital one. Though life is no longer a present reality to modern science, the memory of it remains as a retrospective object of desire. Vitalism, like the hero in a quest narrative, has ended up becoming that which it sought. Vitalism in its search for an occult force, by unveiling and thus demystifying those occult forces, has in the end become an occult force itself, hidden in our images of life and death (Foucault, 1991, p. 18).

The image electric

> I had two pair of wires that were connected to the current, and I touched them and they would explode .... I love electricity because I think it is very mysterious.
>
> (Burden, 1999)[31]

Today, electricity and life are understood in radically different ways from what they were at the time of the inception of the Humane Society's Method. Yet, the relationship forged between electricity and life in the eighteenth century, though changed, persists in our images of life and death. Electricity, the last of the imponderables, has become the gift of the modern Prometheus, bringing heat and light, power and plenty to industrial society. Electricity is become not only a dominating image in modern life, but the dominant image of life for the modern. Electricity, from the animation of Dr Frankenstein's monster in 1818 to the introduction of AEDs in *Guidelines 2000*, not only bestows life on the dying but displays it to the living as well. Visible evidence of electrical phenomena in the heart, brain, nerves and muscles remains our strongest indicator of the presence or absence of life. The eerily glowing waveform that marches across the cardiac monitor, the electroencephalograph's (EEG) trembling stylus, the convulsions of the flaccid body energized by the brutal power of the defibrillatory shock continue to reassure us that there is such a *thing* as life. And the absence of electrical activity – the infamous 'flat line', the motionless stylus, the absence of a response to defibrillation – continues to reassure us of the certainty of death. The flat line on the cardiac monitor and the strict choreography of the clear-shock-clear sequence are as familiar to today's television audience as the scythe and death-rattle were to past generations. It is in the image electric, which identifies and defines death, that an occult vitalism keeps the mysterious vital-force active.

The QRS complex: the flat line

The QRS complex is the deflection of the baseline on the screen of a cardiac monitor. It indicates the electrical excitation causing ventricular contraction. Less technically, but accurate enough for our purposes, it is the 'blip' on the ECG that indicates a heartbeat. The absence of QRS complexes reflects the absence of any electrical activity in the heart and is the infamous 'flat line' on the cardiac monitor.

The electrocardiograph is a specialized type of galvanometer recording the minute electric currents generated by the heart's action, invented by Willem Einthoven in 1903. As a recording device, the ECG's distant predecessor was the kymograph, invented in 1846 by the German physiologist Karl Ludwig. The kymograph, a pen and drum used to record the pulse, was the first graphic recorder. It provided a direct analogue mode of recording, measuring and comparing physiological parameters. It gave us a different way, a visual means, to see and think about what were in fact quantitative variations in a set of data. Pathology could be translated into a recording made by an instrument. The course of a disease could be read at a glance. By the turn of the nineteenth century, it was possible to understand a patient not only through his or her medical history, not only through pathological signs established by the 'medical gaze', but also via constant physiological monitoring. The continuous oscillating line was to be the parent of all medical monitoring systems and a symbol of the potency of twentieth-century medicine (Canguilhem, 1991, p. 105). Respiratory motion, blood flow in arteries and the electrical activity of the heart were all recorded as oscillating lines that signalled life. Conversely, death became a flat line (K. Arnold, 1997, p. 19). Today, the QRS complex, a line of light twisting rhythmically across the darkened monitor screen, is a potent image of life. The flat line registering cardiac standstill is the media's definitive image of death. Multiple electrical spirits haunt the QRS and the flat line – the subtle electrical impulses that drive the heart, the electrical current that powers the defibrillator, the thin bright line of electrons dancing across its phosphorescent screen. These create an image of physiological function that becomes confounded with the fantasy of Life. Via a series of subtle slippages, the medium does indeed become the message.

Defibrillation: clear-shock-clear

The emphasis on defibrillation in *Guidelines 2000*, though it has valid therapeutic justification, is not unconnected to the need for an electrical proof of death. The heart's response to electrical shock is used as an index of life, and its absence, death. This electrical proof is a form of violence, only too evident from the clear-shock-clear sequence of the ACLS protocol seen in the flashing discharges and convulsing bodies of television resuscitations. The importance of the violence of this proof will be explored in chapter 6.

EEG: brain death

I have less to say about the electrical silence of the electroencephalogram. Although the EEG partakes of the same electrical imagery as the QRS and flat line, I am forced, by constraints of space, to forgo a discussion of the concept of brain death and the practices surrounding it. Brain death and the tests for it are crucial in a very limited (though highly controversial) number of deaths. These are, by and large, problems for the 'other' paradigm – the death-with-dignity.[32] For the present, I acknowledge that the issue is an important one, certainly influences current resuscitative protocols and needs to be dealt with in more detail at another time and place.

*

Vitalism's choice of the imponderables – air, heat and electricity – was precisely because they were phenomena declared distinct by their absences. Strange objects of touch, not sight, their very lack of visuality is what made them suitable as candidates for an occult force, for the life-force. Science has deprived us of the *vis vitae*, and of its potential for representation. Nevertheless, in the modern, life has its iconic representations, though they are, like the concept of life itself, somewhat attenuated and of a second order. And the absence of these – the loss of the QRS resulting in the flat line, the lack of movement on administering a shock, the electrical silence of the EEG – express the flight of life: an entity we know as a fantasy, but still cannot grasp as non-existent. The modern iconography of death struggles, and perhaps ultimately fails, to make present the absence of the nonexistent.[33] However, there is, in contemporary representations of the deathbed in film and on television, a traumatic excess attempting to fill this void – something to which I shall turn in chapter 7. For the present, I only wish to point to the flash of electricity arcing across the convulsed chest as a glimpse of life, and the flat line sliding silently across the monitor screen as death.

5
Mouth-to-Mouth: The Lips of a Corpse

> People generally have great fear of the moribund and would probably hesitate to apply mouth-to-mouth resuscitation to persons who were cyanotic, vomiting, etc.
>
> (Eisenberg, 1997, p. 277)

The Baltoro glacier is a 62 km long river of ice. It flows down from K2, the world's second highest mountain. The trek to base camp at 18,000 feet is ten days in and ten days out, all of it above tree line, most of it on the glacier itself. It is devoid of trees, animals and insects; the only sounds the wind and the creak of the ice. It is a world of thin clear air, hard blue sky, and sheer, ice-capped granite towers. It is magnificently sterile. We were on our way out, about four days down from base camp. The night previous there had been a three inch snowfall, but that morning the sky had cleared and the sun on the snow was near blinding. I, and the friend who had invited me on the trek, were trudging along the path tramped through the snow by the long line of porters. In front of us, we saw a small group of three porters moving very slowly. In a short time, we had drawn near to them. One of them, apparently sick or injured, was being helped by his two friends. When we caught up, we stopped them. The affected porter was probably in his mid-twenties, and, though he didn't look particularly ill, was having some trouble breathing. I wasn't the trip doctor, he was miles ahead with the medical kit, probably already in the next camp, nevertheless, I had a look. The disabled porter told us his name was Iftikar. His colour was good. His respiratory rate, about 20, and pulse, about 80, were a little fast. We stripped off layers of clothing so I could examine his chest. None of us had been out of our clothes for about two weeks. But that morning, in the sun, in spite of being surrounded by snow and ice, the air was warm. There was no evidence of injury. He had good movement to both sides of the chest. You could see his ribs beneath his skin, but he was well muscled and looked generally healthy. I had no stethoscope, so I put my ear against his back and listened to his lungs – on the right, on the left. I could feel his skin hot against my cheek, perhaps a low-grade fever. When I listened to the front of his chest he had good heart sounds with no murmurs or evidence of failure. On the right, low down, at the back, there were a few rattles present on deep inspiration. My buddy, who was also a doctor, then examined him. We decided he probably had the beginnings of a small pneumonia. Though I didn't have my medical kit, I had a film canister with a small selection of pills in my day pack. I dug out a couple of Keflex, perhaps not the ideal antibiotic, but it would do for now, and a couple of aspirin. I had him take these. We indicated that we would continue with him to camp and there examine him in more detail. But he waved us on with a smile. His friends said they would continue down slowly, stopping and resting as necessary. OK, fine, there really wasn't much more to be done, so we made arrangements to see him as soon as he got to camp, and went on. We arrived in camp at about four in the afternoon. We had something to eat with the rest of the group; then went and lay in the sun, dozing on some large boulders at the edge of the glacier. Six o'clock, no sign of the sick porter and his friends. Eight and they still weren't there. We began to worry. Myself, the trek leader, and four porters set off back up the glacier to find them. Nine o'clock and it began to get dark. Still no sign of them. Because of the new snowfall and the possibility of stumbling into a crevasse, we decided it would be unwise to continue. We turned around and headed back to camp. We hoped they'd taken another route and would be waiting for us when we got down. It was pitch black when we got back. They weren't there. I didn't sleep much. At daybreak, we started back up the glacier. At about ten in the morning, we found them. They'd not had a tent, but had bedded down in sleeping bags. The sick porter was now wrapped in all three sleeping bags, and the other two porters were brewing tea on a small stove. We went over to the man in the sleeping bag. I felt my stomach drop. This could hardly be the same man we had left behind yesterday. He was awake, breathing very hard. His lips were blue, his skin cold. His chest now, through the stethoscope, sounded like a pot of boiling water, like a spring bubbling up through the ground, like the last of a milkshake being sucked though a straw. In a hospital, back home, with oxygen and 24 hours of antibiotics, he'd be out of danger. Here in the middle of glacier, at least five days from even a stone hut with dung fire, he was a dead man. I started an IV on him and began to run in IV Kefzol. We sent one of the porters back to camp to bring up a tent, food, fuel, whatever we would need to set up camp here. There was nothing to do but sit beside him and keep watch. It was another magnificent day. The sun moved across the valley, firing the snow. When it reached us, it was so warm we stripped him naked and rub him with snow to bring down his fever. I gave another dose of antibiotic at two. At about four, he began to perk up. His breathing was a little easier, his colour had improved and he asked for some water. We sat him up and gave him a few sips. Then he began to cough. The first paroxysms brought up a little phlegm. Then he took a deep breath, coughed, and a fountain of blood erupted from his mouth and nose. As he turned his head away, blood sprayed out over me, over the porters supporting him, and out in a semicircle to the distance of what must have been ten feet. Blood lay beaded and streaked on the snow, bright red in the sun. I won't say that I've never seen so much blood, because I have, coming from lacerated femoral arteries and oesophageal varices and postpartum haemorrhages, but I had never seen so much blood come from someone's lungs. I was still looking at the blood shining on the snow, when he just fell over dead. That was it, no movement of his chest, no pulse, no heart beat. He was, incredibly, dead. Still looking at the blood and snow, I tore the knitted hat from my head, wiped his face, and blew air into is mouth. But my breath went nowhere. It came back to me in a mouthful of blood. I spat it out and tried again. There was no point. There was but blood where air should be. There was nothing to be done. Nothing even to say. The porters fetched water from the stream that ran along the edge of the glacier; I took a couple of dirty T-shirts from my pack, and the porters used them to wipe the blood, as best they could, from his body, then they wrapped him in the blood stained sleeping bag. The porters and I went over to the little stream, stripped down and washed the blood off ourselves. All glacial melt-water carries large amounts of dust, 'rock flour', milled out of the stone over which the glacier has been grinding for centuries. Here in the Baltoro, the underlying rock contains large *quantities of mica, and thus the water is not the usual dirty grey, but shining silver. Beautiful, like sparkling metallic paint. As we stood in the sun, using aluminium cooking pots to pour the water over ourselves, little specks of mica caught in our hair and the fine lines of our skin. Even when we dried off, it remained. When you turned your hand this way and that, it sparkled like sun on snow.*

Artificial respiration

Mouth-to-mouth is the 'P' of the acronym, CPR – cardiopulmonary resuscitation, and within that resuscitative protocol, it is the B, breathing, of the ABCD mnemonic. The Humane Society recommended mouth-to-mouth ventilation in its founding document of 1774. Yet the technique was abandoned in the late 1780s, replaced by bellows ventilation, which in turn was dropped in the 1830s, replaced by a succession of manual ventilatory techniques. In the late 1950s, mouth-to-mouth was reinstated. In 2000, mouth-to-mouth again demonstrated its potential for problem behaviour in *Guidelines 2000*.

The Method

Mouth-to-mouth ventilation has been documented as being employed by midwives in the resuscitation of newborns as far back as the fifteenth century, but it is likely that as a folk practice it is so ancient as to be undateable (Baker, 1971, p. 337). 'And the Lord God formed man of the dust of the ground, and breathed into his nostrils the breath of life; and man became a living soul' (Genesis 2: 7). In Exodus (1: 17) the midwife Pu'ah 'breathed into the baby's mouth to induce the baby to cry'; and in the Talmud 'The newborn is held so that it should not fall on the earth and one blows into its nostrils' (Shabbath 128.b-4).

In the sixteenth and seventeenth centuries, bellows ventilation was used to keep animals alive during vivisection. Andreas Vesalius, in *De humani corporis fabrica* (1542), described the use of tracheotomy, endotracheal intubation and bellows to revive dogs that had been strangled. Paracelsus attempted, unsuccessfully, to resuscitate a corpse using bellows. Sporadic reports of its use can be found through the mid-eighteenth century (Physician, 1746, p. 68). However, though there was continued use of mouth-to-mouth by midwives and accoucheurs, and bellows by anatomists, neither technique became widespread in orthodox medicine.

The first documented English language case report of the use of mouth-to-mouth ventilation in an adult was by William Tossach, a surgeon from Alloa in Scotland (Tossach, 1752, p. 108). On 3 December 1732, a group of miners entered a pit, which had been closed for a fortnight, in order to extinguish a fire that had broken out in the coal. The miners were overcome by fumes and quickly returned to the surface coughing and short of breath, but one, James Blair, was brought up pulseless and not breathing. Tossach sealed his mouth over Blair's and blew into his lungs:

> He was in all Appearance dead. I applied my Mouth close to his, and blowed my Breath as strong as I could ... I blew again my Breath as strong as I could, raising his Chest fully with it; and immediately I felt six or seven very quick Beats of the Heart; his *Thorax* continued to play, and the Pulse was felt soon after in the Arteries .... After about an Hour he began to yawn, and to move his Eye-lids, Hands and Feet .... In an Hour more he came pretty well to his Senses, and could take Drink; but knew nothing of all that had happened after his lying down at the Foot of the Ladder, till his awaking, as it were, in the House. (Tossach, 1752, p. 110)

Little attention was paid to this report until 1744, when John Fothergill cited it in an essay on resuscitation (1782, pp. 110–19). In 1740, between Tossach's report and Fothergill's reiteration of it, Réne-Antoine Ferchault de Réamur published *Avis pour donner du secours a ceus l'on croit noyez* (*Notice in Order to Give Help to Those Believed to Be Drowned*) (1990). The recommendations in Réamur's and Fothergill's essays were very similar. Fothergill states:

> There are some facts, which in themselves are of so great importance to mankind, or which may lead to such useful discoveries, that it would seem to be the duty of every one, under whose notice they fall, to render them as extensively public as it is possible .... Anatomists, it is true, have long known, that the artificial inflation of the lungs of a dead or dying animal will put the heart in motion, and continue it so for some time; yet this is the first instance [referring to Tossach's report] I remember to have met with, wherein the experiment was applied to the happy purpose of rescuing life from such imminent danger .... It is not easy to enumerate all the various casualties, in which this method might be tried not without a prospect of success; some of them are the following: – Suffocations, from the sulphurous damps of mines, coalpits, &c. the condensed air of long unopened wells, or other subterraneous caverns; the noxious vapours arising from fermenting liquors received from a

narrow vent; the steam of burning charcoal; sulphurous mineral acids; arsenical effluvia, &c. Perhaps those, who, to appearance, struck dead by lightening, or any violent agitation of the passions, as joy, fear, surprize, &c. might frequently be recovered by this simple process of blowing into the lungs, and by that means once more communicating motion to the vital organs. Malefactors executed at the gallows would afford opportunities of discovering how far this method might be successful in relieving such as may have unhappily become their own executioners, by hanging themselves .... But this method would seem to promise very much in assisting those who have been suffocated in water .... To conclude, as I apprehend the method above described may conduce to saving a great many lives, as it is practicable by everyone who happens to be present at the accident, without loss of time, without expense, with little trouble, and less skill; and as it is, perhaps the only expedient of which it can justly be said, that it may possibly do great good, but cannot do harm; I thought it of so much consequence to the public, as to deserve to be recommended in this manner to your notice. (1782, pp. 110–19)

Fothergill's recommendation of mouth-to-mouth was followed in the 1760s by that of the Swiss physician Samuel Tissot, and his Scottish pupil William Buchan, but these recommendations were to lie fallow until Fothergill's student John Coakley Lettsom assisted in the founding of the Humane Society in 1774. The Humane Society found that mouth-to-mouth was easily performed and easily taught. The equipment necessary, a pair of lips and a pair of lungs, was always available; it was reasonably safe; and when it was effective it was dramatically so.

From air to oxygen

The learned Grubelius ... informs us, that whilst a Physician was preparing the Remedies proper to restore to Life, a Woman, who had fallen into such a Syncope, that she was thought dead, her own Servant, who had a great Attachment to her, restored her to Life by blowing in her Mouth. But 'tis probable, that this Method produces its happy Effects, rather by restoring the Motion of the Blood and Lungs, than by Means of that vivifying Principle, which some superstitious Authors suppose to be lodg'd in the human breath.

(Physician, 1746, p. 80)

During the period immediately preceding the Humane Society's institution, notions of air and of respiration were undergoing radical change. For most of the eighteenth century, the mechanical theory of lung action held sway. In this, the lungs were no more than a conduit to allow blood to get from the right to the left sides of the heart. As seen from the above quote, the mechanical theory quite specifically condemned the Aristotelian-Galenic idea that air might be a vehicle for some type of vital quality or force. This mechanical theory of lung function was the basis of the apoplectic theory of drowning discussed in chapter 3.

Mechanism had sought to alter the status of air, transforming it from an occult force, the *pneuma* of the ancients, to a material substance whose qualities might be subject to measurement. Vincenzo Viviani and Evangelista Torricelli discovered that air had weight. Otto von Guerke demonstrated that along with weight, it had mass. Joan-Baptista van Helmont coined the term 'gas', but it was Robert Boyle's concept of gas as matter in an expanded state that enabled him to explain the behaviour of air as a material substance.

One of the most startling discoveries to come out the scientific investigation of air in the eighteenth century was that atmospheric air was not a single substance. John Mayow postulated that the heat of living organisms, the combustion of gunpowder and the processes of fermentation were all dependent on 'nitro-aerial particles' in atmospheric air. This aerial nitre was responsible for the scarlet colour of arterial blood and irritability. This vital substance in the blood enabled it to enliven the other organs. It gave muscles, including and especially the heart, movement (R. Porter, 1999, p. 221).

In 1766, Joseph Black identified 'Fixed Air', as a gas produced by respiration and combustion that would support neither.[1] In that same year, Henry Cavendish isolated hydrogen, and in 1772, Daniel Rutherford, nitrogen. It was in 1774, the year of the Humane Society's inauguration, that Joseph Priestley identified 'dephlogisticated air',[2] and in 1774–5, Antoine Laurant-Lavoisier explained the same phenomena through the qualities of a gas he labelled '*oxygène*'.[3] In 1778, Lavoisier published what is now accepted as the correct explanation of the process of respiration, postulating that *oxygène*, a component of atmospheric air, was absorbed by the lungs, and carbonic acid gas, a product of the body's metabolic process, was excreted by them. *Oxygène* was the cause of the florid colour of arterial blood and was what induced irritability or vitality in the recipient organs. He and

Pierre Simon Laplace gave convincing evidence that respiration was to the living body what combustion was to the inanimate world; both required *oxygéne*, and both produced carbonic acid gas and heat (R. Porter, 1999, pp. 246–54).

The Humane Society kept a close eye on the discoveries of Priestley and Lavoisier, commenting on them in its *Annual Reports*. John Hunter recommended that 'perhaps the Dephlogisticated Air, as described by Dr. Priestley may prove more efficacious than common air' in the resuscitation of the drowned (Hunter, 1837, p. 79). Anthony Fothergill waxes lyrical:

> [Vital Air] might be procured on moderate terms from common nitre, which yields it in a very considerable quantity – an article, unless in time of war, generally to be obtained remarkably cheap. How many thousand tons of nitre has Europe consumed of late, in making gun-powder, and that with the avowed intention of DESTROYING thousands of its inhabitants?[4] Might not a small portion be spared for another purpose, at *least* equally humane and laudable, *viz.* that of PRESERVING a remnant of our unfortunate fellow-creatures! Is it not singularly curious, that a substance of such very humble pretensions as common nitre (or salt-petre) should possess properties on which hangs the fate of the most powerful empires! since by chemistry, it may either be converted into a fulminating engine, to overturn fortified cities, or to enable the garrison to launch out death and destruction on the besiegers! Or, that by a different process, it may be made to pour forth Vital Air – that VIVIFYING FLUID diffused through the atmosphere, which breathes in the zephyrs, which whispers in the breeze, and which cheers and supports animated Nature! (1795, p. 116)

Fothergill recommends it be kept in bell jars in the receiving houses of the Society for use in resuscitations.

The Humane Society was quick to incorporate new developments as they came along. It validated its protocol by citing advances in the chemistry of atmospheric gases. The union of the chemistry of atmospheric gases with physiological experiments in respiratory function yielded knowledge that found practical application in drowning protocols. This seemed an ideal example of the emerging scientific method – experiment and theory wed so as to give birth to rational therapeutics (Goodwyn, 1788, pp. 1–98). Unfortunately, this marriage was not to last.

Good airs and bad

Mouth-to-mouth

The above advances in natural philosophy and medicine seemed to hold out the hope of a rational and effective therapeutics. It is thus somewhat paradoxical that the advance of science that encouraged mouth-to-mouth's inclusion in the Humane Society's protocol in 1774 were also responsible for its expulsion from the protocol in 1812 (Royal, 1812, p. 27). When the discoveries of Priestley, Black, Lavoisier, Cavendish and Rutherford concerning the composite nature of atmospheric air and the characteristics of its component gases were related to the discoveries in respiratory physiology of Hooke, Lower, Mayow and Laplace, air became valorized into a 'good' gas, which supported life – vital air (oxygen) and a 'bad' gas, which stifled life – fixed air (carbon dioxide). The use of the rescuer's breath, containing increased quantities of the bad gas and decreased quantities of the good gas, was seen as tantamount to poisoning the victim. The division of atmospheric air into component parts, labelled good and bad, corroborated the already longstanding belief in miasmas, that is, unhealthy airs as the cause of disease.

Anthony Fothergill, supporting the use of bellows, declared, 'Others deny that air, already vitiated by respiration can be fit for the purpose [of ventilation], to say nothing of the indelicacy of the operation, and therefore justly prefer atmospheric air' (1795, p. 112). Struve added, 'Most physicians are of the opinion, that [the blowing in of air by the mouth] is injurious' (1803, p. 192). Between 1782 and 1788, the Humane Society tolerated mouth-to-mouth, preferring the use of bellows where available. In 1812, it condemned mouth-to-mouth outright: 'as the air expired by the most healthy is not pure air, but chiefly carbonic, or what arises from burning charcoal, it is more likely to destroy than to promote the action of the lungs, and hence should be avoided' (Royal, 1812, p. 27). Benjamin Waterhouse bluntly declared that, 'To blow one's own breath into the lungs of another is an absurd and pernicious practice' (1790, p. 17).

Exhaled breath and vital air became the polarized ends of a crude moral continuum based on physiological effect. Exhaled air was waste, impure, soiled by its contact with man's animal nature. Atmospheric air, at a midpoint in the continuum, was the untainted gift of nature, part of the cosmic equilibrium that nourished man. Best of all was vital air – nature's bounty refined by man's genius into its perfect form. Like the *aether* of the ancients, vital air was the ideal to which terrestrial air aspired. Vital air was pure and good, supporting life and giving warmth.

> When pure Oxygene Gas can be procured, and the Lungs inflated with it instead of Common Air, there can be no doubt of its superior efficacy. It can be conveniently carried to any requisite distance in an oiled silk bag, having a stop-cock fitted to it; and this bag may be used instead of the bellows. (Curry, 1815, p. 52)[5]

If some vital air was good, more was better: if some fixed air was bad, more was worse.[6] Exhaled breath became poison. By the beginning of the nineteenth century, mouth-to-mouth was in the process of being banished to the same hinterland of shady medical practices as tobacco smoke enemata and emetic tartar.

Bellows

Bellows ventilation had, since the early 1500s, been used in the preparation of animal specimens for vivisection, and there were advocates of its use in the resuscitative situation:

> Whenever a proper machine can be obtained for inflation, it must ever be preferred, as respirable or Vital Air will bid fair in a number of cases to prove more efficacious than air blended with contaminated vapours from the respiratory organs of an assistant. (Royal, 1789, p. 91)

Cullen, Monro, Kite and Hunter all published their own designs for bellows, and Savigny supplied bellows in the resuscitation kits he manufactured for the Humane Society. Bellows, in allowing the use of atmospheric or vital air, avoided the danger of poisoning the victim. Nevertheless, bellows ventilation in its turn was discredited and dropped from the protocol in the early 1830s (Royal, 1849, p. 68).

The use of bellows had always been somewhat problematic. Frequently they were not to hand at the scene of an accident and their use was considered rather complicated for the layperson. Bellows ventilation came under severe criticism in 1821 in a series of lectures on asphyxia by Sir Benjamin Brodie, president of the Royal College of Surgeons. He pointed out that once breathing stopped, the heart stopped, and the inflation of the lungs alone would not restart it. This was true enough, but Brodie seems to have been almost intentionally misunderstood, for he did not say that the inflation method was useless in all cases; he was only pointing out its futility in cases of complete cardiac standstill. As late as 1862, Brodie continued to recommend the inflation method when respiratory intervention was deemed necessary (1865, p. 407). A more serious concern over the use of bellows developed in 1829 when Leroy d'Etoiles demonstrated that it was possible to rupture the lungs of animals by sudden and forceful inflation. This experiment was much quoted in the English literature, and the unfortunate d'Etoiles has been blamed for severely setting back the cause of artificial ventilation (Keith, 1909, p. 748). In fact, d'Etoiles did not condemn the use of bellows, he merely cautioned their use. He himself continued to use them, but adjusted their volume to the age and size of the patient. The Humane Society's rejection of bellows *appeared* to be based on a careless, even wilful, misconstruction of the work of Brodie and d'Etoiles. As with mouth-to-mouth, there was an almost unseemly eagerness to be rid of the technique.

Manual ventilatory techniques

In the 1830s, mouth-to-mouth and bellows ventilation were replaced by the manual ventilatory techniques that were to remain standard practice until the late 1950s. Over 100 eponymous manual 'methods' were developed over that 100-year interval – the Leroy Method, the Dalrymple Method, the Marshall Hall Method, the Silvester Method, the Pacini Method, the Bain Method, the Howard Method, the Schultze Method, the Schroeder Method, the Shucking Method, the Schuller Method, the Bowles Method, the Laborde Method, the Schafer Method, the Holger-Nielsen Method, and so on (Keith, 1909, p. 748; Gordon et al., 1951, p. 1447). It would be tedious to go into all these in detail. Most involved some form of chest or abdominal compression, associated with manipulation of the arms or shoulders,[7] although there were also some imaginative permutations – swinging the patient between one's legs, bouncing them up and down on a pole, yanking repeatedly on the tongue (Keith, 1909, p. 828). Manual ventilatory techniques offered the advantages of neither poisoning the patient with the vitiated breath of the rescuer, nor threatening to blow their lungs out with the excessive pressure of bellows, and, moreover, 'Inducing respiratory movements, by which air is drawn into the lungs without apparatus [is] entirely in harmony with that of Nature' (Silvester, 1858, p. 576).

Throughout the first half of the twentieth century, mouth-to-mouth was occasionally championed, but its proponents were few. The Silvester and Schafer Methods dominated. There were regional variations, and rival life-saving institutions pushed their preferred techniques with missionary zeal. In 1909, the Humane Society was using the Silvester Method; the Royal Life Saving Society the Schafer Method; and the National Lifeboat Institution the Marshall-Hall Method. In 1932, Colonel Holger Louis Nielsen developed the Holger Nielsen Method. Gordon, in his 1951 study of manual techniques, provided evidence of the superiority of the Holger Nielsen Method over the other manual methods (1951, p. 1444). In 1951, at a conference attended by the American Red Cross, armed forces, Boy Scouts, Campfire Girls, Girl Scouts, AT&T, Bureau of Mines, YMCA, American Medical Association and public utility and civil defence organizations, the Holger Nielsen Method was adopted as the preferred technique of artificial ventilation (Dill, 1951, p. 171).

Unfortunately, manual ventilatory techniques had one big disadvantage: they did not move enough air to support life (Gordon, 1951, p. 1444; Dill, 1958, p. 317; Safar, 1958, p. 671). This lack of efficacy was, of course, not apparent at the time. In 1950, Archer Gordon published his study on the tidal volumes generated by the various manual ventilatory techniques.[8] He found that most were grossly inadequate and that even the best, the Holger Nielsen method, was borderline (1950, p. 1447). A number of studies followed disproving the claim that mouth-to-mouth was ineffective because expired air contained too much carbon dioxide and too little oxygen (Elam, Brown and Elder, 1954, p. 749; Johns and Cooper, 1957; Safar, 1958, p. 671; Cooper, 1975, p. 487; Timmermans, 1999, p. 220).

IPPV

Intermittent-positive-pressure-ventilation (IPPV) was at the time being introduced successfully in Scandinavia for the short-term management of patients with respiratory insufficiency caused by poliomyelitis or barbiturate overdose (Nilsson, 1951, p. 1; Ibsen, 1954, p. 72).[9] James Elam had been using mouth-to-nose respiration in the late 1940s on patients with acute paralytic polio. He demonstrated that expired air was fully capable of maintaining arterial oxygen levels and, furthermore, the various manual ventilatory techniques currently in practice were not. In 1952, Elam remarked to Gordon that manual ventilation methods were doomed (Elam, Brown and Elder, 1954, p. 749). Researchers were given the opportunity to prove this by the

US Department of Defense, who were interested in the use of mouth-to-mouth in treating soldiers paralysed by nerve gas (Cooper, 1975, p. 487; Johns and Cooper, 1957). These studies, published in 1954, demonstrated the clear superiority of mouth-to-mouth over manual ventilatory techniques, but the National Research Council-National Academy of Sciences and the American Red Cross were not impressed, and refused to endorse the technique (Safar, 1989, p. 53).

In 1956, Elam teamed up with Peter Safar in a series of experiments (Safar, Escarraga and Elam, 1958, p. 671; Safar, Escarraga and Chang, 1959, p. 760), which, Safar said:

> convincingly demonstrated that the manual methods of artificial respiration were virtually worthless and mouth-to-mouth ventilation the most effective means of respiration. And, perhaps most important, anyone (rescuers from ten years to old age) could perform effective mouth-to-mouth respiration, even on adult victims, after only minutes of instruction. No bags, masks, or tubes were required. (Eisenberg, 1997, p. 97)

After more than 100 years of disgrace, mouth-to-mouth began its return. In March 1957, the National Research Council-National Academy of Sciences recommended the use of mouth-to-mouth in the resuscitation of infants and children. The evidence of benefit was equally convincing in adults, but it was thought that the public would be unwilling to perform the technique on adults. However, in May of that year, the US Army adopted mouth-to-mouth in adults, and, in 1958, the American Medical Association, the National Research Council-National Academy of Sciences and the American Red Cross also endorsed mouth-to-mouth in adults (Dill, 1958, p. 317). The Canadian Red Cross, alleging that it would be difficult for 'a layperson to place his lips against the lips of a corpse', did not give its approval until 1960 (Eisenberg, 1997, p. 102).

When, in 1960, the resuscitative protocol that was to become CPR was given its first public airing at a meeting of the Maryland Medical Society in Ocean City, there was still resistance to the inclusion of mouth-to-mouth. Some delegates expressed the hope that the second component of the protocol, external cardiac compressions, might provide an adequate means of ventilation (Benson, 1961, p. 398). However, evidence of mouth-to-mouth's superiority was overwhelming and mouth-to-mouth was included in the official protocol formalized by the American Heart Association in 1963.

Reasons and rationalizations

In explaining the long period of mouth-to-mouth's disgrace, medical commentators (meaning medicine, not history of medicine) shake their heads in wonder at what they see as the imprudence of abandoning a simple, safe, effective technique, supported by intuition, tradition and a strong physiological theory, for a series of complicated manual manoeuvres that are, at least in hindsight, none of the above (R. Lee, 1972, p. 418; Eisenberg, 1997, pp. 92–102). What they hint at is folly, though pleading mitigating circumstances – low patient numbers, poor communications and confusion over pathophysiology. Eisenberg places the blame for the abandonment of mouth-to-mouth on over-confidence in an immature, insufficiently sensitive and insufficiently rigorous empirical methodology (1997, p. 19). In his view, the dropping of mouth-to-mouth and retention of less effective techniques, such as friction, was the result of a poorly systematized and anecdotal approach.

On the other hand, historians of medicine perceive eighteenth-century physicians as falling prey to a different, though complementary, error: that of the over-rigorous application of theory. The spectacular advances of Enlightenment physics and mathematics are seen as giving medicine a desire for a similar Newtonian unity of theory, making it overly dependent on the rationalist approach and thus overly dogmatic (Bynum, 1994, p. 17; Canguilhem, 1991, p. 107; R. Porter, 1999, p. 246). The apparent folly of mouth-to-mouth's abolition is thus, at least in part, seen as due to the clinical misapplication of the discovery of the compound nature of atmospheric air and the valorization of its components. Furthermore, the particular developmental stage of science and medicine at the turn of the eighteenth century, that is, the 'immaturity' of the scientific method, is blamed for allowing deductive reasoning to override clinical experience and empirical evidence. In this way, the same scientific process by which respiration was proved essential to life, and thus artificial ventilation essential to resuscitation, is thought to have resulted ultimately in mouth-to-mouth being condemned.

Certain amounts of folly, lax empiricism and overweening rationalism undoubtedly did contribute to the suppression of mouth-to-mouth, just as they do to errors in medicine today.[10] However, I would maintain that, though contributory, these are not sufficient causes for mouth-to-mouth's banishment. Significant as they no doubt are, the cause appears inadequate to the effect. When iatrochemistry, by valorizing the components of air, made possible a condemnation of mouth-to-mouth based on physiological theory, one could almost hear a collective sigh of relief issue from the clinical literature. The facility with which the technique was dropped and the vehemence of its detractors gave the concept of 'bad air' more the appearance of an excuse than a reason. Science was telling the scientists, the doctors and the public exactly what they wanted to hear – that it was no longer necessary to place one's 'lips against the lips of a corpse'.

The lips of a corpse

Life is not inexhaustible; it can be damaged, squandered, stolen. Life and the 'life-force' have always been intimately linked to breath. To place one's lips against the lips of a corpse puts one in danger – danger of losing one's own life. Mouth-to-mouth is an effective technique, yet it is a technique that has always had problems maintaining its presence in the protocol. The belief that the breath of the rescuer was capable of poisoning the victim has been discussed above. In addition to that fear, the 'indelicacy' of the procedure was often mentioned in the protocols of the Humane Society. And there was, of course, also, the ever-present fear of contagion. As we shall see, the fears of poisoning, disgust and contagion point to a much deeper fear – the fear of death.

The fear of infectious disease remains, today, the most common reason given for reluctance in performing mouth-to-mouth (Becker et al., 1997, p. 2102). The mouth, the respiratory tract and breath have always been deeply implicated in both the imagined and actual spread of disease, whether consumption in the eighteenth century or AIDS in the twentieth. Germ theory has been cited as the major cause of the demise of mouth-to-mouth (R. Lee, 1972, p. 418; Eisenberg, 1997, p. 87). This claim, though not entirely incorrect, is somewhat misleading. Mouth-to-mouth was abandoned long before 1878 and Pasteur's announcement to the French Academy of Medicine. Germ theory certainly contributed to mouth-to-mouth's continued exile after that date, but germ theory was but the latest recension of a very ancient fear, the fear of contagion. As early as 1546, Giralamo Fracastro had revived Epicurean and Lucretian notions of *seminaria contagiosa*, 'seeds of infection'. The contagionist model of epidemic disease was given a considerable boost in the late seventeenth century by the discovery of tiny 'animalcules' under the microscopes of Athanasius Kircher and Anton van Leeuwenhoek and was further bolstered by the success of vaccination in controlling smallpox and of quarantine in controlling the spread of plague.

Alongside, and in competition with, contagionist ideas of epidemic spread was the miasmatic theory of disease. Ancient in origin and particularly strong in the sixteenth to the nineteenth centuries, it explained epidemic disease as being caused by unhealthy exhalations (miasmas) from plants, animals and people, from the effluvia of swamps and drains (*mal-aria*: bad air), from maleficent elements in the soil and from putrefaction (Lloyd, 1978, p. 272; Longrigg, 1993, pp. 25–33). 'Bad airs', or miasmas, when brought into contact with persons of suitable constitution, produced illness. In 1831, Asiatic cholera dramatically invaded Europe. The failure of quarantine to contain cholera's spread strengthened the miasmatic model. Nineteenth-century sanitarians, such as Edwin Chadwick and Florence Nightingale, believed in miasmas, equating stink with disease. The black smoke belched from the chimneys of the factories that fed the growing cities of Europe and America and the corrupted breath of the poor made ill by working in them were virulent poisons endangering the health not only of the poor, but of all, threatening the well-being of the economy and empire (D. Porter, 1999, pp. 124–5). Miasmatism and the sanitarians saw little that was good in exhaled breath and thus in mouth-to-mouth.

In 1854, cholera was proved by John Snow to be water-borne. This dealt a serious blow to miasmatism. In the latter half of the nineteenth century, the resurrection of contagionism and the triumph of Pasteur's germ theory further damaged miasmatism, but did little to exculpate mouth-to-mouth. 'Bad air' was quite easily co-opted into the new contagious disease model, going from being the aetiological agent to the vehicle of transmission. Nor did exhaled breath relinquish its status as poison, for the increased carbon dioxide in it remained a major concern. Exhaled breath was doubly damned as both poisonous and germ-infested. It is hardly surprising that it was in this period that manual ventilatory techniques proliferated. The nineteenth century's obsession with bad airs and the twentieth's with germs, in spite of being legitimate fears about real phenomena, remain manifestations of the atavistic, but ever present, fear of contagion.

Infection

> Fear of catching AIDS or some other dread disease deters many laypeople from performing cardiopulmonary resuscitation, especially the mouth-to-mouth breathing part. That fact prompted researchers at the University of California Davis Medical Centre to wonder whether doctors and nurses are any more willing to do CPR on strangers. After all, they're trained

to save lives, and they should know that HIV is not transmissible through saliva. A lot of good that education does them. In a survey of health professionals trained in cardiac life support, the UC Davis researchers found that fewer than half would perform CPR on a stranger who collapsed in a supermarket. And only about a third would do CPR on an adult hospital patient whose HIV status was unknown. As potential CPR candidates, homeless people fared worst of all. Little more than a fifth of the healthcare workers said they'd perform CPR on a homeless adult. Like lay people, doctors and nurses say fear of HIV, hepatitis, tuberculosis and herpes would keep their lips sealed in such situations. But 84 per cent said they'd do CPR on a neighbor, 88 per cent on a child they knew at the swimming pool, 93 per cent on their own parents and 94 per cent on a spouse. (Which makes one wonder about the other 6 per cent).

(Rubin, 2001)

Between 70 and 100 per cent of health care workers say they would refuse to do mouth-to-mouth on a known homosexual and 50–100 per cent on a stranger, though only 20–40 per cent would refuse to do it on a child (Mannis and Wendel, 1984, p. 15; Hew et al., 1997, p. 279; Horowitz and Matheny, 1997, p. 392; Brenner et al., 2000, p. 1054; Melanson and O'Gara, 2000, p. 48). The fear of infection is the most common reason given for failing to do mouth-to-mouth. The main fear is of HIV transmission, despite the fact that there are no reports of the transmission of HIV through mouth-to-mouth ventilation.[11]

Though the fear of infectious disease is the reason given for failing to give mouth-to-mouth, the two most significant factors in terms of willingness to do mouth-to-mouth are 'familiarity' and age. 'Familiarity' amounts almost to kinship status (see quote from Rubin above). Age turns out to be a particularly interesting criterion. The younger the victim, the more likely we are to be willing to perform mouth-to-mouth. As already discussed, when mouth-to-mouth was being re-introduced in the 1950s, the initial recommendations were for its use in the resuscitation of infants and children only. The reason given was the revulsion of rescuers at its use on adults, supposedly because of 'aesthetic' considerations. It is somewhat debatable which is the more 'aesthetic' experience: giving mouth-to-mouth to a mucousy, meconium- (foetal faeces) smeared neonate or an adult covered in vomit. Aesthetics aside, our culture valorizes childhood and because of the positive value placed on children, people appear to be willing to make a greater sacrifice for a child than for an adult. There is also a perception of childhood 'purity'. Children are considered, by default, to be pure and good. They are not seen as bearers of contagion (though anyone who has ever worked on a paediatric ward can set you straight on that). Unsullied by long contact with the world, they are considered bacteriologically clean and morally incorrupt. However, there is a darker side to the child's innocent status, for as well as being innocuous, they are also impotent. In the ancient world, the child and especially the infant lacked a fully developed soul. Roman funerary rites for children dying before the age of puberty, when the *genius* was thought to develop, were often very perfunctory. Without the full power of the life-force, children are both less than 'human' and less of a threat.

Our aversion to mouth-to-mouth is considered a serious problem by the AHA, for it was found that reluctance to do mouth-to-mouth prevented bystanders from initiating the other techniques contained in the ABCD sequence.

> Despite three decades of promulgation, CPR is not performed for the majority of victims who require lifesaving care. Studies have identified reticence to perform mouth-to-mouth ventilation as a significant barrier to more frequent performance of bystander CPR .... Above all, aesthetic and infectious disease concerns by the public and healthcare providers appear to be major barriers to provision of basic CPR. (Becker et al., 1997, p. 2102)

Guidelines 2000 has responded to these findings. Though IPPV in the form of pocket mask or mouth-to-mask ventilation remains prominent within the BLS protocol (and in the form of bag-valve mask or endotracheal tube ventilation within the ACLS protocol), rescuers, though not encouraged to abandon mouth-to-mouth, are given dispensation to forgo it.[12]

> Mouth-to-mouth rescue breathing is a safe and effective technique that has saved many lives .... If a person is unwilling or unable to perform mouth-to-mouth ventilation for an adult victim, chest-compression-only CPR should be provided rather than no attempt at CPR made. (American, 2000, pp. I.22–I.59)

Professional healthcare providers are instructed:

> Never use mouth-to-mouth or mouth-to-nose techniques without barrier protection, in general use either mouth-to-face shield, or mouth-to-pocket face mask, or bag-mask device. (Cummins, 2001, p. 19)

> Under these conditions [where there is no barrier device] the provider will have to decide whether to provide mouth-to-mouth ventilation without a barrier device or to forgo ventilation and provide chest compressions only. (Cummins, 2001, p. 208)

The use of a barrier device, when available, is the preferred approach to mouth-to-mouth, but failing that, it appears that it is permissible to forgo ventilations entirely. This is despite the fact that elsewhere in the same document the rescuer is warned:

> The ACLS Approach teaches that whenever an assessment step reveals a life-threatening problem; go no further until that problem is solved. The obstructed airway is a common clinical problem that dramatically illustrates the point. Rescuers who fail to open a victim's airway or to provide proper ventilations must not proceed to chest compressions, defibrillation, or medications. *They must open the airway.* To do otherwise condemns the patient to certain death. (Cummins, 2001, p. 9)

It is apparently permissible to forgo ventilation, despite the fact that:

1. the risks of infection are nil (American, *Guidelines* I.22–I.59),
2. current barrier devices are ineffective in preventing cross-contamination and various mask devices are difficult to use (American, *Guidelines* I.22–I.59), and
3. failure to ventilate 'condemns the patient to a certain death'. (Cummins, 2001, p. 9)

The argument used by the AHA in dispensing with mouth-to-mouth is, in the end, social and psychological rather than physiological. The tensions resulting from this are evident in the conflicting advice given in *Guidelines 2000*.

Indelicacy

In the Humane Society's literature, even as mouth-to-mouth was being strongly recommended, the disagreeableness or indelicacy of the operation was inevitably mentioned (A. Fothergill, 1795, p. 112):

> The blowing into the mouth may, upon an emergency, answer ... but the difficulty of getting people to continue it will be easily conceived, on account of the operation being so extremely disagreeable and troublesome. (Kite, 1788, p. 140)

Attempts were made to make the procedure less disagreeable and troublesome through the use of specially designed boxwood or ivory tubes (Kite, 1788, p. 271). Should such instruments be unavailable, a handkerchief, tobacco-pipe, quill, pencil-case, wine-strainer or the rolled-up sole of an old shoe were recommended – anything to avoid the indelicacy of mouth-to-mouth contact (A. Fothergill, 1795, p. 117; Curry, 1815, p. 48). As late as 1944, the textbook *Medical Physics* mentioned mouth-to-mouth as a technique infrequently used, because 'the medical profession considered it a vulgar act' (Fisher, 1944, p. 1241). Even today:

> What about the unpleasant and disagreeable aspects of doing CPR either in hospital or out of hospital? Would you really be able to do mouth-to-mouth rescue breathing on a stranger? What if the victim is bleeding from facial injuries that occurred when the victim collapsed? (Cummins, 2001, p. 43)

Concepts of decorum and indelicacy, historically and culturally-specific as they are, conceal the more profound emotion of disgust.[13] The mouth is a liminal area, a zone of transgression, an area of contact between self and other, between the subjective and the objective, a conduit for the impure and a reservoir of the erotic. Of course, none of these is an entirely unconnected concept. The mouth, for a number of reasons, is a danger zone (Bakhtin, 1984, p. 325; Bataille, 1985, p. 59; C. Turner, 2000, p. 10).

One need hardly be a psychoanalyst to appreciate the hesitation felt on being asked to administer mouth-to-mouth to an unconscious, possibly dead, drug addict covered in vomit.

> Three paramedics and a security guard sit in the harsh fluorescent light of the ER coffee room waiting for a call:

Older Paramedic: 'So there I am. This junkie got something jammed 'tween his teeth. Now none of these junkies want to give mouth-to-mouth. It was a blowdrier. So I pulls it out. His body was cold, 'cept for his throat. It'd been blow dried for about an hour. Junkie had second degree burns o' the tongue. Mmhm.'
Rookie: 'Didja' ever give mouth-to-mouth?'
Older Paramedic: 'Yeh. Long time ago when I was your age, boy. Never again. Chances are, ya end up with a mouthful of puke. Junkie puke.'
Rookie: 'I'd do it if I had to. Y'know it's part of the job. How 'bout you?'
Frank: 'What?'
Rookie: 'Didja' ever do mouth-to-mouth before?'
Frank: 'Once. On a baby.'
Security Guard: 'Babies? Now babies are a whole different thing entirely.'
(*Bringing*, 1999)

'Junkie puke', the mere words raise a shudder of disgust. We see the reluctance of the older paramedic to give mouth-to-mouth contrasted to the rookie's enthusiasm. Expressed in their conversation are fears of impurity, contagion, poisoning and death. Even today, despite the strength of its empirical, experimental and theoretical justifications, mouth-to-mouth remains 'a custom more honour'd in the breach than the observance'. Its use, when it is used, as it is later in this film, is made exceptional because of its more frequent absence.

A kiss is generally thought to be an expression of care or desire, but the physical intimacy involved in kissing also places it high on the list of acts with a potential for disgust. Though a kiss may be a demonstration of love as a type of altruistic 'caring', the kiss is also an erotic act. The lover's kiss is a controlled transgression. Whatever the relations between love and lust might be, they do at least coincide in their ability to surmount disgust. In the lover's kiss, the dangers of overly close personal contact are limited by being hedged in with numerous taboos. If we obey the rules, we will be safe. The 'kiss of life' violates almost every one of those rules. Mouth-to-mouth requires that we perform an intimate act in the public arena, with a stranger, perhaps of unsuitable gender, and, even worse, a stranger of uncertain vitality, possibly even a corpse. The 'kiss of life' is not consciously erotic. It believes itself altruistic. It aspires to saving the life of the victim.

However, in the touching of lips, disgust and the dangers of the erotic are always present.

> It can be pretty yucky .... When people practice CPR on a dummy they imagine Cindy Crawford or Tom Cruise, but the guys who drop in the supermarket tend to resemble Rodney Dangerfield [the portly American comedian]. I think that's yet another reason bystander CPR is already far too rare and is becoming even less common. (Becker, quoted in Easton, 1997)

The word 'disgust' is, etymologically, an expression of distaste. Charles Darwin maintained that the mouth not only experienced, but also came to express disgust. He postulated that man lost the power his ape-like ancestors possessed to voluntarily vomit, and replaced it with the facial grimaces of disgust, which were our first form of representation and speech. Language originated in the interjections that one makes when disgusted, such as 'ugh!' and 'ach!' (1998, pp. 246–58). The acquisition of speech meant that man could now communicate with words what was edible and what was poisonous. In Darwin's formulation, disgust becomes the founding moment in which nature produces culture out of itself. Ian Miller maintains that such arguments based on the etymology of the English word are misleading (1997, p. 7). Nevertheless, regardless of the developmental mechanics of the emotion of disgust, there is a line running from Lessing to Darwin to Freud to Bakhtin to Lacan to Bataille that has invested the mouth with a primary role in the generation of disgust (C. Turner, 2000, pp. 10–70). For Mikhail Bakhtin, the image of the gaping mouth 'is the open gate leading downward into the bodily underworld. The gaping mouth is related to the image of swallowing, this most ancient symbol of death and destruction' (1984, p. 325).

Certain low, impure, polluting objects – such as faeces, blood and the corpse – and certain areas of the body – such as the mouth, anus and genitals – possess (except in very specific circumstances, understood to be exceptional) an extraordinary power to disgust (Miller, 1997, pp. 10–44; C. Turner, 2000, pp. 1–10). The disgusting object is variously described as dirty, low, unclean, impure, unruly, disordered, evil, ugly, diseased and just downright bad. Darwin interpreted disgust as a strongly aversive emotion which, in its rough contours, could be seen as a form of defence warning us of objects that might harm us. Though not all objects that threaten danger are disgusting (the tiger may provoke terror, but seldom disgust), all that disgusts is, in a very specific way, dangerous. Disgust flags the special threat of contagion.

Contagion

In ontological theories of disease – such as the animistic belief in possession by evil spirits or our own germ theory – disease, death and infection are understood as the result of an external agent, entity or power invading, possessing and destroying the purity of the soul or the body.[14] Contagion is the process by which the pure is made impure (Longrigg, 1993, pp. 25–33). In mouth-to-mouth contact, though the chance of an infectious disease being acquired is small, albeit real, pollution, on a symbolic level, is absolutely guaranteed.

Disgust flags contagion; they are inextricably bound each to the other. Disgust distinguishes the contagious from the merely dangerous – shit from shotgun. That-which-disgusts enacts contagion as a progressive series of movements transgressing the border between the self and other, and transforming both in the process:

Transgression

'Contagion' is derived from the Latin *con-* (together) + *tangere* (to touch) = to touch together. The pure becomes impure through contact of the former with the latter. The threatening object is brought 'too close for comfort'. Immanuel Kant saw the essence of disgust as an excessive proximity between subject and object (1978, pp. 99–110). The agent of contagion is capable of a proximity so extreme that the borders between it and me begin to blur. Contagion does not stop at the border. It invades. It transgresses. The agent of contagion has the ability to invade what should be whole and holy, to violate what should be inviolable, what should stay outside enters within.

Transformation

Contagion not only transgresses, it changes. That is, contagion alters the transgressed object in such a way as to reverse its value, transforming it from a-thing-desired to a-thing-shunned. This metamorphosis of the object is accomplished by a malevolent addition. The pure becomes impure. A stain, a possessing spirit, a germ are added, compromising the object's distinct and independent being. It destroys being's integrity as a self-sufficient whole. It destroys its purity.[15] Contagion, through malignant addition, fragments and degrades the object making it 'bad'.

Contagiousness

Contagion requires transgression and transformation, but its most characteristic and important element, the power for which this malevolent process as a whole is named, is its contagiousness. Contagiousness or infectivity is an aggressively generative power. It spreads and multiplies. The stain not only enters and spoils, but, most importantly, it transfers to the object spoiled, the power itself to spoil. What is infected is also infective – like the vampire: not only dead, but deadly. We fear not only being violated but also in turn ourselves violating. The fear of contagion is the fear of evil proliferating in an endlessly extending chain of pollution. It is the fear of becoming ourselves the agent of evil.

Omnipotence

To transgression, transformation and contagiousness might be added a fourth element, though, in fact, it is not so much an operative characteristic of contagion as its aspiration. The ideal agent of contagion aspires to omnipotence, in that it would have no object capable of resisting its power. It is the threat or promise of omnipotence that disgust guards against. While humanity supposedly aspires to the pure, the beautiful and the good, it is the polluted, the disgusting and the wicked that appear to have power. In terms of desire, there is a valorization of the high over the low, the good over the bad, the pure over the impure; but in terms of potency, there is a paradoxical elevation of the second term over the first. Purity is always vulnerable to the defiling powers of dirt, because any stain, no matter how small, destroys purity. 'A teaspoon of sewage will spoil a barrel of wine, but a teaspoon of wine will do nothing for a barrel of sewage' (Rozin, quoted in Miller, 1997, p. 9). The impure is not merely passively inferior; it is a constant threat to the superiority of the pure. There is no contact of the high with the low without contagion destroying the former through the latter.

Agents of contagion (whether evil spirits, miasmas or germs), by invading and transforming, threaten the borders of being, threaten the victim's identity, integrity and existence. Even worse, the agent of contagion threatens to make us like *it* – infected and infectious, with a destructive power over which we have no control. It threatens to make the self other. Disgust warns us of this threatening transformation. It attempts to protect the integrity and the purity of the body and the self. The frontier that disgust establishes and patrols is that of being (C. Turner, 2000, p. 84).

Disgust

Disgust marks the generative power of a transgression that has always already occurred. It is in this that the omnipotence of contagion lies: we are compromised before we are even threatened. To explain this somewhat obscure pronouncement, we need to look within, at what is most obscure to us: our selves. That which we like to think brings us near to the divine (or differentiates us from the animal or at the very least makes us human): our soul, our consciousness, our reason, our self – that which produces order and envisages form – must share our bodies with the messy processes of life. Our bodies betray us. Whatever entity we consider our pure and distinct 'self' must share the interior of our bodies with shit. Polluting substances such as blood and shit find their origin in the processes of life. Eating, fucking and living end in shit, decay and death; then rise again from them. Though contamination by the outside world threatens us with impurity and death, we are already contaminated by the very living processes that make our being possible – death is already within us; we are already contaminated by existing.

Being is never as well defined as we would wish. There is always anxiety over the congruence of self and body. Our fear is that the body does not quite contain the self; that we spill over into the world and it into us. The body is compromised by those things that open into or escape from its occult depths – by its orifices and wounds, by its secretions and excretions. Anuses, mouths and genitals are points at which the integrity of the body is betrayed by its very construction. They are holes in our being by which *things*, brought close, slip past the barrier of surfaces, insinuate themselves into what lies beneath and contaminate it. They are wounds leaking shit, piss, spittle, snot, semen, blood and pus into the outside world. On gaining access to the outside, that-which-should-be-inside becomes contagious, threatening those who come too close, making us fear each other and doubt ourselves (Miller, 1997, p. xiv).

This conflation of internal corruption and external contamination engenders an anxiety that the threat from without is always already there. Disgust is an admission that the border between self and other is always already breached, that our integrity is always already compromised, that there is no distinct malevolent other to fight or fly from. The enemy is already and has always been within, busily undermining the ordered boundaries we have constructed between our selves and the world, threatening to precipitate us into disorder and formlessness – threatening being.

According to Lacan, the birth of the order that allows the subject to develop its own subjectivity (an individual identity and borders to self) and a world in which to exist (a set of object relations) necessitates giving up the pleasure of undifferentiated existence, of the child's blissful unawareness of his or her existence outside the mother. The renunciation of this undifferentiated state preceding consciousness becomes the loss around which the ensuing symbolic system is built. It is the one thing that the formal system of symbol cannot articulate – for it precedes it and is formless (1988, pp. 154–5).

The ordering of the world is never complete and definitive. Borders are never inscribed as boldly as we would wish. The formless is that which is left over from our first assay of the inside/outside. It is those things which could not be included in self and which did not quite fit in other. It is those things from which it is impossible to parse out a definite and distinct form. These objects cross physical boundaries as in Freud's constitutive formation of inside/outside. They confuse categories as in Mary Douglas's concept of dirt (1966, p. 165). They blur ontological boundaries as in Julia Kristeva's abject (1982, pp. 1–9). They threaten power relations as in Ian Miller's concept of the 'low' (1997, p. 180). They transgress category boundaries calling the structure of order itself into question, revealing the residue of the formless at its core. The formless are the 'leftovers' of the imposition of order, reminders of the primal loss and threat from the flux of the world. Chris Turner equates the formless with Derrida's 'dangerous supplement' – that which any account of reality fails to include – and with Lacan's idea of the 'Real' – the 'lack' or constitutive void at the centre of any discursive formation (2000, pp. 17–21). This loss, this lack, this void is always already there, developmentally, ontologically and logically, for it is what being is constructed around.

The dirty, the abject, the disgusting – those objects and acts that resist classification and blur ontological boundaries; that are anomalous and ambiguous, partake of the formlessness of that state prior to the symbolic project of bringing order and meaning to the world – of that state prior to the development of consciousness. They are what is 'left over' from the state of undifferentiated existence that was sacrificed in the acquisition of order, symbol and language. The very existence of the formless, hidden and silent within these objects, threatens to break down the protective barrier erected around the fundamental interpretive frameworks of language and symbol, precipitating the subject into the abyss of non-being, which is also the pleasure of unification with the lost object, the pleasure of the erotic (Lacan, 1988, pp. 154–5).

Disgust is a fundamental constituent of the erotic, charging it with an irresistible energy. The erotics of the kiss contain the hope of a union with the beloved that might ascend to an ecstatic loss of identity. However, inextricably bound to that desire is the fear that in achieving it we shall cease to be. In the lover's kiss, existential fear revels in the dangerous attraction of blissful oblivion. The erotic and disgust are inextricably bound as forces pulling us toward and warning us away from the edge of oblivion. All objects or acts that disgust are the focus of coexistent compulsions to look and to turn away, an ambivalent gaze that both desires and rejects its object.

Disgust is the marker and contagion of the generative power of the pre-conscious void around which being is constructed. The emotion of disgust raises a warning flag over the incomplete integrity of being, all being and especially our being. The fragile self is threatened by the aggressive flux of the world, which lacking integrity itself, threatens to destroy ours. But our integrity is always already compromised, and it is to this that disgust bears witness. Disgust warns us of, and is the only possible reaction to, a transgression that has always already occurred (Cousins, 1994, p. 62). Disgust resists articulation because the transgression it flags is prior to the imposition of order, before symbol, fundamentally inaccessible to language. It is that 'something faced with which all words cease and all categories fail, the object of anxiety *par excellence*' (Lacan, 1988, p. 182). It is the point of collapse, where meaning is obliterated and language fails. Lurking in the depths of contagion, and flagged by disgust, is the inarticulable void that is the origin and source of human life.

Contagion exists as a real process in the real world, as epidemics throughout the centuries bear witness. However, contagion also exists in the realm of the symbolic, not as a superstitious misinterpretation of reality or some form of neurosis but as a force in service to the inarticulable reality of being. Failed by language, being is apprehended through the channelling of this force by ritual. Ritual re-enacts the transgressions, transformations and generative powers of contagion in an attempt to master being. In the methodology of ritual, the same substances that pollute are the substances that purify. Fighting fire with fire, that which has been made impure is by impurity made pure again. The blood of the sacrifice washes clean the bloody stain of guilt.

Kiss of life, kiss of death

Shit and piss are, in many ways, good, honest filth. Even spit and vomit are reasonably straightforward. Breath is more problematic. Air's formlessness, invisibility and invasiveness allow it unusual powers of transgression. Air, which 'envelops the earth and is breathed in by all land animals' (OED, 1992), has a subtle inside/outside quality that allows it to transgress the subject/object boundary without rupturing it. This makes it a powerful and dangerous substance, for the body in its physiological necessities and for the mind in its heuristic ones.

Air's otherness enfolds us entirely and intimately, and then penetrates via the respiratory tract to our very heart – penetrates so deeply that its qualities, good and bad, become our own. Breath transgresses not only the physical borders of the body, but the metaphysical frontier between body and soul. As discussed in chapter 4, breath is like unto the vital-spirit that animates being. Breath carries life with it. The breath of the rescuer inflating the lungs of the victim and providing vital oxygen to the bloodstream is, even today, at some deep level, still the living *aer* of the Greek cosmos and the life-giving *pneuma* of the *psyche*. But, this vital air once breathed in is corrupted by the processes of life hidden deep within our bodies. It is then breathed out, carrying with it the potential for corrupting others. The breath of the rescuer, far short of the perfection of *aether* or oxygen, carries within it the poison of carbon dioxide – carries not only the benefits of life, but its corruption as well.

It is far from a one-way street. It is not only the victim who is placed in danger, so too is the rescuer. The death-damaged *psyche* of the victim is a vehicle of contagion. It moves out from his or her body to pollute what comes too near. We fear the dead as deadly. Expired breath threatening infection and death in the real world threatens contagion and impurity in the symbolic. In mouth-to-mouth ventilation, there is hope and fear in every breath – hope of communicating life to the breathless corpse; fear of death being communicated to the rescuer. What saves also destroys. Mouth-to-mouth puts one in danger – danger of losing one's own life. The 'kiss of life' is also the kiss of death.

The disgust engendered by mouth-to-mouth flags contagion, warning us of an existential threat. Mouth-to-mouth ventilation, encouraging a hazardous proximity to death and the annihilation of self, challenges the rescuer to put his or her own life-force, manifest in their breath, at risk of being blighted, squandered or stolen. On a physical level, we endanger our health, even our life; on a symbolic level we endanger our purity and integrity; on a metaphysical level we endanger our *psyche* or soul. One opens oneself up not only to corporeal death but also to existential oblivion. Mouth-to-mouth ventilation forces a powerful conjunction of sign and object. The symbols of life suddenly meet the reality of death – we place our lips on the lips of a corpse.

To what purpose? The conquering of disgust, enabling us to face the dangers of contagion, disease and death, that is, the risking of the existence and integrity of self, both in physical and metaphysical terms, is the price paid for our valorization of life and society. The CPR protocol works on psychological and social levels by encouraging the heroic – the sacrifice of oneself for the good of others. The rescuer, through the good act, becomes the good citizen working to build the good society.[16] Not only is the life of the individual victim saved, but life in general is valorized as a social good. The heroic use of resuscitative protocols in general and mouth-to-mouth in particular is not only proof of the value we place on life and culture, but is necessary for their very existence. The necessity of the social bond, the supreme value we place upon life, any life, and our love of humanity will, supposedly, sweep aside all the fears I have so tediously outlined.

I do not discount that such altruism and philanthropy are real, powerful and necessary forces. They operate quite openly and laudably in the actions of rescuers, be they eighteenth-century Thames watermen or twenty-first century CPR providers. However, as we have seen, they do not operate quite as often as we would wish, and mouth-to-mouth yet remains 'a custom more honor'd in the breach than the observance'.

Recap

In the late 1700s, we have the unearthing, development and application of a therapeutic technique, mouth-to-mouth, by the newly emergent scientific method. Yet this same methodology discarded mouth-to-mouth in the early 1800s, only to re-institute it 150 years later. On examining the historical unfolding of respiratory physiology, certain reasons for what initially appears to be the folly of abandoning mouth-to-mouth become evident. In the last years of the eighteenth century, the discovery of the compound nature of air and the roles of oxygen and carbon dioxide in life processes led to the valorization of air into 'good' and 'bad' airs, and to the demonization of expired breath as a poison. Furthermore, it has been argued that, at that point, the particular developmental stage of the scientific method might be seen as being immature – operating with less than rigorous empirical methodology and with an overweening confidence in deductive reasoning. These factors allowed the above valorization of 'good' and 'bad' air to determine practice – the result being the dropping of mouth-to-mouth. Nineteenth-century Romanticism's recourse to nature as a criterion of value exalted the 'naturalness' of manual compression techniques over the 'unnaturalness' of mouth-to-mouth, and then in the last half of that century, germ theory reinforced already well-established fears of contagion. These factors form a recognizable logic, which, though in hindsight we may consider flawed, is none the less understandable.

Nevertheless, as I have implied, this narrative is not entirely satisfactory. The explanation seems inadequate to the result. In an attempt to rectify this, I have countered that a deep psychological aversion to the technique made science's disproof of mouth-to-mouth not just possible but welcome. The 'indelicacy' of the procedure and its affront to propriety clothed the atavistic emotion of disgust and the equally profound fear of contagion. However, as with the arguments based on the history and progress of science, the emotion of disgust and the powerful fear of contagion do not take us quite the full distance in explaining mouth-to-mouth's disappearance in the nineteenth century or opposition to its reinstatement in the twentieth. Here again, the cause is inadequate to the effect.

It is seldom that one can explain the disappearance of any therapeutic technique solely on the basis of its failings, whether they be empirical, symbolic or psychological. In the case of mouth-to-mouth, the technique was dropped not merely because of its perceived disadvantages, though of course those played a large part, but because it was actively displaced by another technique – the technique of manual ventilation. Manual ventilatory techniques not only appeared to satisfy the practical requirements of ventilation, while allaying the fears implicit in the abandoned procedure of mouth-to-mouth, but, more importantly, they satisfied a repressed, though inescapable, imperative issuing from the deathbed – that of deathbed violence. To explain this, we will need to examine the third component of the CPR protocol, external cardiac compression.

6
External Cardiac Compression: Beating a Dead Horse

> The Royal Humane Society would be rooted out like a horde of assassins ...
>
> (G. K. Chesterton, *Heretics*, 1919, p. 1)

The patient was an elderly Hasid. When he collapsed at home his son started chest compressions, gave his father mouth-to-mouth, did what he had been taught in the 'Heartsaver' classes he had attended at the community centre. The paramedics arrived. Took over chest compressions. Intubated. Attached the old man to a cardiac monitor. Defibrillated – normal sinus rhythm. Started an IV. Gave drugs. Loaded him in the ambulance and sped to the ER. The electrocardiogram in the emergency room showed an inferior MI. The standard coronary protocol was commenced. The old man was agitated and trying to pull out his ET tube and IV. We sedated him with morphine. Put him on a ventilator. Put in a central line, arterial line, urinary catheter, and nasogastric tube. Transferred him to ICU. He was coded three more times in the ICU and survived. The son sat in the ICU waiting room and wept. Tears of shame for the sin he had committed. It was Shabbath.

External cardiac compression

An incorrigible act

Folk therapies

As we saw in chapter 3, many of the folk therapies employed in the resuscitation of the drowning victim involved the use of considerable physical force in an attempt to rid the lungs of water and excite the fading life-force back into action. Victims were hung by the heals and beaten with sticks, rolled back and forth over a barrel, jogged up and down on the back of a horse, and so on. 'Successive concussions ... incite the hidden springs of life into action' (A. Fothergill, 1795, p. 143). One of the primary goals of the Humane Society was to mitigate the more violent of these 'pernicious' practices: 'It is natural to imagine that these [medical] Gentlemen ... will be more cautious not to employ these pernicious and justly-exploded methods' (Humane, 1777, p. 100). The Society justified its prohibition on beating victims on two grounds: one empirical, the other theoretical.

Many of the more violent efforts of rescuers were in an attempt to expel water from the lungs. Post-mortem dissection of drowning victims in the mid-1700s had shown that, unless they had been long dead in the water, their lungs were not filled with water. As discussed in chapter 3, it was understood that the asphyxia of drowning was due to small amounts of inhaled water causing laryngospasm, excluding air from the lungs (Goodwyn, 1788, p. 98; Curry, 1815, p. 41). The second justification for abandoning these violent techniques was theoretical. At that time, though the theory of apoplexy was being replaced by the theory of asphyxia, apoplexy remained an important consideration in many physicians' minds (Physician, 1746, p. 45; Kite, 1788, p. 130). The apoplexy theory ascribed the proximate cause of death in drowning to a surfeit of blood in the head, causing compression of the brain. Hanging by the feet, rolling over a barrel and beatings were thought to increase that already life-threatening congestion. The Humane Society portrayed the various aggressive methods used to remove water from the lungs as worse than useless; because they aggravated cerebral congestion, they were dangerous. The Society thus expunged from its protocol the more abusive forms of stimulation (Cullen, 1776, p. 8).

However, it proved difficult to bring this violence completely to a halt. The Society's *Annual Reports* recount instances of barrel rolling, chest beating, abdominal compressions and agitations well into the nineteenth century (Royal, 1812, pp. 25–6). The Society's own protocol, though mitigating the severity of the violence perpetrated on the dying, certainly did not abolish it entirely. In the place of overt beatings, the Method employed agitation, friction, volatiles, electrical shocks, tobacco smoke enemas, oral stimulants, and so on – all in an attempt 'to incite the hidden springs of life into action'.

As the apoplectic theory of drowning gave way to the asphyxial, so its underlying doctrine, mechanism, gave way to vitalism. Vitalism adheres to the homeopathic dictum of sympathetic action – like responds to like. Life is a force, and the revival of a force – the life-force – requires force – physical force. Thus, as the vitalistic view gained strength, more aggressive therapeutics began to creep back into the protocol (if they had ever really left):

> Stimulants of the most violent kind ... are administered with a view to excite, if possible, the inert vitality. (Struve, 1803, p. 85)

Violence directed against the body was used to rouse the life-force. It was believed that the life-force dwelt most tenaciously in those organs most directly concerned with movement, that is, in the muscle fibres, especially the muscle fibres of the heart (Physician, 1746, p. 39). Physical force was thus directed to 'excite the latent principle of irritability, on which the motion of the vital organs immediately depend' (A. Fothergill, 1795, p. 15). Chest and abdominal compressions, which had previously been justified and then condemned as methods of clearing the lungs of water, were reassigned the job of stimulating the 'irritability' of the heart. Chest compressions might also stimulate the heart indirectly by moving blood from the liver, great vessels and lungs into the heart, where blood, the vehicle of the life-force, might stimulate cardiac contraction and thence circulation and respiration (Physician, 1746, p. 51). The idea of the stimulatory effect of chest compressions, direct or indirect, was to become less prominent in the nineteenth century, as electrical shock was put forward as a more deeply penetrating, powerful and efficacious stimulant. However, chest and abdominal compressions did not disappear for, as we have noted in chapter 5, they were transformed into the manual ventilatory techniques replacing the by then disgraced technique of mouth-to-mouth.

Manual ventilatory techniques

Justification for beating on the body shifted from the straightforward folk practice of clearing the lungs of water to a belief that it might stimulate the *vis vitae* by encouraging muscular irritability then on to a means of mechanically moving air in and out of the lungs (Curry, 1815 p. 49). Therapeutic violence debunked within one organ system and physiological theory, fled to another, then another, then another. Chest compression was a technique that refused to die. Looking back at the demise of mouth-to-mouth in the early nineteenth century, it becomes apparent that mouth-to-mouth was dropped not only because of the possible untoward effects of 'bad air', not only because of fears of contagion and the emotion of disgust, but because an organ system and a theoretical doctrine were required as vehicles for the continuing practice of beating on the body. Mouth-to-mouth didn't jump, it was pushed. When in the late 1950s mouth-to-mouth was re-instituted and manual ventilatory techniques were forced out of the protocol, therapeutic violence did not disappear but survived by adopting yet another physiological justification and organ system – external cardiac compression was put forward as a means of maintaining circulation.

External cardiac compression

In the eighteenth century, compression of the chest to augment blood flow to the heart had been given some credence within the vitalist theory of irritability; however, in the early nineteenth century, it was subsumed under chest compression's use as a manual ventilatory technique, but the use of chest compression as a means of augmenting circulation was never entirely discounted and resurfaced as a means of dealing with chloroform induced pulselessness (Robiscek and Littman, 1983, p. 569). In this context, external chest compressions met very limited success and failed to be taken up generally. Rather, *open* chest cardiac massage began to be used to deal with anaesthetic-induced ventricular fibrillation (Hake, 1874, p. 241). Open chest cardiac massage became the standard technique for artificially supporting circulation until the late 1950s (Green, 1906, p. 1707; Stephenson, Reid and Hinton, 1953, p. 731). This technique, which required a thoracotomy in which the chest was opened surgically, was, as one can imagine, somewhat problematic. Messy and prone to complications, it could be performed only in the hospital by a skilled professional, and, if it was to be successful, had to be performed with extreme dispatch.[1] When, in the 1950s, mouth-to-mouth was re-instituted and manual ventilatory techniques were forced out of the protocol, external chest compression again became (in a way of speaking) available for circulatory support. Jumping from the respiratory back to the circulatory system, external chest compression was put forward as a means of maintaining circulation thus avoiding the excessively invasive trauma of internal massage.

In 1958, Kouwenhoven, Jude and Knickerbocker, doing research on electrical defibrillation, developed defibrillator paddles that, as a safety feature, required significant pressure on the chest before they would discharge. They found that in fibrillating dogs applying this pressure to the chest resulted in a transient increase in femoral artery blood pressure, in other words, compression of the chest produced a palpable pulse in the pulseless animal. If they repeatedly applied the paddles to the chest, they were able to extend the period of time that the dog's heart could be in fibrillation and still be successfully defibrillated (1960, p. 1064). They realized that hands were as effective as paddles for compressing the chest and so applied the technique to patients experiencing cardiac arrest induced by halothane anaesthesia (Jude, Kouwenhoven and Knickerbocker, 1961, p. 1063). External cardiac compression appeared to buy time until electrical defibrillation could be accomplished. 'Anyone, anywhere, can now initiate cardiac resuscitative procedures. All that is needed are two hands' (Kouwenhoven, Jude and Knickerbocker, 1960, p. 1064). As has been outlined in chapter 2, Kouwenhoven, Jude and Knickerbocker's findings were united with Safar and Elam's research on mouth-to-mouth and presented at the 1960 meeting of the Maryland Medical Society in what is now considered the 'birth of CPR' (chapter 2, p. 34).

A controversial act

Even at its introduction into the modern CPR protocol, there were doubts as to external cardiac compression's efficacy in maintaining circulation. Safar, a strong advocate of CPR, referring to Kouwenhoven's seminal article, points out that:

> It was known from the start that carotid blood flows and cardiac output during VF and external CPR may range unpredictably between trickle flows to 30 per cent normal .... [CPR is] meant only to be a stopgap measure to maintain borderline oxygen delivery until spontaneous circulation is restored, as quickly as possible, with epinephrine and defibrillation. (Safar, 1996, p. 5s)

Experimental evidence for the efficacy of external cardiac compression was weak. The two target organs of CPR, the brain and the heart, have metabolic requirements well beyond what external cardiac compression is capable of providing. Even in optimal conditions, external cardiac compression produces coronary artery flow rates of only 20–35 per cent of normal. Animal experiments have shown that flow rates of even as high as 60 per cent of normal are inadequate in maintaining high-energy phosphate (ATP) levels during ventricular fibrillation (Paradis et al., 1989, p. 361; Angelos et al., 1999, p. 583). The inability to maintain ATP levels is the start of cell death.

External cardiac compression also has difficulty maintaining brain function. Normal cerebral cortical blood flow is 55–75 ml/100 gm/min.

The minimal blood flow required to maintain cortical function is 20 ml/100 gm/min. Most animal studies show flow rates during CPR of closer to 5 ml/100 gm/min (C. Brown et al., 1987, p. 491).[2] Granted, fractional blood flows may be adequate in maintaining metabolism for very limited amounts of time, and CPR was never meant to be more than a temporizing measure, but its discouraging survival rates demonstrate that it struggles to accomplish even that (Lombardi et al., 1994, p. 676; Stiell, 1999, p. 1175).[3]

Furthermore, a convincing physiological theory of why external cardiac compression works is also lacking. The predominant theories at present are the thoracic pump and cardiac compression theories. In both, the valve system of the heart is thought to allow forward blood flow when a pressure gradient is created between the ventricles of the heart and the arterial system. However, both theories have more critics than supporters and many of those who strongly endorse external cardiac compression admit that they do not know how it works.

Finally, the Hippocratic dictum *Primum non nocere* ('First, do no harm') applies. External cardiac compression has complications, especially when done improperly – broken ribs, lacerations of the liver and spleen, marrow embolism, cardiac trauma and gastro-oesophageal damage. All of which might be excused if a life is saved. However, what is now of greater concern is the delay external cardiac compression may cause in initiating defibrillation, potentially effective for those patients who are in ventricular fibrillation. In animal experiments, the use of external cardiac compression prior to defibrillation, resulting in a delay of defibrillation by as little as 90 seconds, has a marked negative effect on the success of defibrillation. In one animal study, no CPR prior to defibrillation produced a 65 per cent termination of ventricular fibrillation on the first shock. Prior CPR for 90 seconds gave an 18 per cent termination of ventricular fibrillation on the first shock (Niemann et al., 1999, p. S4). Other animal studies have demonstrated the opposite: decreased short-term survival if external cardiac compression is delayed to allow for defibrillation (Berg et al., 2003, p. 458). In *Guidelines 2000*, external cardiac compression has been demoted, and the emphasis is on early defibrillation through the use of AEDs (American, 2000, pp. I.22–I.59).

> Because decreases in defibrillation response time interval were usually associated with a greater increase in survival than were increases in bystander CPR, we propose… if a defibrillator is available near or at the scene, then the sequence of actions should be to call 911, defibrillate, then initiate CPR. (Nichol et al., 1999, p. 522)

Despite its poor clinical results, an experimentally proven inability to accomplish its physiological goals and the lack of an adequate theory to explain its supposed effect, efforts continue in an attempt to salvage external cardiac compression. The last 40 years have seen a succession of external cardiac compression techniques – anterior chest compression, lateral chest compression, interposed abdominal compression, high-frequency CPR, active compression-decompression, phased thoracic abdominal compression-decompression, simultaneous ventilation compression, vest compression, mechanical compression, and so on. Despite these many alternatives, anterior chest compression, as originally recommended in the 1960 protocol, 'remains the mainstay of artificial circulation during cardiac arrest because of its simplicity, non-invasiveness, and the lack of sufficient evidence for improved outcome for other methods' (Neumar and Ward, 1998, p. 40).

The multiplication of variants of external cardiac compression is reminiscent of that already witnessed in the nineteenth-century proliferation of manual ventilatory techniques. Whenever one sees a therapeutic technique spawn a large number of variants, all aimed at the same effect, one can be certain that none of them works or, at the very least, as is probably the case with external cardiac compression, that their efficacy is extremely limited. One can also be pretty sure that one is dealing with a crisis in which it is important to try anything, and so anything is tried. This was true of manual ventilatory techniques and is probably true of external cardiac compression.[4] The accumulating evidence that early defibrillation is by far the most important factor in improving survival rates and the increased emphasis on AEDs in *Guidelines 2000*, though it does not deny, at least implies less than complete confidence in external cardiac compression's effect (see chapter 2).

A persistent act

The persistence of chest compressions might be seen as an example of technique persists; theory changes. Bynum observed this phenomenon in relation to bloodletting, justified under both humoral and iatromechanical theories (see chapter 3). When one sees an unsound technique, such as chest compression, in the face of empirical failure, change theoretical justification – in this case jumping from the vitalist theory of irritability in the neuromuscular system to mechanical theories of negative pressure ventilation in the respiratory system to the thoracic pump theory in the circulatory system – one has to ask whether the survival of the technique is based less on its physiological effect than on some other factor, perhaps ignorance, secondary gain, custom or some other external influence. Techniques often persist because there is nothing better. Neve gives the example of nineteenth-century physicians who remained tied to the therapeutic techniques of humoralism long after the theory supporting them had been invalidated (1995, p. 491). Though this was in part due to the inherent conservatism of the profession and the privileged clientele it served, it was also due to the fact that the new theories of iatromechanism and iatrochemistry, though philosophically attractive, offered little in the way of effective therapy. Therapeutics are frequently a case of making do.

Undoubtedly, some acts persist because they are of political and economic advantage to certain groups in society – greed for power and greed for money. Control of the time and manner of death may be used to exercise social control for purposes that have little to do with the well-being of the patient. Timmermans makes the point that large segments of the medical system have a heavy investment in resuscitative techniques and reap significant rewards from their participation in them. This applies not just to the balance sheets of drug companies and equipment manufacturers, but to the survival and proliferation of EMS systems, ERs, ICUs and those professions who staff them (1999, p. 97). There is no doubt that the organization of the deathbed is, whatever else it is, also a manifestation of a particular institutional order based on a particular structure of power (Seale, 1998, p. 67).

In 1792, Curry pointed out that therapeutic practice is often tied to tradition:

> Letting blood ... does not appear to have been founded upon any rational principle at first; and it has been continued more from the force of Custom, than from any experience of its good effects. (1815, p. 62)

Any act that becomes routine cannot help but develop into a custom with an historical tradition. Customs persist and tradition is innately conservative; that is their nature. If not, they would not be custom and tradition. They are the building blocks of culture. Particular ways of doing things are preserved and perpetuated so that there might be a distinct group identified as a society, and a culture to communicate and sustain those things. Culture requires that, though conditions change and individuals are born and die, some *thing* or *things* remain.

However, ignorance, greed and force of habit are but contributory factors to the persistence of technique. Medical techniques supposedly stand or fall by their accompanying physiological theory, but some techniques – bleeding, chest compressions, electrical shocks – persist in spite of changes in their supporting theories. Fair enough when empirical effect is obvious, but when a purportedly practical therapeutic act with uncertain empirical effect persists through multiple theoretical changes, surviving, not so much in the face of changes in theory, but in fact because of them, one should suspect that the act's efficacy is not so much in the realm of the practical as in that of the symbolic – in the realm of myth and ritual. 'Gods withdraw, but their rituals live on .... Ritual is usually older than the myth by which people explain it, and has deeper psychological roots' (Dodds, 1951, pp. 244, 270). Myth may be seen less as an explanation than as an excuse for a rite whose history has been forgotten by the culture and whose reasons lie buried deep within the psyche of the individual. Rite transcends its myth and technique transcends its theory, when technique is rite and theory myth.

Protocol and ritual

The suggestion that the therapeutic protocols of modern medicine bear some similarity to ritual practice is not likely to be welcomed. Still, it is at this intersection of the practical and the symbolic that I should like to site CPR. I am by no means the first to make such a suggestion. Seale expresses no doubts as to the ritual aspect of deathbed therapeutics:

> The medical procedures that accompany death ... have both a technical rational and a ritual aspect, in that they frame and box experience, create new objects from anomalous or dangerous entities, and place individual deaths in the context of a progressive, scientific-rational system. (1998, p. 75)

He goes on to point out that in a society distanced from the certainties of traditional religion, medicine acts as a vehicle for some of the most fundamental classificatory ideas of culture, dividing the healthy from the diseased, the normal from the pathological, the pure from the polluting, the living from the dead. We should not be surprised that in taking over much of religion's work, medicine has filched some of its tools (pp. 75–8). That modern medicine does much of the front-line work formerly done by religion is certainly no secret to physicians.

One need only spend a night in a busy emergency department to observe the time and effort spent counselling the hopeless, absolving the careless and chastising the guilty. Indeed, medicine and religion have always been more closely bound than either would care to admit, and the dual nature of the shaman as healer of body *and* soul has never entirely deserted the physician or the priest.

Before we get too carried away, it must be pointed out that ritual and protocol do differ. Protocol is usually perceived as operating within the realm of science, ritual within that of religion. In protocol, both action and result, cause and effect, are meant to occur in the same register, that of a unitary, material, mundane world. For example, the actions of CPR-as-protocol direct the manipulation of the physical body and the physical environment to accomplish a return to some kind of physical equilibrium. In contrast, the authority of ritual derives from the transcendental or supernatural. Ritual takes one into the realm of what, for want of a better term, is called the sacred. It reaches beyond its own frame of physical enactment, drawing its power from outside the mundane world of its effect. It employs transcendental agency – spirit, God, even the symbolic, depending on one's frame of reference – to accomplish a transformation aimed at establishing order in the mundane world. Protocol is science and as science is discursively redeemable – that is, its questions, methods and answers must all be found within its operating frame of reference.

However, ritual and protocol are analogous, but though analogous, are not identical, for it is analogy itself that divides them. Ritual translates metaphor into action so as to transmit the changes wrought in one register, the symbolic, into change in the parallel system, the physical. In protocol, the practical act accomplishes the practical effect. In ritual, it is the power of the sign within the magic circle of analogy that accomplishes the practical effect. Ritual manipulates symbol in a performance that generates a subjective experience giving the participant access to a transcendent power (spirit, God or symbolic structure), transforming both those involved and the world in which they live, constructing society, individual identity and an interpretive framework for identity and society, that is, constructing culture. Ritual provides meaning by imposing the order of culture on chaotic nature. It creates community through shared acts and feelings, integrating the individual into the society. It is the means by which the microcosm of the individual and macrocosm of the community are writ one upon the other (Lévi-Strauss, 1966, pp. 217–44; Durkheim, 1995, pp. 325–9; D. Davies, 1997, p. 14).

Protocol and ritual, united and divided by analogy, are complementary. Both protocol and ritual are performed in response to crisis, with the intent of restoring order and function. Both are mnemonic devices that seek to navigate ambivalent states where cause and effect are unpredictable. Both allow us to act in the dark, to exercise power without knowledge. Physicians resort to medical protocols when failure (of the body and of therapeutic response) is imminent and judgement is suspect because of paucity of facts and time constraints. Ritual is called on where the uncertainty of an enforced change threatens the stability of social relations. Both are a means of exercising power. Both direct the flow of power between the individual and the community and allow the qualities of each to shape the other.

Given these similarities of intent, similarities of form should come as little surprise. The algorithms of protocol set out instructions for the performance of a highly scripted series of formal acts aimed at a particular result; in much the same way that liturgy directs religious ritual. Protocol is justified by theory, ritual by myth. Both are formulaic, relying heavily on repetition. Though both use language, the emphasis is on action. Both are enacted by participants assigned to roles whose incumbents may vary. On a practical level, both provide the knowledge necessary for action. On an ethical level, they bestow the authority to act. On a psychological level, they distance the participant from the necessary transgressions perpetrated by the act. The replacement of incumbent by role and judgement by technique shifts responsibility for the act from the person acting onto the act itself. Both allow the individual access to power. Both allow a proximity that would otherwise be forbidden. Both allow for action in crisis.

Denial and death

'Death ... is not an event in life or outside it, but rather a structural component and an inherent force constituting and shaping life' (Carel, 2000, lecture notes). However, this does not exclude our reluctance to die or have those we love die. We value life. Resuscitative protocols and deathbed rituals are defences against death. Dominion over death, some would argue, is the whole point of ritual, all ritual – in fact, the whole point of society and culture (Malinowski, 1974, pp. 51–9; D. Davies, 1997, p. 16). The anthropologist Maurice Bloch asserts that all ritual, not just deathbed or funerary ritual, is a re-enactment of the fundamental drama whereby life triumphs over death (1992, pp. 4–7). All ritual enacts a transformation, using the biological transition from life to death as a powerful natural symbol (Seale, 1998,

p. 66). When a major transformation in circumstances or identity must be expressed, when a passage must be symbolically navigated, then the example of the passage from life to death is close to hand. As a paradigm for a 'rite of passage', death is formulated not as irrevocable loss but as transformation. On going through any and all ritual, one emerges 'as one who has died and, through contact with some higher power, now possesses some of that higher power to insure that ordinary life is ordinary no longer' (D. Davies, 1997, p. 178). The deathbed is the point at which death – the biological paradigm for ritual – and ritual – the re-enactment of death – face each other, as in a mirror, and are forced to look away.

Society, on a very practical level, denies death by attempting to assure, through cooperative activity, the survival of its all too perishable members. Resuscitative protocols operate at this somatic level by seeking to deny death its victim. Complementary to practical action, deathbed ritual aspires to deny death by giving the impression that death is under control – proof of the triumph of culture over nature. The individual body, both the physical unit and the symbolic microcosm of society, cease to exist, but society, the permanent macrocosm, continues in the culture brought into being, at least in part, by ritual. Deathbed ritual transforms the dying into the dead and the victim of loss into the survivor, so that the continuity of community might be maintained in the collective life that triumphs over the individual deaths of its members (Seale, 1998, p. 66).

This necessary denial of death is not, as is sometimes implied, a passive forgetting, something that merely slips our minds when we are not in its presence. The denial of death is the active process of repression that brings community and culture into being. Society is a tautological practice. Continually threatened by the loss of its members, it is constructed precisely out of its reaction to the trauma of loss. The very existence of 'culture' can be seen as a series of bids for symbolic immortality. Mourning, that is, the active construction of shared grief through ritual, constructs community, so that culture might defy death by reinforcing the desire for life. The enactment of death helps constitute life as a concept, life as a value and life as a pattern of living. CPR's chain-of-survival is not merely a device for ordering the protocol of revival. It is a ritual project, generating a concept of being that constructs the social structures necessary for survival, its own and ours (Danforth, 1982, p. 31; Bloch, 1992, pp. 4–7).

Seale points out that the psychological repression of death is routinely conflated with the 'hiding away' of death in the hospital and hospice, and that, although these are related things, they are not the same thing (1998, p. 70). The exile of the dying and the dead to specialist institutions may help or hinder the active and necessary process of repression. The consensus appears to be hinder. This sequestration cuts us off from the rituals we use both to deny death and channel the return of the repressed into the sublimated form of culture. In a seeming paradox, the denial of death, in the sense of its institutionalized invisibility, hampers the process of the active repression of death that is (some would argue) the inevitable and necessary loss around which culture is built.

Death and violence

Death is a threat. To the dying patient, there are the immediate threats of pain, suffering and existential terror. To the individual survivor, death threatens the loss of love. To society, the loss of the individual threatens the functionality of the group. On the metaphysical level, the loss of another pushes consciousness to acknowledge what it cannot grasp – its future non-existence. Death negates being. It violates what we see as our right to exist. Death tears life from the body, the beloved from the lover, the self from the world. This violation and the violence involved in its realization is especially prominent in the unexpected, the premature, the sudden death – the mode of death with which resuscitative protocols deal.

The sudden death is always seen as a violation of life. Indeed, the sudden death often is, quite literally, violent. Motor vehicle accidents are the leading cause of death in the 1–34-year-old age group. Gunshot wounds, stabbings and poisonings come second (CDC, 2004). However, even if fragments of bone do not pierce the surface of the skin, even if death is a silent blood clot in a coronary artery, sudden death is still a violent disruption of our ideas of propriety and order. Sudden death is death at the wrong time, in the wrong place, for the wrong person. It threatens the dying person and the survivor, the individual and the group, the body and the soul. It threatens order. The threat of violent death produces an especially strong call to action.

In ritual, violence counters violence. Violence, both symbolic and actual, towards the dying body and towards the corpse, is an integral component of deathbed ritual in many cultures (Hertz, 1960, p. 78; van Gennep, 1960, p. 164; Lévi-Strauss, 1963, p. 181). Bloch has gone as far as saying that violence is an integral component of *all* ritual in *all* cultures (1992, p. 7). Violence at the deathbed works at practical, symbolic and psychological levels. On a psychological level, violence may be a manifestation of the guilt and anger of survivors. On a symbolic level, violence is often used to encourage the dead soul in its journey from the tribe of the living to the tribe of the dead. On a practical level, violence is useful in identifying the dead: they don't hit back.

Practical violence: diagnosing death

One of the major fears hovering over the deathbed is the fear that the dead are not actually as they appear: dead. The diagnosis of death is not always straightforward. 'Obvious signs of irreversible death [are] decapitation, decomposition, rigor mortis, or significant dependent lividity' (Neumar and Ward, 1998, p. 35). However, most physicians and families are unwilling to wait for decomposition to set in and would no doubt baulk at decapitation before considering the patient dead. Rather, the declaration of death has long been made on the basis of the absence of 'vital signs' – pulse, breathing, neurological reflexes and consciousness, along with dilated pupils, coldness and rigor (Honigman and Armstrong, 1998, p. 200). These are signs of 'clinical death' and, except in unusual circumstances, though not absolute signs of death, are considered good enough.[5] They are good enough for those deaths where death is, to some extent, expected (usually in the chronically ill or elderly) and straightforward (no complicating factors such as hypothermia or drug effects). In these straightforward, expected deaths, time of death is usually recorded as the moment of the permanent cessation of respiration and circulation. However, it has never been quite that simple, as evinced by early nineteenth-century anxieties over premature burial.

Life in the modern era, no longer dependent on the soul or some non-existent vital-force, is 'the sum of the functions, by which death is resisted' (Bichat, 1827, p. 10). Thus, death is loss of function, and function is only visible in its enactment. As a loss of function, death is demonstrable in the body's response, or rather lack thereof, to the act of resuscitation – no response, no function, no life.

> The process above-mentioned [the Humane Society's Method] should be continued the full space of 3 hours, with very few intermissions, unless the vital functions should be restored sooner. If, at the end of that period, the unfavourable symptoms instead of diminishing should increase, attended with other evident signs of the extinction of life, the case may be considered as utterly hopeless and therefore the process should be discontinued. (A. Fothergill, 1795, p. 165)

The failure of revival becomes the successful identification of death. Formal resuscitative protocols for the restoration of drowned sailors came into being, at the time they did and in the place they did, not only because of the growth of a mercantile empire dependent upon rivers and oceans, not only because the great ritual edifices of religion were in decay, not only because of the remarkable scientific advances of the Enlightenment, though all these were contributory, but because death was ceasing to be what it had been: the beginning of a journey into the transcendent. A new functional definition of death had come into being and with that a new means for identifying death – failure of the resuscitative protocol:

1789:

> The incontrovertible testimony of a series of experiments for several years, has demonstrated the impossibility of ascertaining any other *criteria* of a perfect extinction of a vital principle in the instances of its sudden disappearance, than the ineffectual application of resuscitative means. (Royal, 1789, p. 67)

1993:

> Excluding patients with persistent ventricular fibrillation, resuscitative efforts can be terminated ... when normothermic adults with unmonitored, out-of-hospital, primary cardiac arrest do not regain spontaneous circulation within 25 minutes following standard advanced cardiac life support. (Bonnin et al., 1993, p. 1457)

Every therapeutic act, like the Roman god Janus, has two faces, one looking forward to the future the other looking back to the past. The first is its therapeutic face, in which the validity of the act as effective therapy is confirmed by the occurrence of the predicted positive result. The second is its diagnostic face, in which the validity of the diagnosis, that is the presence of the imputed disease, is confirmed or disproved by the effect of the act. In this latter case, even a negative result can have a positive consequence in that it furthers the diagnostic process. (A practical example of this is the routine use of intravenous glucose in the treatment of an unconscious patient. If the injection of glucose reverses the coma, then one has successfully diagnosed and treated the cause, hypoglycaemia. If it does not, one has at least ruled out hypoglycaemia as a cause, and needs to get busy looking for other causes.)

As will be remembered from the discussion of therapeutic bloodletting in chapter 3, alongside bleeding's therapeutic use there was its diagnostic purpose, where the absence of a brisk bleed on opening a vessel and a dark colour to the blood were indications of the patient's moribund status. Further, the custom, which required the opening of a vein prior to consigning the corpse to the grave, not only made certain that the diagnosis of death was correct, but should that diagnosis be wrong, the opened vein itself would insure that, in due time, it would be made right. If the victim were not dead, he or she soon would be and thus be spared the horror of waking in the grave.

The metaphor of two-faced Janus is thus effaced to be replaced with that of three-headed Cerberus. In the context of the deathbed, bleeding fulfilled a triple role: as a therapeutic manoeuvre, it might restore life; as a diagnostic test, it helped diagnose death; and ultimately, as a dark form of insurance, it guaranteed death. As a last-ditch therapeutic manoeuvre, it sought, rather paradoxically, both to save life and insure death. In the opening of a vein on the deathbed, we see the sinister extension of a terminal medical technique's therapeutic and diagnostic functions – its attempt to correct not only the pathological cause it set out to cure but, failing that, to insure that pathological cause's end: death. What does not cure kills. This is the paradox of terminal therapeutics.

Bloodletting is not the only form of terminal therapeutics made to this pattern. Like the opening of a vein on the moribund, the violence of CPR fulfils a triple role: it might restore life, it helps diagnose death and, failing all else, it insures it. Though the physician has the authority to declare the patient dead without all the rigmarole of CPR (and he usually does so in patients in whom death is, for any number of reasons, expected or 'appropriate'), in the case of sudden or unexpected death, death is usually declared only after resuscitative protocols have been exhausted.[6] Death, defined as a loss of function, is diagnosed by the inability of the protocol to restore function. Furthermore, as with the opening of a vein, the violence of the resuscitative protocol is a final remedy, for death and for life. What does not cure kills. Within the hospital, resuscitative protocols, though aiming to revive life, much more commonly end up diagnosing death. How does the intern know when the patient is dead? When the patient has failed to respond to CPR. There is some point in beating a dead horse – to ensure that it *is* dead.

Symbolic violence: rites of passage

> A *Totenweib* [female mortuary attendant] ... had once seen a 'corpse' that tried to crawl out of its coffin. The *Totenweib* ... struck him with a broom and shouted, 'Go back in there! What do you want with the living – you do not belong with us!
>
> (Bondeson, 2001, p. 91)

The newly dead are feared. As the corpse becomes an unclean and impure source of contagion in the physical world, so also, in the metaphysical, the spirit of the dead hovering between this world and the next becomes a malevolent agent, harbouring a grudge against the living (Hertz, 1960, p. 77). These malevolent spirits may be seen as reifications of the unfinished business of those who die while still socially engaged (Seale, 1998, p. 52). Ghosts are the jealous reproaches of the dead to the living for their continued existence (Freud, 1985c, p. 116). The ghosts of the dead are angry at being torn from life, angry with their kin for allowing them to die and angry with survivors for living while they are dead (D. Davies, 1997, p. 163). One must be careful in asserting that the only relationship the living have to the dead is one of fear. Relations with the dead are intensely ambivalent. As already discussed, ancestor spirits and saints in heaven may be benevolent, intervening for the good of those still living. Nevertheless, fear is a significant factor in relations with the dead, particularly with the newly dead.

The reanimated living we can celebrate; the dead we can mourn. It is those who are neither – the non-living yet undead – who dangerously haunt us. Deathbed ritual aims to resolve this threatening ambivalence one way or another. Ritual resorts to violence, both symbolic and actual, to assist the dead soul in its journey from the tribe of the living where, if it lingers, it may cause mischief, to the tribe of the dead where it now belongs (Smith, 1894, p. 370; Gorer, 1965, p. 362; Bloch, 1992, pp. 4–7; D. Davies, 1997, pp. 2–16). Ritual removes the dead from the world of the living so that the survivors and society may get on with the necessary activities of life.

Ritual marks the biophysical transformation of living flesh to rotting meat. It encourages the moribund to become the dead and mourners to become survivors; each taking up new identities in a cosmos altered by loss. It enacts the translation of the self from the register of physical to that of metaphysical being. In myth-based societies, this journey is from the mundane world to a transcendent afterlife; in secular societies (or if you prefer, at a psychological level), it is the translation of the dead from being to memory.

Bloch claims that these transformations are accomplished through a ritual sequence of destruction, transformation and return.[7] The process begins with the violent destruction of categories – self and other, individual and community, immanent and transcendent, physical and metaphysical, living and dead. This precipitates the players into a transcendent realm of power from which they are then rescued, brought back into the mundane world, but brought back changed. Ritual moves its objects, agents and subjects out of the mundane world of the here and now, a world in which I am constantly under threat from outside powers, into the transcendent realm from which those powers threaten. In that transcendent realm, I undergo a metamorphosis where in exchange for something – my youth, my foreskin, my cattle – I am given power. The transcendent power that had threatened me is acquired by me. In a process of virtuous contagion, violated by power, I become infected with it, to become an agent of it, capable of its control, use and spread. I am then returned to the mundane world, changed by the acquisition of power – no longer a victim of outside forces, but master of them. In Bloch's words, I am transformed from 'prey into hunter' (1992, p. 4).

The power to order, control and change the world is an exercise in violence and can be acquired only through violence – violence suffered and then exercised. Bloch stresses that all ritual uses violence to accomplish its transitions. He calls it 'rebounding violence' because it is a two-stage process. Violence must be perpetrated upon the victim to translate him from the mundane to the transcendent realm. Then, once power has been 'caught', violence must be perpetrated by the new-born agent to return himself to the mundane (1992, pp. 4–7). I do not have the space here to go into the details of Bloch's schema; what I wish to emphasize is his contention that agency must be acquired through the exercise of violence.

Violence is not confined to the victim. All who participate in ritual are violated and through violation transformed. All who participate – victim, agent and witness – are translated and transformed, each in his or her own fashion. At the deathbed, both the dying person as the victim of death, and the survivors as the victims of loss, undergo transformation. The dying person once dead is subject to deathbed ritual to ensure the destruction of their mundane, corporeal self so that they can be reborn into their new life in the transcendent realm of the dead. This, successfully accomplished, gives them peace and their survivors safety. However, this translation of the dying into the realm of the dead would appear, in Bloch's terms, to be incomplete, because, for the victim of death, it is a one-way journey. The point of deathbed ritual is that the dead should *not* return to the mundane world of the living but remain in the transcendent realm of power.

However, return does occur, not for the victim of death but for the victim of loss. By actually dying and by being ritually constructed as dead, the dying person ceases to be a victim threatened by death and becomes the sacrificial object whose proper and permanent place is in the transcendent. This transformation of the victim from present subject to lost object triggers a second shift. On the 'successful' death of the victim, it is the survivors who become victims, victims of loss. (This is recognized, if not articulated in the same way, in the emergency room, where on the cusp of resuscitative failure – at the point of the transformation of patient to corpse – 'As soon as you declare death for the arrest victim, you immediately acquire a new set of patients – the family, friends, and loved ones of the person who dies' [American, *Guidelines* I.136–I.165].) It is the survivors who now become the subjects of ritual transformation. It is they who must complete the cycle of destruction, metamorphosis and return. It is they who undergo the full process of ritual. Being violated by loss, they perpetrate the violence of sacrifice and expose themselves to pollution, so as to enter a realm of power in which, by enacting death, they acquire power over life, so that they might return to and recoup a world changed by loss. And through participation in sacrifice, community is brought into being.

Psychological violence: catharsis

On a psychological level, violence may be a manifestation of the guilt and anger of survivors.

> My obligation is to call 911 [emergency telephone number in the USA] and initiate CPR. I'm not sure I have an ethical obligation, though I know it is a societal expectation. Personally, I would do CPR for a friend or stranger simply because I would feel too guilty if I didn't. (Eisenberg, 1997, p. 252)

In the above, practical efficacy, though assumed, is almost irrelevant. The speaker claims that the obligation he is under is not ethical, nor even social, though he acknowledges it is an expectation of society.

Rather, his reason for initiating the procedure is triggered by guilt. Even in the admitted absence of a transcendent morality and social censure, death imparts guilt. I am alive and she is dead. I let her die and she abandoned me. By living, I condemn myself to death. I am guilty not only of death but of life. Guilt impels me to 'do something'.

The loss of a valued individual threatens the integrity of the lover's ego and the viability of community structure.[8] The dead are a threat. They are a threat to our ordered categorization of the world, a threat to the identity of the individual survivor and a threat to the society that has been destabilized by their loss. Loss generates anger. Anger at loss is easily projected back onto the lost object. The dead are always, at some level, seen as being guilty of their own deaths: 'Why did you leave me?' Furthermore, the death of one is an unwelcome reminder of the mortality of all. This anger at the dead engenders guilt in the survivors – guilt at the anger they cannot help but feel, which is displaced and transformed into guilt over their own past behaviour towards the deceased. Guilt in turn becomes anger directed against the self, other survivors, medical staff and, again, against the dead themselves. The dead bear and project back our anger at their loss. Others have picked apart this vicious circle of anger and guilt much more thoroughly than is done here; all I wish to point out is its inevitable presence at the deathbed (Kübler-Ross, 1973; Freud, 1985c, p. 116; Homans, 1989; Saunders, 1990; J. Davies, 1994, pp. 25–39; Walter, 1994).

The mourner may be seen as a kind of container filled with guilt and anger requiring release. In traditional societies, guilt and anger are purged through ritual cleansing – catharsis (καθαρσις) (Hertz, 1960, pp. 71–8; Lévi-Strauss, 1963, p. 18). In modern Western society, the progress of secularization and science, privileging fact over symbol, and logic over analogy, entails the transposition of catharsis from the realm of magic to that of reason. Ritual becomes psychology. In modern psychoanalysis, catharsis – the opening of a stopcock, allowing trapped emotion to flow out – is accomplished through abreaction, the reliving of the traumatic experience via the 'talking cure' or therapeutic discourse (Freud, 1955, p. 3; Laplanche and Pontalis, 1973, p. 1).

The earliest form of catharsis was the scapegoat, the *pharmakos* (φαρμακος) – 'a victim ... on whom collective sorrow and anger can be discharged' (Durkheim, 1995, p. 404). The pain of loss is projected onto an external object, which then assumes the guilt for the loss. The guilty object becomes the expiatory victim, which then is sacrificed to atone for the loss (Dodds, 1951, p. 43). The scapegoat is the 'other':

another species, another tribe, another person. Both the corpse and the newly released soul qualify as 'other', indeed, as the most threatening kind of other, because they are so easily recognized as also being self. In Durkheim's formulation, the pain engendered by the loss of death is projected outwards onto the soul of the expired victim. The pain experienced at loss is then seen as a malevolent imperative issuing from the disgruntled soul. 'Thus is explained the metamorphosis that makes a dread enemy out of yesterday's relative' (1995, p. 405). The corpse, left behind as the ambivalent representative of both the beloved self and the malevolent other, bears the brunt of the anger directed against the dead. It becomes the scapegoat.

Catharsis, as the ritual cleansing of pollution, relies on the homeopathic doctrine of like curing like: fighting fire with fire, violence with violence. It is the impure made pure by impurity. It is the expulsion of a violating force by a similar force, violent and violating. The purging of blood with blood.[9] The re-enactment of the crime as expiation for it. Ritual takes unacceptable emotions and channels them into socially acceptable modes of action. In this way, guilt and anger are expunged so as to initiate the process of grieving, which is the work of rebuilding identity – the deceased's in the realm of memory and the survivor's in a world changed by loss. This process of rebuilding identity is an active process, and it might be argued that it is initiated by an act of murder.

Recap

In the early eighteenth century, folk therapies aimed to beat back life into the drowned. The violence central to the folk therapies, when limited by The Method of the Humane Society, did not stay long repressed, but re-emerged in the manual ventilatory techniques of the nineteenth century. When, in the 1950s, these manual ventilatory techniques were forced out of life-saving protocols, violence did not disappear but survived in the form of CPR's external cardiac compression. In the year 2000, chest compression, though not disappearing, ceded lead position in the protocol to AEDs and a form of electrical violence, defibrillation. The recent changes in the CPR protocol have done little to mitigate the inherent violence of the act, rather, that violence has again merely changed form and theoretical justification.

Violence is necessary in both the revival of the moribund and the survivors' redemption from loss. Revival, operating through CPR-as-medical-protocol, uses violence in a straightforward attempt to breach the boundaries of the body to gain access to its interior (in its own way an occult, transcendent space) so as to repair the damage that has been inflicted upon it by nature. In protocols for the resuscitation of the trauma victim, there is an axiom: 'A tube for every orifice, and an orifice for every tube' – nasogastric tube, endotracheal tube, urinary catheter; where there is no handy orifice, we make one – IV, central line, chest tube, peritoneal lavage catheter. We violate the body's surface, that is, the fantasy of the body as a unitary entity, to operate on its parts, that is, the body's physiological functions, to transform it from its dangerously dysfunctional state to one of safe functionality.

In the redemptive act of moving the victim, agent and witness into the realm of transcendent power that is the source of 'life', deathbed ritual violently transgresses the body's boundaries, culture's categories and society's rules. This violence, though it is destructive, is, at the same time, creative. Destruction is the prelude to transformation. There is in ritual, always, a violation of boundaries as a prelude to the elision of the set categories of the mundane world. It is this elision which allows us to slip across the border into the transcendent realm where body and soul, life and death, protocol and ritual, act and performance are confounded one with the other in the process of infecting us with power.

Underlying CPR's overt therapeutic purpose is a complex of occult acts – identification of the dead, rite of passage for the dying and catharsis for the survivors. Each, at some point, at some level, in some form, utilizes violence. The violation of the body that is death and of the community that is loss is countered by the violence of the protocols of revival and the rituals of redemption. Violence counters violation in an attempt to acquire power, or at least the illusion of power, over death. Few corpses go to the grave unbeaten. No one dies – everyone is, in a sense, murdered.

A gang of murderers

> We are ourselves, like primaeval man, a gang of murderers.
>
> (Freud, 1985b, p. 86)

On an intellectual level we recognize death and our inevitable end in it; yet it is hard to believe that we will die. For the unconscious, there is no death. This paradox is difficult to sustain, and Freud suggests that one of the mechanisms by which we maintain it is through murder – actual, ritual and symbolic. One's fantasy is that it is only other people who die and that they do so at one's will. This implies that, because death is dispensed and controlled by human agency, it is not an inevitability. If one can control death, then one might be immune to it. To control death is to become an agent of death, that is, to become, to at least a certain extent, a murderer. However, civilization prohibits the unbridled extension of the ego to do as it wills. The first moral commandment according to Freud was 'Thou shalt not kill'. The sense of triumphant survival gained by killing others is thus tempered by guilt. Civilization forces us, if we kill, to take up the guilt of the murderer. We are thus caught in a powerful ambivalence when faced with the death of another (Seale, 1998, p. 59). Grieved by loss and frightened by our own mortality, we rejoice in our personal survival and revel in the specious immortality we gain from being not merely passive spectators to death but active agents in its unfolding.

There is no rationalization of this guilt; it can only be transcended. One means of accomplishing this is through the cathartic release of emotion in the ritual act. Ritual becomes the means of inducing a state in which reason, time and material existence are transcended in what Freud describes as the 'oceanic feeling' (1985a, pp. 252–3). This 'feeling' binds the individual to the group and the ego to life, creating a powerful alliance for effecting denial. Jung saw this alliance not as the denial of death but as a transcendence of it, bestowing upon each man and woman a symbolic tie with all other humans, affirming the value of life over death. Death is not merely an occurrence but a ritual sacrifice, the necessary sacrifice of the past to the present and the present to the future – the sacrifice that those living before us made so that we might live, and that we must make to those who follow (Seale, 1998, p. 59). The continuity of 'life' becomes the prime valorization of the sacrificial death. The community enacts death through deathbed ritual so as to transform the accident of death into sacrifice. The sacrifice valorizes life by allowing community to construct its own being through the translation of nature into culture.

Exorcising daemons

> Resuscitation is the ultimate life-affirming act …. 'It implies a commitment on the side of Life'.
>
> (Safar, quoted in Eisenberg, 1997, p. 253)

Ritual, which is above all gesture, takes up at the point words fail. Incomprehensible and incommensurable, death dwells in a void beyond speech. Analysing the deathbed is not the same thing as dealing with death. Any analysis, including my own, falls far short of giving us the resolution we desire. It merely frames the paradox of living to die. Words, the vehicle of reason, will always be inadequate to the experience of the deathbed. Neither myth nor therapeutic discourse nor critical analysis satisfactorily comprehends death.[10] We can only gesture towards it. Ritual performance 'is one of the few mechanisms at man's disposal that can possibly solve the ultimate problems and paradoxes of human existence' (d'Aquili et al., 1996, p. 132). Any resolution to the paradox of death – the attempt to bridge the immanent and transcendent, the physical and the metaphysical, the individual and the collective, being and belonging, the living and the dead – can only lie in the same register as its generation, the realm of the act. Everything that ends, if it is to have an end, ends in movement (Bachelard, 1983, pp. 106–8). It is in his actions that man most easily obtains knowledge of the divine (Dodds, 1951, p. 271).

Death is enacted, not described. Ritual enacts death so as to construct life – as function, as being and as community. The rhythmic violence of external cardiac compression attempts to resurrect life, hammering it back into the body from which it has fled, while at the same time, beating the life out of it, chasing that-which-was into the transcendent realm of heaven, hell or memory.[11] Only by enacting death do we purge ourselves of the daemon of life. If the violence of external cardiac compression is sacrifice and the violation of mouth-to-mouth is redemption, then the shock of defibrillation is, perhaps, epiphany: in the flash of electricity arcing across the chest, one apprehends life.

The fears surrounding mouth-to-mouth ventilation, the excessive violence of chest compression and the vital spark sliding across the monitor screen are evidence of an occult vitalism that, though denied by science, still drives medical therapeutics and the popular imagination. Hidden within the protocol of CPR is the reification of living as life. Life, in the ritual of CPR, ceases to be a set of scientifically determined functional relations and reverts to a real and valued entity binding the individual to the world. Life becomes suspiciously like unto the soul. In the enactment of CPR, life is instantiated as a fact and valorized as good. In a secular society, in which there is no afterlife or *telos* to give meaning to life, life becomes the secular *telos* that is also the transcendent *arche*.

Life is the desired condition of being, which the dying victim is revived back into by CPR-as-protocol. Even more crucially, life is the *daemon* that is purged from the dying body by CPR-as-ritual. Life is that which we desire to possess and, at the same time, must sacrifice to secure possession. This sacrifice enshrines the dead in the transcendent realm of memory and life in the transcendent realm of value. In the enactment of death, loss is lived by the performers, such that the ontological foundations of their own existence, both as individuals and as a social group, that is life and culture, are apprehended, strengthened and given value. The ritual performance of CPR on the street and on the screen is, to paraphrase Barthes, our attempt at producing death while trying to preserve life (2000, p. 92).

Death rescues life from the mundane. Our modern scientific concept of life is not substantive. It has no reassuring material form. No longer the transcendent soul of religious tradition, nor even the vital-force of Enlightenment natural philosophy; in the modern, 'Life consists in the sum of the functions by which death is resisted' (Bichat, 1827, p. 10). Life is the routine functioning of the organism. Routine function fails to draw our attention. 'Health is life lived in the silence of the organs' (René Leriche, quoted in Canguilhem, 1991, p. 91). Life has become a silent absence, a void at the centre of being. It is less death that modernity fails to apprehend than life. It is less death that sends a chill down our spines than the absence of life. Ritual precipitates the performer into existential awareness. In CPR's construction of death, the frailty of the existential status of life is compensated for by traumatic excess. Lacking the ability to articulate 'being' through the language of the transcendent, transgression replaces transcendence (D. Porter, 2003). Death, as constructed by ritual, is experienced as a kind of erotic transcendence, filling the empty concept of life with an awareness of subjectivity well beyond the power of words. In lieu of meaning, the experience of death fills life with affect in order that it might have value.

Though science no longer recognizes the substantial existence of life, it persists yet, as the daemon that haunts being. Without some kind of substance, no matter how subtle, without some kind of form, no matter how vague, without some kind of movement, no matter how occult, without some kind of being, life is too hard to handle. Life is too hard to handle in physical terms, thus the resuscitative protocol, and too hard to handle in metaphysical terms, thus deathbed ritual. It is in the enactment of death that we purge ourselves of Life – and, in so doing, conjure life out of death.

The erotics of death

> The breasts of those of [the Humane Society's] members who have rescued the prisoners of death, have experienced sensa-

tions, the very idea of which the powers of description are too feeble to convey.

(Bartlett, 1792, p. 6)

The algorithms are intended to lead the clinician along the path of assessment and intervention during the resuscitation experience.

(American, 2000, pp. I.136–I.165)

For the rescuer, the sensation of a successful resuscitation is something not soon forgotten. Accused of playing God, is it possible that the rescuer, like the method actor, 'feels like a god'?[12] It would be disingenuous of me to deny the emotional 'high' one rides throughout 'the resuscitation experience'. This feeling of manic self-intoxication, though rarely acknowledged, exists. The paramedic hero in the film *Bringing Out the Dead* proclaims: 'Saving a life is the ultimate rush.' As we will examine in the next chapter, much of the *mise en scène*, camerawork and editing of television shows such as *ER* and *Rescue 911* are attempts to reproduce a hyper-real, adrenalin-stoked, omnipotent rush. This ecstatic, intoxicated state is the madness that confers power, and, though holding no place in the execution of a protocol, is an essential part of ritual.

Throughout history, intoxication and intoxicants are entangled with medicine as both pathology and therapy. We should not be surprised that they emerge at the deathbed – opium for the victim, the ecstasy of ritual for the rescuer and the catharsis of dramatic performance for the spectator. Each gives access to the realm of transcendent power. Each transports one into a subjective state confounded with objective reality. Intoxication is 'a feeling of an indissoluble bond, of being one with the external world as a whole ... the boundary between ego and object threatens to melt away' (Freud, 1985a, pp. 252–3). It is a return to the pleasure of undifferentiated existence: child/mother, self/other, one. As the boundary between ego and object melts away, the altered subjective state of intoxication becomes indistinguishable from change in the objective world. In this elision, the change in one's self is confounded with the power to change the here and now. It is from this experience of chaos that order is born. It is from here that the subject develops his or her own subjectivity (an individual identity and borders to self) and a world in which to exist (a set of object relations). Subjective state and objective act, self and world, cause and effect, slide towards each other in an attempt to transform both the world and oneself. This return to the creative, undifferentiated state preceding consciousness is not the work of words but of acts. Rational discourse is powerless because the renunciation of that state, in our coming into self and order, in our coming into culture, is the loss around which the ensuing symbolic system of language is built. The erotic is that thing that the formal system of language cannot articulate for it precedes it and is formless (Lacan, 1988, pp. 154–5).

In the *Phaedrus*, Socrates speaks of the telestic madness induced by the *orgia* (οργια) as the means by which Dionysus confers power (249e–55d). Communion with the god, through ritual, invests man with power and man knows, through his experience of intoxication, that he has acquired the power of the god – power over life and death. By inducing a state of common identity with the gods, by submerging our individual identity in the intoxicated madness of the herd, Dionysus 'the Liberator' sets us free to act (Dodds, 1951, pp. 66–77). Dionysus is the cause of madness and the liberator from madness. Dionysus is the god of the cathartic cure – the impure made pure through impurity; the purging of blood with blood. The *oreibasia* (ορειβασια), the Bacchic dance, culminates in the tearing to pieces, and swallowing raw, of the sacrificial victim. It is experienced as a mixture of supreme repulsion and supreme exaltation, at once horrible and holy, both pollution and purification (Dodds, 1951, p. 278). The Maenads drink and dance and violently rend the victim so as to induce an erotic ecstasy in which a sense of transcendence over the ordinariness of things both invites and challenges death. This piacular sacrifice binds the community together in a shared subjective state, a communion of consciousness (Durkheim, 1995, p. 392). The violence of the Bacchic dance offers a purging of guilt, fear, anger and sorrow. Indeed, it removes one from the realm in which these things have meaning. Meaning is submerged in action. There is nothing but the act, uniting being, admitting of no distinctions of time, space, self, other, life, death. All are confounded in a state of pure being existing solely in the violence of the act.

Access to grace is not though words nor explained by words. Argument breaks down; language fails; ritual triumphs. The strange act of CPR induces, not always, but often enough, a subjective state that the delicacy of modern science hesitates to label. There is no place for epiphany in medicine. Nevertheless, as histrionic as it sounds, to resuscitate a cold, blue, pulseless, hypothermic child *is* to feel like a god.

> Saving someone's life is like falling in love. The best drug in the world. For days, sometimes weeks afterwards, you walk the street

making infinite whatever you see. Once, for a few weeks, I couldn't feel the earth. Everything I touched became lighter. Horns played in my shoes. Flowers fell from my pockets. You wonder if you become immortal. As if you've saved your own life as well. God has passed through you. Why deny it? And for a moment there, why deny for a moment there, God was you. (*Bringing Out the Dead*, 2000)

Thus the erotics of death.[13] Plato recognized Eros as the experience of divine madness and the operation of divine grace. Eros is the one mode of experience that brings together the two natures of man, the divine and the bestial. Eros is rooted in what man shares with the animals: life, death and sex. Yet, Eros is also the dynamic impulse to consciousness, driving the soul forward in its quest for knowledge, experience and satisfaction beyond the mundane being of the individual creature alone as itself. The erotic is the phenomenal bridge between the human as he or she is and humanity as it might be (Plato, *Phaedrus*, 249e). What is at stake in the eroticism of ritual is not merely excitement, sexual or otherwise, not merely the enjoyment of transgression and power, but the channelling of forces that, should they not find controlled release, would destroy both individual identity and society.

To resist Dionysus is to repress the elemental in one's nature; the punishment is the sudden complete collapse of the inward dykes when the elemental breaks through perforce and civilisation vanishes. (Dodds, 1951, p. 273)

What the Greeks called *ecstasis* (εχστασις) and Dodd's labels 'a subjective state of common identity with the god', Durkheim interprets as the human experience of 'society' (1995, p. 382). Bloch emphasizes the increased social power that accrues to those whose contact through ecstasy with transcendent power changes them from victims of life into agents of death (1992, pp. 4–7). Eliade describes shamanism as a 'technique of ecstasy', which accessing a supernatural world, gives the shaman power not only over death but also over the tribe (1957, p. 4). What is at stake in the cathartic excesses of deathbed ritual is the relation between the individual and society, what might be and was labelled 'humanity'.

Dehumanization and humanity

CPR is accused of dehumanizing the dying, treating them little better than a slab of meat. And from a common-sense point of view, this is a valid accusation. But then, death *is* dehumanizing, in the most straightforward, non-pejorative, unemotional sense of the term. Death makes us other than human; it makes us a corpse. Though the return of life to the patient and the return of the patient to humanity may be the point of resuscitative protocol, the point of deathbed ritual *is* dehumanization – to transform the man or woman into something no longer human, to strip our humanity from us so that we can progress towards another state of being. As death transforms the living body into a corpse, so deathbed ritual transforms the dying person into a sacrificial victim, and the sacrificial victim into an ancestor and into a memory. Each step dehumanizes, moving the object of its actions further and further away from membership in the community of agents perpetrating those acts of transformation. Deathbed ritual engineers, in Seale's words, our 'final fall from culture' (1998, p. 170).

We are probably (though we have no way of knowing) the only species that actively constructs death and the only species that actively constructs its own identity. In constructing death, we are also constructing its opposite – 'life'. If life is to be anything more than animation, that is, more than animal function, then it must be human life as part of humanity – the community that comes into existence through its active construction of death. Out of the violence perpetrated on the body of the sacrificial victim loss is negated and community is born as a transcendent and immortal form. On the failure of the protocol to save life, the resuscitative act, as deathbed ritual, binds victim and rescuer together in the work of constructing life in the abstract by purging life in the physical. Paradoxically, the dehumanizing violence perpetrated by CPR upon the dying body, transforming it into a corpse, destroys in the individual and in the somatic what it constructs in the community and in the imaginary – 'humanity'.

The transcendent power of community, what Durkheim called the social bond, and the Rev. Pratt, humanity, flows through the hands of the rescuer in an attempt to save the victim's life, construct an appropriate death and transform the inevitability of loss into culture. The rescuer proves (that is, both tests and demonstrates) his or her humanity, even love for the victim, in an act of violent compassion. The heroic use of resuscitative protocols is not only proof of the value we place on life and humanity, but is necessary for their very survival, both biologically and socially. Without this valorization of life over death, culture would be impossible; as the vehicles for it, individual living humans, would cease to exist. The Humane Society and the American Heart Association see themselves as institutional manifestations of the praiseworthy goal of building an inclusive social structure that recognizes and values each individual human life:

> It is true that only a few will be resuscitated. But we must also acknowledge a greater truth: the effort of resuscitation is ennobling .... As Peter Safar eloquently wrote about resuscitation, 'Its moral impact and the commitment it represents may have a much broader influence in a world where life has too often been regarded as cheap.' Resuscitation is the ultimate life-affirming act. 'Medicine imposes compassion, reason and decency on a random universe,' says Safar. (Eisenberg, 1997, p. 293)

However, our performance of CPR is not merely about restoring life to the apparently dead, ennobling the rescuer and valorizing life. The fantasy of rescue is also the fantasy of sacrifice, two sides of a single coin. It is death, the loss of life, that makes redemption necessary. It is sacrifice, the taking of life, that makes redemption possible. Redemption, in the modern, is no more than our accession to the human state, which in Bloch's terms is the transformation of prey into hunter. To become human is to accede to power through violence. We act so as to demonstrate that we are capable of acting, as well as being acted upon. We act to redeem our involvement in the mortality of others and, ultimately, the guilt of our own mortality. It is out of the act of murder as an act of creation, as a re-ordering of a world of unrelenting loss, that society is born and the individual is redeemed. There is no redemption without sacrifice. Without having killed, we are not fully human. Without experiencing the guilt and the ecstasy of murder, we cannot 'feel the pow'r of soft HUMANITY!'

The ecstatic intoxication of deathbed ritual is the manic re-creation of the pre-linguistic paradise where self and the world existed as one, in unity out of time. It is our mutual defence against the violence of being in world. Levinas maintains that participation in death is the primary ethical responsibility of the human being, that human existence is based on the sociality of death (2000, pp. 16–21). The ecstatic madness of the deathbed is an attempt to encompass the impossible relations between self and society and the impossible situation of living to die. Without a means of encompassing these paradoxes, there is neither human being nor humanity.

The terminal paradox revisited

Though the initial goal of any resuscitative protocol is to restore life, at a certain point in its enactment, we go from saving the moribund to determining whether or not the deceased is indeed dead. Caught up in the violence of the deathbed, we move beyond even that. We go beyond diagnosis and therapy to create what we initially wished to deny. We construct what we fear, because that is the only way we can, if not comprehend, at least apprehend it. We create death by enacting it.

The fear of death and our challenge to it are realized in the acts of mouth-to-mouth ventilation, external cardiac compression and defibrillation. These practical therapeutic acts, having erased from consciousness their connections to the symbolic, and thus repressed their connections to the past and to history, borrow from what is to hand, in this case contemporary science, the justifications necessary for their continued performance. Within the materialist perspective of modern medical science, there is a necessary occultation of ritual by protocol. That is, ritual must remain hidden behind protocol, magic behind science. It would not do for the physician to admit that he or she is manipulating signs rather than objects. Exposure would destroy not only the credibility of the protocol, but the scientific faith upon which the effectiveness of its ritual aspect depends. Thus, for the act of murder to be tolerated, it must disguise itself as diagnosis, the diagnosis of death, and for the diagnostic act to persist it must hide behind its therapeutic claim to restore life. Behind these façades, the enactment of the symbolic proceeds, producing the subjective state that allows us, if not to obliterate, then at least to endure the paradox of living to die.

CPR neatly pulls together the protocol of revival and the ritual of redemption in an effort to effect a transition from a state of danger to one of safety. CPR-as-protocol attempts to revive the victim, saving him from death, and, in preserving his life, save the community from loss. CPR-as-ritual enacts a mythic narrative of sacrifice and redemption: turning the body into a corpse, the beloved into an ancestor, the past into memory, while at the same time, generating images, words and gestures to act as signifiers binding together victims of loss into a community of survivors. Ritual, through the controlled exercise of violence, gives the dead peace, survivors safety and the community coherence.

One begins to suspect, in light of problems involved in the implementation of advance directives (see chapter 8), in the growing use of CPR by the laity, and in the ubiquity of CPR's portrayal in the media, that it is less the public who are incensed with the violent ritualization of the deathbed than the professionals who fashioned it, promulgate it and are now forced to perform it. Though there is a great deal of public support (and rightly so) for hospice and palliative care, the public has yet to take up Chesterton's call to root out 'like a horde of assassins' paramedics, ICU nurses and emergency physicians. The equation of a 'good' death with a death-with-dignity and a 'bad' death with the resuscitative protocol is, I believe, not nearly as straightforward as is usually maintained. Though most people express the desire for a quiet, pain-free, dignified death, most also find comfort in the positivist ideal of redemption through action: 'I did all I could'.

> You should be proud of the fact that you are learning to become an ACLS provider .... Of course, these emergencies can have negative outcomes. You and other emergency personnel who arrive to help in the resuscitation may not succeed in restoring life. Some people have a cardiac arrest simply because they have reached the end of their life. Your success will not be measured by whether a cardiac arrest victim lives or dies but rather by the fact that you tried. Simply by taking an action, making an effort, just trying to help, you will be judged a success .... What is important is to take action and to try and help another human being .... If the person you try to resuscitate does not live, take comfort from knowing that in taking action you did your best. (Cummins, 2001, pp. 41–3)

Salvation is no longer the redemption of an afterlife. For the victim revival is redemption. For the rescuer it is in 'taking an action, making an effort, just trying to help'. Modern medicine, in fact, modernity itself, bestows an intrinsic value on action.[14] Unfortunately, this demand for action often violates the dying body with what may be painful and degrading acts. Worse, it razes the dying person's self-directed construction of self by denying them autonomy in their final act (Gruman, 1978–9, p. 237). So it is that medical practitioners, accused of being blinkered by the technological imperative of positivist science, are condemned for passing the sentence of life: if something can be done, it should be done.

What then does CPR amount to? A protocol that justifies itself in the language of science, yet whose effect is more in the realm of the symbolic than the physical; a protocol that has participated in the medicalization of death, moving it out of the home into the hospital, moving it out of the hands of the family and into the hands of strangers; a protocol that stands accused of robbing the individual of dignity in the process of dying. On the other hand, CPR, with its lights and beeps and sparking discharges, provides tangible evidence that there is such a *thing* as life and that life has value. Furthermore, it is the means by which the layperson is allowed to participate in the death drama, preserving within it certain atavistic mechanisms for helping him or her deal with the dangers surrounding the deathbed. It provides an arena for heroic action in a society in which those opportunities have become increasingly rare. It allows the rescuer to demonstrate his or her humanity towards, or even love for, the victim. It allows the rescuer through the good act to become the good man or woman helping to build the good society. And for that society, it provides an imagined model for death, which can be represented and reproduced for the consumption of all.

Over the last 40 years, CPR's most striking success, I would argue, has been less in its clinical efficacy than in its colonization of the media – less in the number of lives saved on the street than in its ubiquity on cinema and television screens. CPR, on street and screen, is a performance, and its performance on the screen is as important as its performance on the street. When, in real life, the physician comes through the doors of the resuscitation room to confront the family with death, the script has, to large extent, already been written. When he says, 'We did all we could', the family, nurtured by images in the media, nods its head in sad understanding. Throughout the late twentieth century, it has been via television, for better or worse, that we experience the deathbed, and so, in the next chapter, we shall examine CPR's portrayal in that medium.

Part Three
The Fantasies

7
The Media: Getting it Right?

> On a bad week, we reach twenty million people: on a good week, thirty-five.
>
> (Morocco, 2001)
>
> *In series 5, episode 2 of* Buffy the Vampire Slayer, *Buffy enters the front door of her Sunnydale home. Her mother is lying on the couch. The camera pans to the mother. Her eyes are wide open, mouth slack, not breathing. Buffy shakes her mother's shoulders. No response. She runs into kitchen. Dials 911. 'Hello. It's my mom. She's not breathing .... What should I do? ... Do you know how to administer CPR? ... It's very simple. You want to tilt your mother's head back. Cover her mouth with yours and breath into her mouth. Give ventilations then ...' Buffy tilts her mother's head back. Pinches her nose. Gives two breaths. Starts chest compressions. '1, 2, 3, 4, 5...' Suddenly a cracking noise. Buffy gasps. 'Oh God! Hi. Are you there? I broke something .... The paramedics should be there in a moment. You might have cracked a rib. It's not important.... She's cold .... The body's cold?... No! My, MOM! Should I make her warm?... No, if she's not responding to the CPR, the best thing is to wait for the paramedics. OK?' Buffy looks out the front window. She hears the ambulance siren. Goes to the front door. Ambulance pulls up. Cut back to mother lying on couch, looking very dead. Buffy sees her mother's skirt hiked up revealing her slip. Hurries over and rearranges the skirt as the paramedics enter. Paramedic feels for pulse. 'Getting no pulse.... How long's she been like this?... I found her... a few minutes.' Cut to flat line on monitor. 'She's cold, man. Call it.' Paramedics quietly begin to*

pack up. 'I'm sorry, but I have to tell you that your mother's dead. It looks like she died a good while before you found her. There's nothing you could have done.' Sound of dispatcher on paramedic's radio: 'Dispatch 7. We have a 206. What's your status? ... We're moving .... Right. I'm going to call this. Now the coroner's office may take a while. In the meanwhile, you should have a glass of water and try not to disturb the body. Do you need anything? Is there someone you can call?' Buffy sees the paramedics to the front door. Cut to commercial break. Return from break. Overhead shot of Joyce's body. Head and shoulder shot directly into dull eyes and slack mouth. A pair of hands emerge from screen left and zip her into a body bag.

(Buffy)

Mediated death

Media portrayals of CPR encompass the pathos of the dying victim, the heroism of the individual rescuer, the shiny technology of a powerful science and the tensions within a society that puts guns on the streets and paramedics in ambulances. In the flashing lights of the ambulance, in the image of the body convulsed by electrical shocks and in the glowing line of the cardiac monitor announcing life or death, CPR stands as a sign of the modern: modern life and modern death.

CPR and television grew up together. Network broadcasting in America began to reach a mass audience in the early 1950s and it was in the early 1950s that resuscitative protocols began to coalesce around studies on artificial ventilation. CPR since its inception has exploited the power of the moving image as a tool for instruction, as a means of propaganda and as a form of entertainment.

Instruction, propaganda, entertainment

After acceptance of mouth-to-mouth ventilation at the Armed Forces Conference on Artificial Respiration and Nerve Gas Poisoning in Denver in May 1957, Peter Safar, with help from the US Army, began to make documentary films of his experiments. In December 1957, on live television from New York, Safar demonstrated mouth-to-mouth ventilation on his own wife, Eva, while James Elam narrated. Elam, supported by the Army's Walter Reed Movie Group, made the film *Rescue Breathing* in 1959. Several thousand prints were made and distributed to the armed forces and life-saving societies. At the meeting of the Maryland Medical Society in 1960, where CPR was given its medical imprimatur, James Jude showed a film of chest compressions on a child and an adult. William Kouwenhoven ran two films: one of a dog's heart in fibrillation and the effect of the application of electrical shocks to it; the other demonstrating how to perform closed chest defibrillation on a human. At the same meeting, Safar used film to demonstrate mouth-to-mouth ventilation on a paralysed volunteer. In 1961, Archer Gordon produced the film *The Pulse of Life*. It was for this that Gordon devised the ABC mnemonic (airway-breathing-circulation). Also in 1961, Jude, Kowenhoven and Knickerbocker, funded by the drug company SmithKline French, produced the film *External Cardiac Massage* (Eisenberg, 1997, pp. 92–132). Numerous instructional life-saving films followed in the 1960s and 1970s, and then, in the 1980s, videos. In the 1990s, CPR began to be 'sold' on television. 'The use of 30-second public service announcements depicting one member of an elderly couple giving CPR to their stricken partner broadcast over a six-month period increased the rate of bystander CPR from 43 per cent to 55 per cent' (Becker et al., 1999, p. 353).

Up until very recently, BLS was taught as a four-hour course by instructors trained and certified by the AHA. The course used a combination of printed material, lectures, demonstration and hands-on practice on manikins. However, rates of the correct performance of CPR following instruction were low and retention of skills poor (Gombeski et al., 1982, p. 849; Kaye and Mancini, 1986, p. 620; Nichol et al., 1999, p. 517: Todd et al., 1999, p. 730 Batcheller et al., 2000, p. 101) (see Appendix 1, pp. 241–3). The AHA began to look at alternative teaching techniques. A study on the teaching of CPR found that a 34-minute instructional videotape was more effective in teaching the technique than the traditional, hands-on, manikin-oriented, AHA 'Heartsaver' CPR course (Braslow et al., 1997, p. 207; Todd et al., 1998, p. 364). Eisenburger and Safar, after reviewing the literature, state that 'Audio-tape or video-tape coached self-practice on manikins was more effective than instructor-courses' (1999, p. 3). Today, video is an essential component of the CPR courses given to healthcare workers and the public. In some situations, it is the course, taking the full instructional load (American, 2000, pp. I.371–I.376). The AHA now endorses a combined approach using videos and instructors – 'a "watch-then-practice" video-based medium, having documented that as the most effective didactic method for skills acquisition' (American, 2000, pp. I.371–I.376).

From instruction to propaganda is but a short step: 'Video has the potential to motivate students by presenting real-life cases' (American, 2000, pp. I.1–I.11). Film was used not only to propagate the protocol at the physical level of technique, but also at the social level, encouraging commitments to personnel, facilities, equipment and finances. Films made by Jude, Elam, Kouwenhoven and Safar in the late 1950s and early 1960s were used in the crusade to get CPR accepted by government, medical and life-saving organizations. These documentary films were used to persuade the authorities responsible to come up with research funding and encourage them to authorize CPR as *the* life-saving protocol.

It was television, however, that brought CPR to the masses, inducting them into the 'chain-of-survival'. In 1970, the current affairs television show *60 Minutes* sent a crew to Seattle to film a segment on the burgeoning citizen CPR programme. They rode with paramedic units, filming several resuscitations. The show stimulated considerable response, with a markedly increased awareness of the protocol and calls for similar citizen programs to be established elsewhere (Eisenberg, 1997, pp. 232–6). However, CPR's successful television career was not confined to news and documentary.

> A Jack Webb TV show may also have helped. In 1970, Webb got interested in the mobile coronary-care units and thought they'd make the basis of a great television series. His producer, Robert Cinader, rode with paramedics from County Fire Station 36 and learned the ropes firsthand. The resulting series, *Emergency*, became a major hit. 'It was a major force in not only legitimizing the paramedics in our county,' recalled [Dr] Criley, 'but also for exporting the idea across the country. People would watch and hear the fire sirens, kids would watch and see all these marvelous things going on. That gave us tremendous impetus.' (Eisenberg, 1997, p. 240)

The above quote implies that the move from instruction to propaganda to entertainment is a cumulative process; elements of instruction and propaganda remaining embedded within medical dramas produced for entertainment.

The medical drama is effective propaganda and it has produced results. Troy, in a letter to the *New England Journal of Medicine*, states that at least half the students attending community CPR classes give as their motivation their viewing of popular medical dramas: 'Students often recount events of a particularly spectacular CPR-based "save" in some episode' (1996, p. 1605). Wallack and Bingle point out that since *ER* first aired, the number of fourth-year medical students at Indiana University School of Medicine enrolling in emergency medicine residency training programmes has doubled. 'Although other factors, such as market forces, may also be involved in this significant increase, the omnipresence of television may now be influencing physician's career choices' (1996, p. 1605).

The first US television, entertainment series featuring medicine as the context, with physicians as central characters, was *City Hospital* debuting in 1952. Previously, in the early 1950s, radio had *Dr. Kildare*, which was, in 1960, moved to television. In that same year, *Ben Casey* debuted. The plots of the episodes usually revolved around the physician's struggle against a specific pathological condition and its associated social and psychological problems. The illnesses presented were most commonly acute problems requiring dramatic therapy that led to complete cure, or, very rarely, death. Death, when it was portrayed, was usually a quiet slipping away, conforming to the death-with-dignity paradigm. The 1970s saw little change in this pattern in shows like *Marcus Welby MD* and *Medical Center*. In the early 1980s, *M*A*S*H*, *St. Elsewhere* and *Chicago Hope* shifted the plotline away from the patients' problems to the doctors'. The clinical situation served as a vehicle by which the physician's personality could be put under stress and the resolution of the tensions engendered drove the plot (Turow, 1996, p. 1242). It was also in this period that the taboos around the portrayal of death on screen began to weaken. However, most deaths were still handled with ellipsis, that is, a gentle fade-out, or bathos, a slow pan to a banal image, such as clouds in the sky. This changed in the 1990s, primarily through the phenomenal success of *ER* and its compelling formula of sex and death.[1]

> Scriptwriters ... are handed a microscope with which to inspect the grislier fundamentals of life. Into the daily regime of a hospital Accident and Emergency department are thrust harrowing stories of life and death, extreme revelations of love and hate riven by grief and vengeance. (Silver, 1998, p. 6)

Nowhere is the power of the doctor-hero more visible than in his or her struggle with death in the arena of CPR. The image of the heroic doctor is, of course, not new. Bynum speaks of 'the cult of the surgeon' in the nineteenth century, 'associated ... with science, drama, and heroics' (1994, p. 137). Today, within the magic circle inscribed by the bright lights of the studio resuscitation room, the doctor, like the epic hero, potent with the force of life, is given the power to master a world filled with danger.

If we look at medical dramas, such as *ER* and *Casualty*, they are composed of long- and short-term story arcs. The long-term arcs are centred on the staff's somewhat sordid personal lives. They act as continuity devises, binding together short-term story arcs comprised of life and death vignettes full of violence, blood and gore:

> What could be more compelling than watching an emergency-room team try to save the life of a critically injured patient? Why, pondering the possibility that two of them will fall in love .... Dr. Doug Ross (George Clooney) and nurse Carol Hathaway (Julianna Margulies) kept the lid on their mutual attraction. But now that her fiancé and his lovers have been tagged and bagged .... will Doug and Carol's repressed passions flat line or finally come back to life? (Rensin, 1995)

It should not come as much of a surprise that sex and death are a winning combination – sex for the staff and death for the patients.

Getting it right

As fanciful and fantastic as the lead characters' personal lives are, their actions in the ER and in resuscitative scenarios are exquisitely accurate – in fact, suspiciously so. The genre has an obsession with 'getting things right'.

> *Casualty*, now in its thirteenth series, continues to move and grip millions of people with its complex, up-to-date plots and vibrant authenticity .... It works because of the strength of the programmes authenticity .... The incidents we see are realistic and horrific .... harrowingly true to life .... reflecting the cut and thrust of a real A&E department .... The watchword for the series is authenticity, which requires scrupulous and far-reaching research .... *Casualty* is very true to life, and the story lines painstakingly researched .... 'My role as a medical advisor ... [is] to make sure that they all get it right.' (Silver, 1998, pp. 6–23)

The obsessive technical accuracy of these shows touches scripts, sets, acting and camera techniques. All are infinitely more 'realistic' than they need be for the sake of entertainment. In the resuscitation room of the medical drama, the real and the represented are consciously confounded by writers and directors, in a process that replaces dramatic verisimilitude with instrumental accuracy.

> At Holby City,[2] the distinction between reality and fiction is blurred .... The stories have got to be real .... If the [medical] advisors say it absolutely couldn't happen, then we don't do it. I think that's why people think that it's real – because it is! (Silver, 1998, p. 48)

This obsessive pursuit of technical accuracy, though it is meant to be reassuring, is vaguely disturbing. There are a number of reasons given by the producers of these shows for the excessive accuracy of the medical drama. These might be sorted under the categories of instruction, documentary and entertainment.

Instruction

The most common reason for accuracy usually given by these shows' writers and producers has to do with a perceived public service commitment to the television audience. *ER*, the hit show from which most of this genre has drawn its format, was initially formulated and produced by Michael Crichton, who based the show on his experiences as a medical student at Massachusetts General Hospital. For Crichton, the accuracy of the medicine portrayed was important and he has said that he feels a responsibility to present medicine 'as it really is'. Mark Morocco, a practicing emergency specialist, and head of the medical advisory unit for *ER* states:

> On a bad week, we reach 20 million people: on a good week, 35. It's entirely possible that there's an entire generation, an entire cohort of people out there whose medical information and interpretation of their medical experience comes from this television show .... The good thing is that we are able to give some accurate medicine to the populace. (2001)

Likewise, the British series *Casualty*:

> *Casualty* pride themselves on producing programmes that are medically accurate. A bonus for the writers is that *Casualty* has encouraged viewers to practice simple first aid. (Silver, 1998, p. 36)

Those who write and produce these shows see them as a means of educating the general public about health, disease and the healthcare system. It is certainly possible to see this altruism as a sop to the Broadcasting Standards Commission, a cynical dose of 'redeeming social value' in order to justify the medical drama's sometimes dubious taste and commercialization of tragedy. Tempting as it is to be cynical, the altruism of those who produce medical dramas should not be discounted. They are genuine in their wish to educate the public. Nor are they the only ones to emphasize the instructional potential of the genre. Dr Ron Walls, chief of emergency medicine at Brigham and Women's Hospital in Boston, points out that:

> Even if TV shows make CPR look too easy or too successful, they're still educating the public about the value of CPR, and that is a very good thing. (Timmermans, 1999, p. 224)

Today, 72–92 per cent of patients report television as their prime source of information about CPR (Schonwetter et al., 1991, p. 372; Schonwetter et al., 1993, p. 295; Murphy et al., 1994, p. 545).

> Completely untrained in the medical technique of cardiopulmonary resuscitation ... she still knew enough from TV shows casually seen and educational broadcasts barely overheard to do the right thing at the right time. (Eisenberg, 1997, p. 5)

The watching of resuscitation on television has been accepted as proof of competence in CPR by at least one US court in its interpretation of Good Samaritan laws (Mercier, 2001). In a postmodern twist, episodes of *ER* and *Baywatch* are now being used to instruct healthcare personnel in resuscitative techniques (Hotz, 2001). The portrayal of CPR on television may thus be seen in the positive light of encouraging the general public to learn a potentially life-saving technique and become involved in a social movement whose goal is the welfare of fellow human beings.

Documentary

A second factor contributing to technical accuracy is that of 'documentary'. Mark Morocco again:

> One of the reasons that the show was a hit is that it was the first 'reality' show. It was a show that allowed people to see into an area

they were familiar with but that they didn't get a chance to see clearly. (2001)

The producers of medical dramas are well aware that the public feels excluded from medicine and has a desire to see what lies behind the curtain. The general public feels particularly excluded from the life and death scenes that 50 years ago occurred in the home and now occur behind the closed doors of emergency rooms and ICUs. The audience's desire to 'look behind the scenes' is answered by the director's attempts to show 'what really happens'. From an internet fan site:

> Patients' wounds are probed, their chests are cut open, bullets are extracted, and babies are delivered. The audience is made to feel like it is watching a documentary of sorts, rather than a cleverly constructed narrative. ('ER', 2002)

This documentary capacity serves to support the plausibility of the dramatic action. John Wells, producer of *ER*, maintains that because most viewers have never been arrested or thrown in jail, cop and lawyer shows can get away with less than obsessive detail, whereas almost everyone has visited an emergency room at some time in their lives. With this experience, there is a good chance they would spot inaccuracies, destroying the plausibility of the scene (Morocco, 2001).

Entertainment

Though these shows have their instructional and documentary aspects, their main purpose is entertainment. Much like the gladiatorial contests of the ancient world and present-day spectator sports, the medical drama attempts to involve us in the action – turning us from spectators into participants. This is done by immersing us in the immediacy of present action. The scenes portrayed are not only meant to be happening in the present, but they are meant to absorb us in action that is happening right *now* and right here. They are meant to induce the adrenalin rush of participation.

How it's done

Though instruction, documentary and entertainment do not exhaust all the possibilities for the medical drama's pursuit of accuracy, they at least provide a place to start in examining how the medical drama achieves its particular version of realism. *ER* employs a full-time, Board-certified, emergency medicine specialist as head of its medical unit, plus four other part-time specialist physician advisers. *Casualty* does much the same. In both cases, a number of the show's writers are physicians, nurses or paramedics. Besides giving technical advice, suggesting story-lines and vetting scripts, there is always a physician on the set during shoots to spot technical errors, such as the incorrect wielding of a needle-driver, and to advise on the 'feel' of the scene. Neil Baer, physician and writer for the show:

> We draw on medical stories (many inspired by my own experience or by incidents related by doctors and nurses throughout the county) .... We try to make the medical care shown in each episode credible and accurate, without sacrificing the story's dramatic impact. We believe we would be doing a disservice to our audience if the material were incorrect .... With medically trained writers working on the show, we have built in checks for accuracy .... We meet with a technical advisor trained in both emergency medicine and internal medicine and resolve any disagreements about therapy or diagnosis – just as in real life. Should we treat the patient with a second- or third-generation cephalosporin? Can we forego a computed tomographic scan of the head? ... We often say that writing for *ER* is like taking care of real patients without ever leaving the computer keyboard. (1996, p. 1604)

The contention is that accuracy supports plausibility, supports dramatic verisimilitude – that is, it helps us suspend our disbelief in mere representation. It is a question of aesthetics – the 'real' as affect.

> In terms of the truthfulness of the medicine on the show, one of the commandments of ER is that everyone who works here ... believes that you produce more realistic drama and affecting drama by starting from truth than you do from artifice .... Medicine in the media has often been portrayed inaccurately, where the people making it say, 'Well that's enough to get the point across. If there's a neurosurgeon or a critical care nurse out there, who cares? They're less than 1 per cent of the audience and we don't really care.' The problem with that is that people who are not neurosurgeons and are not critical care nurses, on some level, do have a sense of what is real, though they may not be able to put their finger on what that is. (Morocco, 2001)

The vignettes of illness and death portrayed in these shows are made less to seem like stories and more like 'slices of life'. As already mentioned, the long-term story arcs, centred on the staff's personal lives, are little more than continuity devices, the grout in a mosaic binding together short-term story arcs comprised of life-and-death vignettes. This narrative technique, really a kind of anti-narrative, is aimed less at telling a tale with a beginning, middle and end, than focusing our attention on short, intense bursts of action that have more the character of image than narrative. Contributing to the 'slice of life' aesthetic is that each episode is usually played out in real-time, or in as close as television can get to it. Few hour-long episodes span more than a few hours in the real-time of a real emergency room. Part of the 'real' feel to the show has to do with the action happening now in the same time scale in which one is viewing it.

On a more concrete level, the set of *ER* is uncannily real, for it is the corpse of a real ER. The set is an actual emergency department, torn from a decommissioned hospital in east Los Angeles and reconstructed on a sound stage at Warner Brothers. This 'set', unlike most television sets, maintains its real-world coherence in that each room has four walls, a ceiling and a floor, and, unlike most sets, the rooms adjoin each other as they did in the hospital from which it was torn. This 'set' has been reconstructed exactly. The flooring is the original cracked and worn linoleum from the late 1950s. The walls have scuff marks, finger smudges and general signs of wear. What makes the use of real space possible is *ER*'s particular use of the Steadicam, with which I'll deal presently.

The props are also real – not models, of respirators, defibrillators, laryngoscopes, and so on, but the real things, obtained from medical supply companies. One of the medical directors of *Casualty* relates that:

> The reps are much more happy to give the stuff to *Casualty* than to give it to the NHS [National Health Service]. I was sorting out props for the first episode of Series 13 and I told the assistant floor manager I would need a particular kind of monitor. 'Oh,' he said, 'we'll get three or four of those.' I sweated blood to get just one into our hospital here. (Silver, 1998, p. 16)

Likewise, for *ER*:

> Our set is much better equipped than any hospital I have ever worked in. I'd definitely rather get sick on the set than in a real ED. (Fong, 2000)

Furthermore, the human 'props' are real. Real medical staff are often used as extras.

> Tubes are stuck into dummies, blood squirts on cue, background nurses (real ones recruited for authenticity) pass scalpels and start IV drips, as the Steadicam operator snakes among them like a Martha Graham dancer. 'Cut! Great!' yells the director. (Scheller, 1996)

Actors are taught not just how to hold a needle driver properly, but how to suture. They are taught how to defibrillate, intubate, put in a central line.

> We usually demonstrate the procedure on the day of filming so the actor can visualize it before getting in front of the camera. It genuinely surprised me how bright the actors are, how fast they pick up things. They seem brighter than medical students in understanding and interpreting medical directions .... Some of these guys, the way they suture, if you didn't know, you'd think they really were physicians! They also ask a lot of questions about what is going on medically, which helps them with their performances because it comes across as more authentic. (Fong, 2003)

Mark Morocco again:

> What that means about a show like *ER* is that when you get down on the set with someone like Tony Edwards [the actor playing Dr Green] whose going to be in front of the camera, Tony is very, very concerned as an actor, as an artist, that he is able to portray what he portrays truthfully through that lens. The only way that he can do that externally is to do it internally. That's kind of an American method actor thing. Even our classically British trained actors like Alex Kingston find there is some solace in the actual real manipulation of these real instruments. (2001)

Though there is an obvious practical advantage in teaching the actors the necessary skills so that they appear technically competent on screen, Morocco hints that there is more going on. It may be no more than a superficial gloss on the Stanislavky 'Method', or it may be something deeper – solace in the manipulation of the real. I'm not quite sure what that means, but I think it is of significance. Perhaps, like Quesalid, the 'sham' shaman famously studied by the anthropologist Franz Boas, in order even to 'act' the part of a healer, one must, at some level, really practise healing (Lévi-Strauss, 1963, p. 175). Even when one knows it is all a sham, one ends up, in some way, suspending disbelief so that acting becomes action. This is not unfamiliar territory for the physician: medicine in the real world is sometimes as much performance as practice. Often bedside manner (arguably a form of performance) is as important as mastery of technique. Practices and performances are inextricably linked. When we, as healthcare professionals, work, we play to an audience. The performance is part of the practice, the acting part of the action.

Script, set, props and actors, all are geared to an accurate reproduction of 'real' life. But what of the medium itself? The 12-, 24- or 36-inch television screen is surely a frame separating reality from representation. I want to look now at the camera work of *ER* as a means of blurring that distinction. A quote from a fan website demonstrates awareness of *ER's* unique shooting style:

> Perhaps *ER*'s greatest quality, alongside its multi-layered characterization and its willingness to explore contentious issues, is its 'cinéma vérité' shooting style. The show's medical emergency sequences are captured with long Steadicam shots that follow the doctors and nurses through the passages, into the emergency rooms, and – even – from room to room. ('ER', 2002)

The Steadicam is a specialized camera plus harness strapped to the cameraman rather than mounted on a tripod or dolly. Its purpose is to isolate the camera from the movement of the cameraman's body. Instead of being stationary or relying on a track or cart to move, the camera can go anywhere a cameraman can walk or run. It transforms the camera and the cameraman into a sort of video cyborg. The operator is free to perform ultra-smooth camera moves – 360-degree pans, booms, and so on – while standing, walking, jumping or running.

Right from its pilot episode, *ER* has been identified with the Steadicam. 'Many have attributed the success of *ER* to this fast paced, reality driven, camera style' (Bouchie, 1999). From a fan-site: 'I tried watching *Chicago Hope* after *ER*, but it just seemed so boring after watching the non-stop Steadicam work in this show' (Mah, 2002). Up to 70–80 per cent of *ER's* footage is shot with a Steadicam. In most television shows, the percentage is less than 1–2 per cent.³

The Steadicam allows the cameraman and the camera to move as a unit, without the jerkiness one gets in home videos. It closely mimics the phenomena of human sight. Our own vision is not jerky, because the brain coordinates the muscles of the eye and tweaks image processing in the brain to compensate for body movement, 'turning a bumpy ride into a smooth flight'. The Steadicam, using a system of springs, balance arms and counterweights, does much the same thing, allowing the screen to reflect more exactly visual perception during body motion. The Steadicam is particularly well suited for certain effects:

Movement: Moving camera shots in tight quarters, where a dolly would bang into walls, door jambs, or trees, and so on. This is what makes it so useful in the enclosed ER that is the set of *ER*. Further, 'For any moving camera shot where the quality of the move contributes to the emotional qualities of the scene, such as the "hardness" of accelerations/decelerations, pans, and so on' (Lapus, 2003). For 'hardness', read 'hard reality'.

Realism: For human or animal points of view, which move through the world realistically. The Steadicam lends itself to an eye-level point of view, which is, in cinematography, considered the 'normal' point of view. It thus mimics, or at the very least marks, presence – that is, the presence of the viewer as an actual participant in the action (Guild, 2002). 'In TV shows like *ER*, Steadicam shots put the audience in the middle of the action, as if they were another character in the show. This simple machine has truly changed the world of filmmaking forever' (Harris, 2002).

Time: The Steadicam is particularly useful in shooting long one-shot-sequences, where the lack of editing, means that the narrative plays out in uninterrupted real-time. It is also used in shots where time is a factor, such as such as during a sunset, when shooting dogs, kids or non-actors, and when shooting VIP's on tight schedules. The Steadicam operator can execute lengthy moves that would previously have consumed inordinate amounts of shooting time to set up. It is useful in situations where changing cameras and bringing in a dolly would interrupt the actors' concentration, or be an unnecessary waste of effort (Lapus, 2003).

I would draw attention to the emphasis placed by directors and cinematographers on the quality of realism that they maintain the

Steadicam delivers. The Steadicam allows real movement in real locations, in real-time, mimicking real ocular physiology. Its aspiration being to make the viewer 'feel' as if they were 'really' there.[4] This aspiration towards the 'real' and the 'present' is not restricted to technique and effect, but also affects the methods of production, as exemplified in the Steadicam's facilitation of the one-shot-sequence.

If you're shooting a sequence in one shot, with no coverage, what you shoot on the day is what you end up with in the final edit. You've done all the editing by choreographing the shot – all the decisions have been made. On the one hand this might seem to be restrictive – locking you into a situation you can't get out of, but you have the advantage of seeing it all in front of you in real-time. What you're doing is to produce there and then what you want to appear on the screen. (Guild, 2002)

The spectacular one-shot sequences that define *ER* are complicated flowing actions, shot in one take with multiple moves and no cutaways. They allow the viewer to run down the hall beside the stretcher, and '[bring] the audience right into the center of the action' (Greene, 1997). The Steadicam wants you *there* and it wants you there *now*.

Accuracy and realism

The medical drama exploits its particular form of realism for a number of purposes. I have identified at least three: image as instruction, image as document and image as entertainment. In each of these, the relation between reality and image, and medium and message, is somewhat different:

Image as instruction

As is evident from the comments of producers and writers and from the research, which shows where the general public gets information about medicine (see below), television is a mode of instruction. The use of representation for instruction requires a form of realism that might be called illustrative realism. This presents a reality distorted by the need to expose the functional relationships and techniques of the portrayed act. This differs from dramatic verisimilitude, which reveals and conceals according to the dictates of narrative structure. Illustration lays the process bare to the dissecting eye, so that it might communicate that information to the constructive hand. In this instructive or illustrative mode, the medium becomes transparent. We need to see through the medium to its content, so that what is seen on the screen might be reproduced in real life. In the case of medical procedures, it requires that we get closer and closer and go deeper and deeper into the human body.

Image as document

Illustrative realism shades into documentary realism, where the value of the image is as a record of what happened. The image is used as an archive of past acts, which then may be used as memento or mnemonic, that is, a fetish for memory. Documentary realism has a claim to some of the same characteristics as illustrative realism. The medium must remain transparent, revealing what actually happened. However, it differs from illustrative realism in that the image is not distorted by the need to understand; all it supposedly portrays is what actually happened. The documentary accuracy of the photographed, filmed or taped image is guaranteed by its indexicality.[5] What the screen portrays is believed to correspond faithfully to reality, because it is a direct record of 'what actually happened'. What is seen is what was, not what is made by the seeing. At least that is the rhetoric of documentary.

Image as entertainment

Though documentary can be entertainment, in drama what counts is that the image should appear plausible, not that it be an accurate reiteration of reality. This is the well-worn path of dramatic verisimilitude. Dramatic verisimilitude, that is, the believability of dramatic representation, demands not precision but plausibility – though the two are not unrelated. Drama need not be accurate, but it must be believable, or at least lead to a suspension of disbelief. This is usually achieved through the classical dramatic devices of consistency, characterization, motivation, narrative flow, and so on. Dramatic verisimilitude relies on the medium being opaque, that is we do not see through it to its content, rather the content is painted upon the medium's surface. In conventional television dramas, the lack of ceilings and a fourth wall, the static point of view, the shadowless lighting are accepted as part of our suspension of disbelief. The medium itself becomes a dramatic convention, signalling the presence of a different world in which we can suspend the laws of the real one so that we might believe what never was or never could be. Dramatic verisimilitude is not about representing the real; rather in conjuring representation into reality, it paints its own version of reality on the opaque screen of the medium.

Though realism and verisimilitude may be complementary, as when accuracy supports plausibility; at other times they may be in conflict, as when aesthetic effect (that is, the production of a specific subjective affect) requires the opacity of the medium and the suspension of disbelief. In classical drama, and most forms of representation, the foregrounded artifice of the medium is the basis of the aesthetic response. The medical drama appears to be a special case, or at least attempts to present itself as a special case, in which aesthetic response cannot exist except as a reaction to the real. All the obsessive accuracy of the scripts, sets and actors, and the intrusive intimacy of the Steadicam, operate to bring us into the action – to turn passive observers into active participants.

What is all this trickery in service to? Certainly, first and foremost, to sell advertising time, and, then, to entertain, document and instruct. However, we need to consider something further – the content of these dramas. Things normally considered obscene, not fit for public viewing: death, suffering, blood and vomit and shit are thrown up onto the screen in an orgy of accurate detail. It is as if the camera's over-determined accuracy will give us the cybernetic vision necessary not merely to penetrate the wounded body but to see through it. But to what? In the modern secular world, we lack an immortal soul, which an image might represent. In the fragmented postmodern world, we lack even a coherent image of the human body. There is no possibility of representation, because there is nothing to represent – beyond the phenomenon of the 'real'. As the show's scripts are, in a way, a failure of narrative, so its camerawork is, in a way, a failure of representation. Forced to forego aesthetics, we are driven to revel in the real.

Only the young die good

Though producers of medical dramas go to extreme lengths to get the medicine right, the TV medical drama is not accurate in all things. Though therapeutic techniques are simulated accurately, their actual outcomes diverge widely from those seen in any real emergency room. In American medical shows of the mid-1990s, there were 75 per cent short-term survival and 67 per cent long-term survival rates (Diem, Lantos and Tulsky, 1996, p. 1578).[6] Most large US centres at that time were reporting long-term survival rates of 2.9–5.2 per cent (Lombardi et al., 1994, p. 678; Stiell, 1999, p. 1175; De Maio et al., 2000, p. 139). Researchers in the social sciences and medical practitioners agree that popular imagination led astray by media misrepresentation has invested CPR with powers of resurrection well beyond its capacities, resulting in unreal expectations in the viewing public (Mead and Turnbull, 1995, p. 39; Diem, Lantos and Tulsky, 1996, p. 1581; P. Gordon, Williamson and Lawler, 1998, p. 780). Diem, Lantos and Tulsky caution that the misrepresentation of CPR on television causes patients to make unwise choices about resuscitation, leading to the overuse of CPR and the indignity of an unnecessarily medicalised death. Thus, it is argued that the false optimism generated by television supports the continued (mis)use of CPR on the streets. It is difficult to deny the contribution of optimistic media-fed expectations to the central imperative to action governing the modern deathbed. The media's co-option of the viewing public into a fantasy of immortality stands accused of denying death and fostering the technological imperative: that all that can be done should be done.

Within the medical profession, there is a great deal of ambivalence about the optimistic media portrayal of resuscitation. The fear is that real-life medicine is judged by the standards of TV medicine and found wanting. Patients (or, more correctly in the case of CPR, patients' families) might be led to demand unrealizable results based on false expectations. Yet, medical staff, as well as families, are appalled by the indignity of aggressive medical technology. Diem makes a plea to the producers of television programmes to 'recognize a civic responsibility to be more accurate' in their survival statistics (1996, p. 1581). Presumably, a more realistic portrayal of CPR and its survival rates on the television screen would result in more sensible expectations on the part of the public, a decrease in futile resuscitative efforts and more death-with-dignity. However, as Diem points out, this is unlikely to happen as the overriding needs of entertainment stand in the way.

Neal Baer (a co-producer of *ER*), in a response to Diem's article, makes the point that, 'Dramatization is at the heart of the question' (1996, p. 1604). One does need to remember that this is entertainment:

> On *ER*, we often present cases of trauma, in which CPR is required because of high dramatic impact. These episodes are fast-paced and visually exciting. If we were to re-enact a minute-by-minute account of actual events in the emergency department, we would

not have 35 million viewers each week. Real life in an emergency room is often quiet, even boring; a television drama cannot be. (1996, p. 1604)

Life snatched from the jaws of death has huge dramatic impact. The medical drama is just that, drama, and producers maintain that audiences are quite capable of distinguishing fact from fiction – that they understand and accept the conventions, exaggerations and distortions necessary in entertainment. Belling points out that the perceptive physician knows that patients may come to him or her with false expectations based on inaccurate media portrayal of survival rates:

> Physicians familiar with those images and able to analyze and interpret them in collaboration with their patients will be in a better position to negotiate the media's rapidly proliferating and often ambiguous representations of health care. (1998, p. 3)

Patients' misconceptions, presumably, can be taken into account and dealt with by a rational presentation of the true figures and frank talk. However, though these mitigating factors do function and are no doubt important, it is not that simple. People's deepest fears and hopes, projected onto the television screen, then re-imbibed in the technical accuracy and statistical fallacy of the medical drama, are not all that easily dispelled by frank talk or critical analysis.

These wildly unrealistic survival rates have been ascribed to modern society's denial of death, to dramatic technique, the requirement for a happy ending and to a cynical manipulation of the media by vested interests within medicine (Diem, Lantos and Tulsky, 1996, p. 1581; Belling, 1998, p. 3; P. Gordon, Williamson and Lawler, 1998, p. 780, Timmermans, 1999, p. 100). Although these are all factors, it is instructive to look at exactly how this sleight of hand is accomplished. The mechanism for the wide discrepancy between survival rates on the screen and on the street rests not on a barefaced lie but on a bias in patient selection (Markert and Saklayen, 1996, p. 1605). On television, 65 per cent of resuscitations occur in children, teenagers and young adults, as opposed to a figure of around 6 per cent in real life (P. Gordon, Williamson and Lawler, 1998, p. 780). On television, 72 per cent of arrests are due to some form of trauma: gunshot wounds, motor vehicle accidents, near-drowning, and so on – 'diseases' of the young and healthy (Crayford, Hooper and Evans, 1997,

p. 1649). Only 28 per cent are due to primary cardiac causes. In real life, 75–95 per cent of arrests are due to primary cardiac disease – a disease of the elderly. In real life, the young and traumatized are much more likely to survive than the old and heartsick. Whereas the survival rate for elderly cardiac patients resuscitated in the intensive care units is around 15 per cent, the survival rate for young adults undergoing resuscitation from trauma is as high as 70 per cent (Markert and Saklayen, 1996, p. 1605).[7] Once selection bias is taken into account, the survival rates portrayed on television are not, in fact, unreasonable. Granted, this bias is hidden from the viewer and thus invites optimistic misinterpretation of survival rates, but we must careful in ascribing this deception solely to ignorance, cynical manipulation or the denial of death. Though these factors do figure in the inflated survival statistics, the sleight of hand produced by patient bias is as much in service to the modern cult of youth, the desire for a particular type of victim and, most importantly, a particularly modern form of death.

'Later the vicar hangs himself ...'

There is seldom an episode of a medical drama in which there is not a resuscitation and/or a death. And, when I say seldom, I mean (almost) never. The following are lifted from the plot synopses of ten episodes of *Casualty*:

- Duncan dies and Jake has a badly injured left leg.
- One of the activists is injured ... though he knows he will die, he refuses treatment.
- An ex-pat, returned from Zimbabwe ... contracted Weil's disease from contaminated canal water, and he soon dies.
- Following a gas explosion at a halfway house for the mentally ill, an injured resident dies in hospital .... After a scuffle, the guilty resident rushes off and throws himself under a train. He is rushed to Casualty but dies.
- Baz is pressured after a man dies after being misdiagnosed by his GP.
- Kate advises a young pregnant girl whose jockey partner has just been kicked to death by a horse.
- Later the vicar hangs himself and is found by his housekeeper: he dies in hospital.
- When the man falls overboard, another suffers a heart attack and dies in the rescue.

- An amateur boxer throws a fight at his trainer's insistence, but collapses and is rushed to Casualty where he dies.
- A drunken driver crashes into the car .... She dies and Kate has to inform the shocked parents.
- An old woman falls downstairs and dies on the way to hospital.
- After attempting to escape from a security van, a Kurdish asylum-seeker finds himself in Casualty .... he runs away and jumps to his death from the hospital roof.
- A building worker ... is distracted on site and accidentally injures a colleague. The colleague dies and his wife leaves him.
- The chauffeur dies and the jogger's legs are crushed.

(Silver, 1998, pp. 60–9)

I could go on. *ER* is even more heavily loaded with death. As already pointed out, the plots of individual episodes and the season's long-term story arcs are to a large extent 'continuity' devices stitching together an hour of resuscitation and death. The fast-paced, episodic format of these dramas, with their sharp cuts and sophisticated editing, is not unrelated to their content. Slick, flashy, hi-tech CPR, straddling the border of life and death, makes for compelling viewing. Unlike classical drama, there is no beginning, middle and end: no *hamartia, anagnorisis, peripeteia, agon* and dénouement.[8] No foreplay and cigarette following, only a rippling succession of climaxes.

It is argued that the unrealistic survival rates of resuscitation on television are a manifestation of our culture's denial of death (Timmermans, 1999, p. 77). I would maintain that optimistic media hyperbole has as much to do with parading death across the television screen as it does with the fantasy of our ability to restore life on the street. Though television's survival statistics give false hope, they do so in service to a morbid voyeurism. Paradoxically, it is the rosy survival statistics that make the ubiquity of the deathbed on television possible. Patients in these television dramas do die, and die frequently. It is important that they die, for the makers of these shows know that a dramatic death is as vital to the survival of the series as a heroic 'save'. Barbara Machin, a writer for *Casualty*, stresses the importance of the Kleenex factor: 'Making people cry is important' (Silver, 1998, p. 27).[9] The fact that, in relative terms, death is the exception rather than the rule serves to increase the absolute frequency of its portrayal and to underscore its dramatic impact. Less is more.

The pornography of death[10]

Return of the repressed

Writers such as Illich (1976), Gorer (1965) and Ariès (1981) have documented the medicalization of death. Death has disappeared down the shining corridors of hospitals to take up residence behind the curtains and closed doors of ERs, ICUs, palliative care wards and hospices. There is little doubt that we as individuals have a much more limited experience of the deathbed than our grandparents did. Death, which is in itself a loss, has also become an absence – absent from everyday life. By and large, the spectacle of the deathbed has gradually been removed from our view. We no longer have public executions. Morgues are no longer open to the curious. People less and less frequently die at home. Today, it is the rare layperson that has touched a body, one minute alive the next dead.

Where then do people get their information about the end of life? Gossip, religious instruction, physicians, grief counsellors, newspapers, books – all contribute, but it has, by and large, fallen to television to broadcast death (D. Davies, 1997, p. 57). For most of us, the contemporary deathbed is, until we lie upon our own, a virtual one. Though the average adult in the West today has never stood in the presence of death, an investigation by the US Department of Justice reveals that, by the age of 18, the average American has seen 40,000 screen deaths (Campbell, 1999, p. 7). For most of us, death is experienced on the screen rather than on the street. It can be argued that representation has stepped in to fill a breach in reality. The experience of the deathbed, once forced upon us by necessity, of which, over the last 100 years, we have been relieved by the modern institutions of the hospital, hospice and funeral home, now returns in the virtual reality of the moving image. Death, like vaudeville, having lost its live audience, has made the canny switch to television. In the twentieth century death abandoned real life for representation. Roland Barthes in 1980, the year of his own death, said:

> Death must be somewhere in society; if it is no longer in religion, it must be elsewhere; perhaps in the image which produces Death while trying to preserve life. Contemporary with the withdrawal of rites, photography may correspond to the intrusion, in our modern society, of an asymbolic Death, outside of religion, outside of ritual, a kind of abrupt dive into literal Death. Life/Death: the paradigm is reduced to a simple click, the one separating the initial pose from the final print. (2000, p. 92)

In the seventeenth century, natural philosophy began to define death in terms of the failure of function. Scientific rationalism's requirement for explanation internal to its operating frame of reference questioned the transcendent, God and heaven as causes of life and as escapes after death. Modernity, in rejecting the transcendent as a source of comfort, also refused it as a source of meaning. In disdaining spiritual worlds and mystical forces, modern death spurns metaphor. There is, for the modern secular humanist, no journey, no choir invisible, no peace which surpasseth all understanding. In the twentieth century, death lost its symbolic function.

We are now in the unprotected position of having to face death as the terminus of individuality. Death can no longer be portrayed as a thing different from but connected to life. Rather, death is a condition of life, its end and negation. As pure negation, it is difficult to embody in metaphor. Like anti-matter, it destroys any metaphorical vehicle that attempts its transport. There are 'No substitutions allowed'. We may no longer hide from death in analogy. 'In effect, in the postmodern world real death becomes an allegory only of itself' (R. Brown, 2000). Bereft of metaphor, there is no delicate turning away from the act, no curtain tastefully drawn before the final scene. Today, physicians, police and social workers are instructed, when announcing a death, to avoid euphemisms and say that the dead 'are dead' – not 'passed away', 'departed' or 'gone'. On TV, in film and on the front pages of the newspapers, death cannot be portrayed but by the dead. Death is not like anything, nor is anything like death. Dead is dead.

Without euphemisms or allegorical images to encompass death, the indexicality of photographic, cinematic and televisual images of dying do something speech cannot – they put before our eyes that which has become unspeakable, that for which we no longer have words. No longer able to comprehend death through language, we attempt to apprehend it through the lens. The failure of narrative in modernity binds us to a kind of morbid voyeurism which compels us to document death as graphically as possible.

Photograph, film and video become documents, evidence not only of death but of witness to that death. As document, the image captured by the camera attempts to convince us that its content is real, that it is unconstructed being, the world as it is. At the same time, the image, by being offered for public consumption, insists that its content is significant, that it is valuable. The indexicality of the camera's image becomes a means of inscribing value upon fact, to convince us that fact and value are the same, that is, to convince us that what we are shown is truth. The traumatic realism of the overly accurate resuscitation scene is conflated with the value of death. It becomes a means of 'outing' death. Publicity for a value judgement that condemns the invisibility of the dying and the denial of death. As described earlier, in my analysis of the mythic constituents of CPR, there are, in those heroic performances on television by Drs Green, Carter and Ross, still traces of the Romantic impulse towards narrative and meaning, but the aspiration of these spectacular resuscitative vignettes is to negate both narrative and meaning in a mediated drive towards immediate experience. The traumatic realism of the resuscitative scene is meant to arouse us. But the camera cheats, for it demands an emotional response not to the life that was lived, but to the spectacle of death – not to the story but to the image. And this elision of image and act carries a particular force – the force of the pornographic.

Existential pornography

> The waning of the twentieth century has been accompanied by a gathering fascination with death. Whether overt or implicit, a preoccupation with transience and extinction runs through much of the work produced by artists today .... they explore the most distressing aspects of existence with cool, alert precision.
>
> (Cork, 2000)

A half-century ago, the sociologist Geoffrey Gorer, in *The Pornography of Death* (1955), argued that because death has become invisible, hidden away by modern society, our thwarted fascination with it emerges in overly graphic and violent portrayals of death in the media. Death repressed in real life as obscene returns in the media as pornography. Pornography, he maintains, requires two things: repression and a medium for the return of the repressed (1965, p. 192). Repression, occurs because something is forbidden, because it is considered obscene, that is, unfit for public viewing. Certainly, the sex act has fallen within that category and it is around representations of sex that most arguments about the pornographic occur. But the actual derivation of the word obscene, from the Latin meaning 'off-stage', *obscaena*, referred specifically to death. Though Greek tragedy is glutted with death, violent death, Aeschylus condemned the portrayal of the actual moment of death on stage. However, in modern culture, as opposed to Greek tragedy, there has been a reversal of obscenity – it is now real-life death that is obscene, not its representation.

For Gorer, pornography was the explicit (the private made public) representation (mediated act) of a forbidden act (the transgression of social norms) for the purpose of arousal (the eliciting of desire) (1965, pp. 192–5). The pornographic is thus determined not only by its content (repressed desire) and its form (the private made public), but by the presence of laws that render the experience transgressive (lawbreaking). However, pornography transgresses in a way that, though illicit, remains tacitly accepted (Kipnis, 1998, p. 155). It performs this sleight of hand via a mediated transgression: a crime one step removed from its actual enactment. It is tolerated, when it is tolerated, because it is representation, because it occurs on paper, film or magnetic tape. Yet this dispensation given by mediation is at the same time a condemnation. Pornography in being representation, image rather than act, is condemned for not being real. It is condemned as voyeurism – second-order experience, where the image replaces the act, where the eye replaces the hand. Pornography's intent is to produce feelings or affects normally engendered by participation in someone who watches but does not act. Affect (in the case of sexual pornography sexual arousal) is induced in the absence of presence. And we find this absence of presence reprehensible. Pornography is a transgression: undoubtedly of social norms, often of the rights of the object of desire and certainly of the border between reality and representation.

In hard-core sexual pornography, sex acts actually take place: 'acting' in the dramatic sense is also the act enacted; the performance is real. Feminists have pointed out that the production of pornography often involves violence to and abasement of the object of desire (Dworkin, 1981; Gubar and Hoff, 1989; Mackinnon, 1993). Pornography, in this formulation, is not really about sex, but about gender relations and power – in most cases, the empowerment of men and the oppression of women. The male gaze is a fetishizing scopophilia that succeeds in naturalizing male power and containing the female body – physically, psychically, socially and politically (Mulvey, 1975, p. 18). Pornography stands accused of inciting men to re-enact the scenes they view. Pornography stands accused of being no mere fantasy but a call to action. Pornography is thus condemned for being produced by a crime and, in turn, inciting crime.

Photograph, filmstrip and video tape are bounded and defined by crimes of production and consumption. As the production of sexual pornography involves the performance of an actual sex act, so its consumption is realized in another act, that of sexual arousal. As the actors in the video cross the line between performing and doing, so in our arousal we slip from being spectators to participants. In the pornographic, aesthetic distance, if one believes in such a thing, dwindles to a fine postmodern line across which representation and reality slip back and forth. Pornography is damned as representation confounded with reality: an image confounded with an act. Pornography is thus accused of transgressing the boundaries of the 'aesthetic experience' (Gorer, 1965, p. 196). Gorer's chief criticism of what he considered the pornographic return of death is that its confusion of aesthetic response with physical and moral responses results in desensitization of the voyeur to the act in the real world. Pornography's violence and lack of concomitant emotional content blunt the viewers' sensitivities to interpersonal violence and the profound implications of death in the real world (1965, p. 195). Spectatorship of the pornographic removes the real-life danger, that, in realizing my own pleasure, if I hurt, I will be hurt back. The confounding of aesthetic, moral and physical experiences, he maintains, leads us to feel the wrong things to the wrong extent for the wrong reasons (1965, p. 195). Of course, the attraction of pornography is that, in the presence of desire and the absence of its object, it allows us to feel something at all.

Over the last 50 years, earlier readings of sexual pornography have been challenged by media, pro-porn feminist and queer theorists. Pornography, some maintain, is not always about gender, power and violence; sometimes, it is just about sex (Kipnis, 1998, p. 154). Norms do shift – what was not so long ago considered obscene now has a PG13 rating.[11] Power relations can be renegotiated – as they have with women taking major production and directorial roles in the porn industry. Pornography is championed as providing a vernacular for a reconstruction of the language of sex, made necessary by the changed sexualities of the postmodern and post-AIDS world. Pornography by holding 'a mirror up to culture, mapping its borders and boundaries through strategic acts of transgression' defines not just the bounds of behaviour, but culture, social order and, ultimately, the social subject. The hidden links between the structures of culture and the structure of the human psyche transfix us in front of the pornographic scene. Pornography distils issues central to culture and to the constitution of the self, and reiterates them through the code of transgression. Perusal of and participation in the pornographic image is an act of free will that goes beyond the bounds of decency, beyond the conventionalized boundaries of the human action, and, as an act outside of the conventionalized borders of humanity, it defines those very borders (Kipnis, 1998, pp. 155-7). Pornography becomes a necessary code attempting to communicate what lies beyond culture and language.

Verisimilitude, violation and vitality

To return to the issue of dramatic verisimilitude and the over-determined technical accuracy of representations of CPR on television, verisimilitude is guaranteed, not by the traditional verities of drama – consistency, characterization, motivation, and so on – but by instrumental accuracy. This is taken to its extreme in the indexicality of 'reality' television, shows such as *Rescue 911* or *Trauma* where real-life ambulance calls, emergency room resuscitations and surgical operations are broadcast as 'entertainment'. Rather than drama representing life, life presents the drama – the relationship between performance and act is reversed. Even in shows such as *ER*, *Casualty*, *A&E* and *Scrubs*, which are obviously fictional dramas, the scripts are written by practising doctors, the actors trained in the skills of physicians and the progress of 'patients' determined by what amount to studio-based morbidity and mortality rounds. The performance is guaranteed by what is accurate rather than what is plausible, or, rather, what is projected as plausible is valorized by its accuracy. Performance is not merely a plausible representation of the act, but its actual enactment. Apparently, whatever it is that is that needs communication can be communicated only by the performance of the act itself.

And, what if the act itself is also a form of performance? I maintain elsewhere that CPR persists because in addition to being a medical protocol, CPR is also a form of deathbed ritual. As ritual, CPR is as much a performance on the street as it is on the screen. This is not to deny that there is a very real difference between pumping on someone's chest in a supermarket and in the television studio, but those who stand watching on the street often comment on how 'unreal' the whole experience is, while those who watch the television screen are often disconcerted by its 'reality'. The pornographic performance communicates the 'reality' of its content via the indexicality of the photographic, cinematic or televisual medium. This slippage between reality and representation results in and is identified by what Laura Kipnis calls a *frisson* or shudder. This shudder, produced by the 'real', equated with the orgasm of the voyeur, becomes the sign or mark of the pornographic.

Linda Williams asks whether sexual pornography is a quest for a truth which cannot be represented, namely, female sexual pleasure (quoted in Kipnis 1998, p. 155). Kipnis goes further, arguing that the pornographic object becomes the signifier for a signified that resists the very boundaries of signification – that is, it expresses that which lies beyond expression (1998, p. 157). In like fashion, the highly charged life-and-death scenes enacted on television fail to articulate death. In the modern world, death is beyond articulation. Rather, these images act as the inexplicable vehicles of a signifier that is suffered not spoken. This signifier is marked by or rather is a shudder: a *frisson*. The *frisson* partakes of the somatic, the aesthetic and the moral, being a physical reaction to a representation of real transgression. The *frisson* engendered by the existentially pornographic conflates the aesthetics of life with the physicality of death and the morality of the human. The *frisson* marks the crossing of forbidden thresholds – and pleasure in that crossing – marking out the very boundaries of the human, as it steps over them.

This pornographic conflation of physical, aesthetic and moral experience transports us into a subjective state that is confounded with objective reality. In it, we experience what is absent from modern life – death – and we experience what is absent from the dead – life. At the juncture where technology fails and discourse falls silent, the camera's lens constructs modern death. We point the camera as we might aim a gun, stopping dead all self-narratives of being. We make of the dead *things*, distancing ourselves from them, not just to achieve the emotional detachment necessary to go on living, not just to relegate the dead to memory, but so that we might apprehend what we as survivors are graced with and sentenced to – life.

As pointed out in the preceding chapter, our modern scientific concept of life is not substantive. 'Life consists in the sum of the functions by which death is resisted' (Bichat 1827, p. 10). Life is a silent absence at the centre of being. In CPR's performance, both on the street and on the screen, the frailty of the existential status of life is compensated for by a traumatic excess that attempts to fill the emptiness of the real, the absence of the objective entities of life and self, with the erotic. Translating the invisible into the visible, the felt into the seen, the relational into the existent, the absent into the present demands excess. Lacking the ability to articulate 'being' through the language of the transcendent, transgression replaces transcendence, marking out a void in the language of modernity.

The pornography of death arouses in us an apprehension of life, not as a physiological concept, metaphysical construct or moral imperative but as inchoate feeling. The *frisson*, the shudder, is both triumph at a life that its very presence substantiates and terror at the absence that lies at its heart. And so we look and turn away and look again, finding pleasure in a brutality we cannot comprehend. This ambivalent gaze, which both desires and rejects the pornographic object, is more than a pathological animadversion. It is the gaze turned in upon itself, the subject as object of its own curiosity. But, what one sees is not what one is looking for, oneself. Rather, what confronts us is an empty space, constituted by the absence of the objective entities of life and self. This void, drawing to itself the gaze it rejects, in the end, must signal its existence through unintelligible affect. In the end, must make do with a mere shudder. In the end, we violate the dead so that we might feel alive.

Street and screen

CPR on the screen, while directly promoting the act of resuscitation, the heroism of medical staff and the dramatic return of life, is, nevertheless, at the same time, the scene through which struts the medical drama's dark star: death. And death is, in turn, re-presented in service to modernity's somewhat tenuous concept of life. If CPR on the street is always ritual as well as protocol, then it is always also performance as well as act.

> Everyone is familiar with defibrillation shocks from television and movies. Everyone knows to expect the 'jump' and muscle contractions whenever a character yells 'clear'.... Often friends and relatives will be at the scene of an emergency. If you respond and take action, these people will look to you to perform precisely and confidently .... Your instructor will encourage you to anticipate many of the scenarios described above. The case scenarios will include role-playing and rehearsals .... practice, is a good technique for improving future performance. (Cummins, 2001, p. 43)

'Characters', 'audience', 'scenarios', 'roles', 'rehearsals' are here used in a straightforward sense, innocent of what they are demanding: performance. Onto the rescuer's shoulders is placed the burden not only of the competent execution of the protocol but also of the convincing performance of ritual as it is practised in 'television and movies'. Though the technique of CPR on the television screen is, as we have seen, obsessively patterned after the protocol of CPR as practised on the street, the application of CPR on the street is now governed, more and more, by expectations of it determined by CPR on the screen. The onscreen confounding of representation and reality in television's pornographic reconstruction of death is complicated by CPR, its chosen image, being ritual as well as protocol, and as such being a form of performance even before it has been fictionalized and broadcast. This circle (vicious or otherwise, depending on one's point of view) of performance on the street and the screen is made possible by the constant elision of reality and representation in both locations.

Whether we like it or not, the media image of CPR determines not only how death is perceived in the real world but also how it proceeds. Without television, film and video, the therapeutic manoeuvres of external cardiac compression, defibrillation and mouth-to-mouth might still be used to correct deficiencies of blood flow, cardiac rhythm and oxygenation; but it would be no secular ritual constructing death. Neither EMS systems, the structuring of critical care around resuscitative protocols nor CPR would exist in the way they do without the media, and specifically without television (Troy, 1996, p. 1605; Wallack and Bingle, 1996, p. 1605). I would suggest that CPR is less a prescriptive medical protocol picked up by television to add colour and excitement to drama (though it is certainly that), than a ritual drama, played out in a medium that has become as real to us as life itself.

8
Conclusion: Modern Living/ Modern Dying

> In a faithless world, the paramedic is the atheist clergyman of the urban emergency, showing up with a bag like a priest ready to administer the last rites.
>
> (Peter Bradshaw, *Guardian* review of *Bringing Out the Dead*, 2000, p. 15)

In the climactic scene of Bringing Out the Dead. *The paramedic, Frank, and his partner, Tom, are slowly cruising the streets in the ambulance. They see Noel – a crazed street person, a regular abuser of the ambulance system. Noel saunters down the street, smashing the windows of parked cars with a baseball bat. Tom, angry at Noel, suggests teaching him a lesson: 'Frank, this is the guy. I've been after him for weeks.... You start talkin' to him 'bout baseball or somethin' and I'll sneak around behind him and get down and you push him. When he falls we get him.' Frank gets out of the ambulance and walks over to Noel. He starts talking to him about the World Series. Noel sees Tom sneaking up on him and runs away. Tom pursues Noel. Frank follows. Frank walks cautiously down a dark alley strewn with garbage. He turns the corner. Suddenly a loud yell. There is Tom swinging a baseball bat down onto Noel's head. 'Nooooooooo!' Frank lunges forward. Pushes Tom off Noel. The bat clatters to the pavement. Noel, face covered in blood, begins to seize. Frank crouches over him: 'Get the kit. We're going to tube him.' 'What the fuck!' 'Get the kit .... You're going to be all right Noel. We're going to save you.' Bloody vomit pours from Noel's mouth. Frank places his left ear next to Noel's mouth. No breath. His left hand goes to Noel's nose, pinches it closed. Frank gulps in air, seals his mouth over Noel's, and breathes. Frank leans* back. *The alley is quiet, just the sound of Frank taking in another breath. He leans forward again, seals his mouth over Noel's, blows. Again. Again. Again. We can hear Frank's slow regular breaths as he blows air into Noel's lungs. The camera now overhead looks down onto Frank's white shirted-back as he bends over Noel, rocking back and forth with each breath. Sudden cut to the exterior of the emergency room. Noel survives.*

(Bringing, 1999)

CPR: the final performance

The climax of the film *Bringing Out the Dead* is the paramedic protagonist's performance of CPR on Noel, the filthy, crazy, disease-ridden 'dirtball', the lowest common denominator of humanity. Prior to this scene, the film had documented Frank's downward spiral into alcoholism and psychosis, occasioned by a fatal error he made in treating a young female asthmatic. Significantly, the girl's death was due to Frank's insistence on performing and then failing to accomplish a technical airway manoeuvre: intubation, when mouth-to-mouth would have sufficed. The dead girl haunts Frank. The scene in which he administers mouth-to-mouth to Noel marks the turning point of the film and Frank's ascent back into the realm of the human. Following this scene, Frank stops drinking and hallucinating, and he begins to sort out his troubled relationship with his girlfriend. Through the heroic act of performing mouth-to-mouth on Noel and by exposing himself to danger Frank sacrifices himself, performing a kind of penance and receiving absolution for his failure to provide the 'kiss-of-life' to the asthmatic girl. Through an act of transgression, he is saved, becoming both priest and sacrifice, redeemer and redeemed.

Though the violence of CPR is decried, it yet remains. As a medical protocol, CPR attempts to save life by the practical application of positivist science. As a deathbed ritual, CPR attempts to counter the dangers that surround the deathbed through the performance of a series of symbolic acts. External cardiac compression – an act of violence, necessary for the identification and translation of the dead – is, for the survivor, both an act of murder and of catharsis. Both the guilt of the murderer and the joy of survivor must be atoned for. Mouth-to-mouth, precisely because of its transgressive nature, hedged in with danger and impurity, is the sacrificial act that atones for the necessary but forbidden violence. If external cardiac compression gives life power over death, then mouth-to-mouth repays that debt by exposing life to death. The impure soul in braving impurity is made pure again. Through an act of transgression, one is saved. CPR has given us a secular narrative of loss, sacrifice and redemption – a story, in the tradition of Vladimir Propp's classic folktale, where the violence of living in the world is countered by and redeemed through transgressive access to a transcendent realm of power. 'In a faithless world', no longer able to save ourselves through prayer, salvation is made possible through action.

The techniques of CPR, having erased from medical consciousness their connections to the symbolic, and thus their connections to the past and to history, borrow from what is to hand, in this case contemporary physiological theory, the justification necessary for their continued performance. The symbolic force of the imaginary cloaks itself in the language of scientific reason to slip past our defences so that we might continue our sacrificial ritual. However, as powerful as ritual and myth are, and despite the fact that they continue to function below the surface of modern medical therapeutics and media representation, there are complications.

Complications

In attempting to fulfil the physical, psychological and symbolic needs of victim, rescuer and survivor, CPR discloses internal tensions that compromise the goals of both CPR-as-protocol and CPR-as-ritual. The most serious of these are exclusion from the deathbed, distortion of technique and indignity.

Medicalization

The technical demands of CPR-as-protocol may overshadow the psychological and spiritual needs of the dying patient and their family. Thus we have the problem of the medicalization of death, blamed to a great extent on the CPR protocol. Medicalization results in the invisibility of modern death and the exclusion of the family from the deathbed. Those who must mourn the dead are prevented from actively participating in those deaths. The act of dying is uncoupled from the act of mourning. However, as discussed, countervailing forces are at work, manifest within that same CPR protocol. The necessity of lay participation in CPR creates an opportunity for agency to be handed back to the rescuer/survivor/mourner. CPR's increasing ubiquity (over 70 million Americans trained) is paralleled by an expansion of techniques available to the layperson (AEDs). These moves are significant in more than just therapeutic terms, for they bring the lay rescuer into a position closer to the deathbed and the moment of death.

Science hindered

In attempting to fulfil psychological, social and spiritual needs, the performance of CPR-as-ritual may hinder the technical advance of the scientific protocol. An example of this is the retention of chest compression, despite lack of evidence for its efficacy. There is a danger that CPR's use as ritual (a universal and unifying response to death) might overshadow and impede its development as therapy (a specific technique to reverse a specific pathophysiological process). Ritual is innately conservative. It constructs and preserves social order by generating meaning, which, to a large extent, means that ritual constructs its own truth. It forms a closed system impeding the process of self-correcting error that is the method of progressive science. Present moves to rationalize the deathbed, both from the psycho-social-spiritual perspective seeking to revive the death-with-dignity and from the medical perspective seeking to de-ritualize CPR by increasing its therapeutic specificity, may be hampered by our apparent need for a comprehensive ritual.

Indignity

Once the protocol-as-ritual becomes a media phenomenon, representational distortion feeds back into the medical system via public expectation to become a social imperative. In this, the physical and psychological needs of the individual dying patient are sacrificed to the symbolic and representational needs of the collective, that is, the family, the medical system and society. The dying become objectified, alienated and dehumanized as sacrificial victims to heroic positivism, redemption through action and the technological imperative. CPR-as-ritual risks violating individual autonomy regarding choice at the end of life – that is, it removes 'dignity' from the dying process. By being swept up into a universal, ritualized response to sudden death, the victim ultimately fails in their completion of the modern project of the reflexive construction of self.

The end-result, unfortunately, is often that many whose condition is well beyond the reach of any current treatment and who may have readied themselves for death are swept away in the enthusiasm of those who surround the deathbed. It has been recognized, since the very inception of resuscitative protocols in the eighteenth century, that not all the dying are fit subjects for resuscitation:

> But lest any, from what has been said on the subject of restoring animation, should wish to have experiments made in cases where there can be no probability of success, it may not be amiss to observe, – attempts cannot be encouraged for the recovery of those who are worn out with age, or die of diseases which essentially injure the organs of the body. (Lathrop, 1787, pp. 17–28)

The same is recognized today by *Guidelines 2000*:

> For many people the last beat of their heart *should* be the last beat of their heart. These people simply have reached the end of their life. A disease process reaches the end of its clinical course, and a human life stops. In these circumstances, resuscitation is unwanted, unneeded, and impossible. If started, resuscitation efforts for these people are inappropriate, futile, undignified, and demeaning to both the patient and rescuers. Good ACLS requires careful thought about when to stop resuscitative efforts – and even more important – *when not to start*. (Cummins, 2001, p. 49)

The death-with-dignity movement, the social sciences and medical practitioners all support attempts to make people's deaths as comfortable and dignified as possible. Few physicians advocate beating the elderly to death in fruitless attempts to revive the unrevivable. It *is* recognized that pursuing life at all costs is not desirable or even possible. Changes to the asystole algorithm in *Guidelines 2000*, reflect this:

> *Asystole: The Silent Heart Algorithm*:
> Asystole is a cardiac arrest rhythm associated with no discernable electrical activity on the ECG ('flat line') .... A large per centage of asystolic patient do not survive .... [It is necessary to] recognize that asystole usually represents a confirmation of death rather than a rhythm to be treated.... In such scenarios, resuscitation fades as a high priority action. Prolonged efforts are unnecessary, futile, often unethical, and ultimately dehumanizing if not demeaning .... The major focus of the asystole case [has] changed from learning the few things you can try to reverse asystolic arrest to learning the care you can provide when you realize that asystole is usually the end of a person's life ...

- To preserve the dignity of the patient and the patient's loved ones at the end of the patient's life, Emergency Departments, in-hospital code teams, and EMS responders should adopt the new AHA criteria for [termination of] resuscitative efforts much sooner than currently practiced....
- To enable EMS professionals to participate effectively and with dignity in the end of the patient's life, EMS systems should develop supportive protocols that ... allow EMS personnel to provide end-of-life comfort and care but free them from an obligation to attempt resuscitation should the victim develop cardiac arrest.
- To enable Emergency Department and critical care unit personnel to provide the therapeutic benefits of having the patient's family present at resuscitative attempts, Emergency Departments, in-hospital code teams, and EMS responders should give thoughtful considerations to this new concept. (Cummins, 2001, pp. 109–10)

As logical and well meant as these attempts at change are, they are not without significant problems. The issue of advance directives is a good example of the difficulties involved in reconciling the conflicting claims of the deathbed. Studies indicate that many elderly and chronically ill patients continue to opt for CPR, despite attempts to convince them otherwise. Rates of those opting for CPR vary from 10 per cent to as high as 90 per cent, with most studies reporting rates at around 50 per cent (Schonwetter et al., 1991, p. 372; Murphy et al., 1994, p. 545). These patients tend to grossly overestimate their chances of survival. This is blamed on the reluctance of patients and physicians to discuss end-of-life issues and on distorted media portrayal of survival rates (Timmermans, 1999, p. 187). When these misconceptions are corrected by providing information about actual survival figures,[1] the number of patients opting for CPR drops, but may still be as high as 40 per cent (Murphy et al., 1994, p. 545). A large multi-centre study (the SUPPORT study) has shown that implementation of the ideally rationalized deathbed, even with the cooperation of medical caregivers and with considerable institutional support, remains exactly that, an ideal. The provision of accurate prognostic data and enhanced physician-patient communication had no measurable effect on the practice of CPR or the implementation of advance directives. Increased awareness of actual survival figures and increased expressed concern for patient autonomy did not alter the use of DNR (do not resuscitate) orders, the number of episodes of CPR, the number of days spent in undesirable states before death and the use of ICU technology (SUPPORT, 1995, p. 1591).

> Because there was no movement towards what would seem to be better practices, one could conclude that physicians, patients, and families are fairly comfortable with the current situation. Certainly most patients and families indicated they were satisfied, no matter what happened to them .... In conclusion, we are left with a troubling situation. The picture we describe of the care of seriously ill or dying persons is not attractive. One would certainly prefer to envision that, when confronted with life-threatening illness, the patient and family would be included in discussions, realistic estimates of outcome would be valued, pain would be treated and dying would not be prolonged. That is still a worthy vision. However, it is not likely to be achieved through an intervention such as that implemented by SUPPORT. (SUPPORT, 1995, p. 1596)

Thus, despite concerted attempts to stop the inappropriate application of CPR, it appears that the practice persists in spite of both physicians' and patients' declared aversion to it.[2] When the moment of crisis arrives and push comes to shove, it appears that it is enormously difficult for family and medical personnel to stand by and do nothing. This is not to imply that the well-managed death-with-dignity is doing nothing. Physical, psychological and spiritual support, the skilled use of opiates, a caring environment, and so on are all *doing* something. But they are not, it would appear, at least in popular culture and in the eyes of many families, doing enough.

In controversies over DNR orders, euthanasia and the rationing of healthcare, the public expresses its wariness of a medical system that, denying an absolute value to life, takes upon itself the task of valuing some lives over others, of determining who should live and who should die. At the deathbed, the ambivalent relationships between protocol and ritual, act and performance, means and ends result in confusion over what is empirically causative, what is psychologically desirable and what is symbolically communicable. The social sciences, while pointing out these confusions and condemning CPR as ritual (at least as a ritual not to their taste), at the same time demands of physicians an increased sensitivity to the spiritual needs of patients. Medicine, taking this to heart, is attempting to rationalize both CPR and the deathbed.

Rationalization

I have argued that CPR survives because it is as much deathbed ritual as medical protocol, and that this synthesis of protocol and ritual has been a neat and useful package. However, it is an unstable alliance. The imperative to 'do everything' is not necessarily welcomed by healthcare professionals:

> Many physicians and nurses experience, at present, a large gap between what they feel they should do and what they feel they are obliged to do for patients at the end of life. (Vancouver, 1996b)

Aside from concerns about indignity, many within medicine resent what they see as undue pressure to waste time and resources on the unsalvageable.[3] Furthermore, medicine's unwitting connivance at the deceit necessary for the practice of what I maintain is occult ritual lies heavy on the medical conscience. Hence the lament 'Why are we beating a dead horse?' Medics dislike being coerced by the practice of futile heroics into betraying the cult of rationality. Medicine prides itself in repudiating ritual and superstition. But it's not easy. Having usurped the priest's place at the deathbed; it's hard for the physician to keep his hands off religion's tools. Medicine's ambivalence towards CPR-as-ritual is perhaps most evident in its frequent practice yet strong condemnation of the 'slow code' (sometimes called a 'Hollywood Code').[4] The slow code is poorly defined, but is essentially going through the motions of CPR – a half-hearted attempt to look as if you are doing something when in fact you are not. 'The practice of responding to a cardiac arrest with a "slow code" is wholly unethical and not acceptable in any circumstances' (Vancouver, 1998). The reasons given for the frequent use of the 'slow code' include fears of litigation, a perverse desire for control on the part of medical staff and expectations of the family. The slow code is grudgingly condoned when it is perceived as being 'done for the sake of the family' and, despite the above imperative, it is a not uncommon occurrence. It should be obvious that the slow code is undisguised CPR-as-ritual and that the healthcare professional is, understandably, uncomfortable with being forced to administer 'last rites' as an 'atheist clergyman'.

Physicians are thus forced to examine CPR critically. Indeed, this book would not be possible had cracks not begun to appear in CPR's façade. As previously discussed, *Guidelines 2000* contains the most sweeping changes to the BCLS and ACLS protocols since their inceptions. The early use of defibrillation made possible by the spread

Conclusion: Modern Living/Modern Dying 227

of AEDs, disclaimers on mouth-to-mouth and moves to honour advance directives are evidence of attempts to rationalize the protocol (American, 2000, pp. I.371–I.376). 'Evidence-based medicine' is promoted as debunking many of the myths surrounding CPR:

> The reputation of the guidelines has been enhanced by the gradual move toward evidence-based recommendations, which provide information about the strength of the scientific evidence behind each recommendation. If the scientific basis for a recommendation is weak and based mainly on accepted practice, it is hoped that the clear indication of a paucity of scientific evidence will stimulate research. (American, 2000, pp. I.77–I.85)

In the case of ACLS arrhythmia algorithms:

> Meticulous, systematic review reveals that relevant, valid, and credible evidence to confirm a benefit due to these [pharmacological] agents simply does not exist.... It was not until the 1990s that researchers discovered the dismal truth that antiarrhythmics drugs were acting more like proarrhythmic agents. Drugs given to prevent VF/VT arrest appear to generate VF/VT arrest. (American, 2000, pp. I.136–I.165)

The ACLS algorithms are thus being simplified by the elimination of many of the complex multiple-drug regimes that were used in the past. More importantly, treatment is being particularized – specific drugs or therapies being recommended for very specific conditions. The emphasis is less on all-inclusive algorithms and more on an increased specificity of diagnosis. An example is the conversion of the single 'Tachycardia Algorithm' of 1994 to the three distinct, though interrelated 'Narrow Complex Tachycardia', 'Stable Ventricular Tachycardia', and 'Atrial Fibrillation and Flutter' Algorithms of *Guidelines 2000* (Cummins, 1994, p. 1.33; Hazinski, Cummins and Field, 2000, pp. 15–19). The first two of these three are still constructed as algorithms, but are considerably simplified, and the third has assumed the format of a table. Though seemingly minor, these changes signal a significant shift from the universal to the particular, from protocol to prescription.

This rationalization of technique works to prise apart the heterogeneous origins, diverse aetiologies and mixed goals that have, since its inception, put the protocol under enormous tension, but also given it considerable power. The neat pattern of the ABCs of resuscitation and the chain-of-survival, which provided such an attractive unified approach to action in the face of the common end-state of death, is being threatened. Instead of a universal protocol particularizing itself through a constantly branching algorithmic progression towards a single goal, we are moving towards multiple therapeutic prescriptions that offer little other than their initiating manoeuvres – defibrillation for ventricular fibrillation, specific drugs for specific arrhythmias, ventilation for respiratory insufficiency, pacing for bradycardia,[5] IV fluids for shock, and so on. This is a continuation of the already established trend of refining the protocol into protocols – CPR becoming ACLS, PALS, NALS, ATLS, and so on. Each therapeutic formula, in becoming more specific to the conditions for which it is used, becomes more limited in the number of individuals to whom it may be applied. Comprehensiveness is traded for specificity. I should emphasize that this is, from the point of view of scientific validity and practical efficacy, no bad thing.

This rationalization of CPR-as-protocol is at the same time the demystification of CPR-as-ritual. The tacit admission of the ineffectiveness of external cardiac compression through the upgrading of defibrillation with AEDs reduces the scope for heroic action to the panache with which one can peel the protective backing off a defibrillator pad. The downgrading of mouth-to-mouth also appears to be a triumph of, if not scientific, then at least psychological fact, in that it recognizes the futility of insisting on the application of a technique, no matter how efficacious, that few are actually willing to do. Advance directives and the substitution of therapeutic discourse for futile heroics point towards an abandonment of atavistic, primary thinking for positive, logical reason. Protocol, by being deconstructed into its specific techniques, appears to be attempting to exorcize itself of ritual. Is this then the end of CPR-as-ritual?

Protocol/ritual

I think not – for a number of reasons. First, as a protocol, the techniques of CPR, though being reconstituted, continue, particularly in its BLS form as practised by the lay public, to hold together nicely as a universal and unified response to sudden death. Also CPR, or rather the concept of the chain-of-survival as realized in CPR, by becoming a structuring paradigm for healthcare delivery, has accrued enormous ideological, economic and political power within medical institutions. The protocol's position is further strengthened by its representation in the media, where, at least for the time being, its ability to sell advertising time makes it unlikely to be withdrawn from our screens. Further, its instantiation as a 'standard of practice' in courts of law and the increased policing of all professions through litigation would make it difficult to dislodge entirely.

Secondly, in its ritual aspect, the proliferation of AEDs, despite their displacement of chest compression, has re-energized vitalist imagery, putting the mysterious power of electricity in the hands of the lay public, drawing them into the ritual structure and nearer to the moment of death. Furthermore, external cardiac compression has not disappeared; it has merely shifted position. Symbolically significant, physically satisfying and representationally dramatic, it yet remains. Likewise, mouth-to-mouth's status, though downgraded, has in reality changed little. It has always been and remains more 'honour'd in its breach' – the seldom practised but constantly fantasized act of heroic sacrifice. The persistent problems involved in the implementation of advance directives, our continued (ab)use of CPR and its unrelenting media proliferation indicate that its ritual aspect has far from disappeared.

Thirdly, protocol and ritual are inseparable. The one is always shadowed by the other. Both allow for action in a crisis. Both are responses to the anxiety induced by a suddenly disordered world, where the macrocosm of a world gone awry is reflected in the microcosm of the subject as anxiety. Protocol and ritual attempt to bring the world and the subject back into order. The very real threat of sudden death is the crisis that triggers the practical acts of CPR-as-protocol in an attempt to recoup life. However, in such crisis situations, the efficacy of any practical act is itself under threat, for the likelihood of success is small. It is precisely because the likelihood of success is small that protocol is brought into play in the first place. Protocols tend to come into play in those situations in which active intervention stands a significant chance of *not* working. Thus, even the authoritative directives of protocol cannot guarantee success and, because the success of the practical act *is* under threat, there is a tendency for its symbolic content to become explicit in the hope that symbol might succeed where practical action has failed.

Protocol, on failing to transform the world through practical action, slides towards ritual, transforming instead the subject through symbol action. This elision of protocol and ritual is inevitable. Protocol is the incarnation of hope within the realm of reason, but hope's origin is always extra-rational, if not it would be judgement. Ritual is the capitulation of reason, in the hope that success, denied in the immanent, might be achieved in the transcendent. Practical acts accrue symbolic import; imperatives become performatives. A threat to the body becomes a threat to the subject. Protocol and ritual unite in the hope of imposing order on chaos. As we slide further into the chaos of the deathbed, the return of life is pre-empted by the construction of death: the power of the act by the power of the sign. The technique is no longer valued for its effect on the object of the protocol (that is, conversion of the patient's ventricular fibrillation to normal sinus rhythm), but for its effect on the subject of the ritual (that is, relief of the survivor's existential anxiety). The revival of the object is transformed into the redemption of the subject. The victim is sacrificed for the good of the survivor. At a critical point, at the point where life becomes death, act and symbol unite, breaching the boundary between causality and analogy, so that the identity of protocol and ritual is realized. Ritual is not contaminating of but coexistent with protocol – not through criminal intent, but of necessity. There is no protocol without ritual; no ritual without protocol.

It is tempting, as I have done, to construct this process as sequential: protocol; on its failure, moving towards ritual; revival that becomes, of necessity, redemption; acts, initially done for the benefit of the dying; on death, ending up being done for the sake of the survivors. There is validity in this sequencing, but these processes are not smoothly chronological. They operate both sequentially and concurrently – revival and redemption simultaneous. One cannot act upon the dying without acting upon the living. One cannot salvage life without constructing death.

CPR necessarily elides protocol and ritual, action and performance, reality and representation, so that it might transform being into belonging, nature into culture, and death into life. None of these elisions can occur without the violence of the category error. It is ritual's commission of this irrationality that allows us to transcend death. Elision is not dialectic. It is not the resolution of paradox, but acceptance of it, and as such, is non-rational and non-verbal. When words fail, action executes. Ritual breaches, elides and confounds the well-established categories of the mundane world in the production of a subjective state of ecstatic intoxication, so that we might apprehend the incomprehensible paradox of living to die. Suffering and loss are inevitable consequences of being living, sentient, reflexive beings – of being human and mortal. Indeed, suffering and loss constitute human being. Triggered by the human condition, the violence of CPR precipitates the rescuer into a subjective experience of death, which if it is not an erotic experience of life, then is nothing. Without that consciousness, we might arguably still be of the human species, but we would hardly be human beings. Humanity, trapped by the paradox of living to die, is compelled to live out the fantasy of the rescue/sacrifice, because that fantasy is what constitutes Humanity, the only thing we have that redeems our mortality.

Dulling the sharp edges

On the one hand, we recognize the futility of beating the moribund to death in fruitless attempts to revive the unrevivable. On the other, as I have pointed out, 'inappropriate' CPR persists because it obeys important deathbed imperatives whose repression seems only to lead to their return in some other form. Surely there must be some form of compromise? Timmermans, though he condemns the technique of CPR in no uncertain terms:

> The major problem is that in the current system most resuscitative efforts are medically unnecessary and socially unwanted .... There exists no justifiable reason to pump drugs, electricity, and oxygen into a biologically dead body. (1999, pp. 185-9)

also grudgingly admits its utility:

> The possibility that a simple medical technique might reverse the dying process – like a *deus ex machina*, which restores order at the end of a Greek play – is too powerful a cultural image to relinquish. Because of the mythical quality of CPR, many deaths will continue to be framed by unnecessary resuscitative attempts. (1999, p. 192)

and offers a compromise of sorts:

> If CPR is here to stay, the way to dull its sharp edges is to turn the procedure into a community-centered event that might ease the transition from life to death, making the needs of relatives and friends the central concern .... a dignified and compassionate sudden death implies that the possibility of death is made explicit, treatment choices are reached with all parties involved, the dying person's wishes are honored, and relatives and friends are included in the last moments, if not as care-providers, then at least as witnesses. (1999, p. 192)

Timmermans makes a number of recommendations about tailoring resuscitative efforts to chances of survival: increased support for families, respect for advance directives, the use of healthcare proxies and something he calls a 'resuscitation will' (1999, p. 188).[6] What he advocates is part and parcel of good clinical judgement, and his recommendations are, for the most part, supported by the death-with-dignity movement, the social sciences and orthodox medicine. The hope is that a rationalization of the deathbed might do away with the barbarism of CPR, to make way for a safe and peaceful passing, managed by a more appropriate form of ritual behaviour. Would that it were that simple.

As was discussed above, most of these initiatives have met with only limited success. Curbs on CPR, the use of advance directives and any number of eminently reasonable attempts at rationalization of the deathbed have all run into resistance. Tony Walter's solution to these problems is a 'more sociological understanding of grief'. Reasonable as the suggestion is, it is the addition of another level of modernist reflexivity to the model of mourning based on therapeutic discourse. I do not wish to imply that this is not a productive approach, but, in the end, analysis, though useful, is neither grief experienced nor mourning done. Though therapeutic discourse may take up much of the labour of mourning, the persistent return of ritual would seem to indicate that discourse is not yet ready to shoulder the entire burden.

Though it may not be possible to relinquish the ritual of resuscitation, it may be possible (as Timmermans suggests and as both Revivalist polemics and *Guidelines 2000* attempt to do) to 'dull its sharp edges'. However, like the attempts by the Humane Society to mitigate the violence of the folk therapies for drowning, dulling the sharp edges of CPR, by removing its violent and dehumanizing content, guts it of its symbolic potency. There is a powerful ambivalence in the violence of resuscitation – beating life into and out of the victim. Ritual does not solve this paradox, rather, it incorporates it, not by negating violence but by shaping and channelling it. That for which CPR-as-protocol stands condemned, its inherent violence, is for CPR-as-ritual essential. The sharp edges are the point. Without them, CPR reverts to the death-with-dignity paradigm – a simulacrum of sleep supported by therapeutic discourse – not an invalid paradigm but, as I have intimated, not a universally effective one either.

I like to watch ...
Following positivism's foreclosure of the transcendent, the necessary congruence between biological reality, social structure and ontological

belief that triangulates the modern border between life and death is achieved by the co-incident termination of biological, social, and ontological being. Such a condensation of death towards an instantaneous present is the goal of a successful negotiation between technology and discourse that is the rationalized deathbed. On the side of technology, medicine is involved in a process of self-critique, attempting to rationalize deathbed therapeutics. The unitary and unified structure of CPR is being broken down into multiple age, condition and place specific prescriptive therapeutic manoeuvres and these are being subjected to evidence based review. Each of them aimed, less to save lives, though that is their ultimate goal, than to produce very specific changes in physiological parameters. Based on these parameters, death then becomes a rational decision about when to start and when to stop. On the side of discourse, there has been considerable success in implementing the death with dignity in hospices, palliative care wards, and even in ERs and ICUs. Modern 'Life' ends, ideally, with the co-incident termination of biological, social and ontological being, that is, the person's body, their personal relationships and their being are all tied up in a neat package that sees their last breath as the final word in all three registers – We call this 'closure'.

Unfortunately, in real life death is seldom that tidy. Having refuted ritual, we find that both medical technology and therapeutic discourse are not quite up to the task of comprehending biological, social and ontological collapse, not quite capable of reconciling our existential desires with biological reality. Try as we may, through technology and discourse, in the real world, it is extremely difficult to manage a precise co-incidence of biological, social and ontological death. Nevertheless, if media theorists are to be believed, the possibility of such an integration does exist.

The leave that postmodernity gives us to elide reality and representation means that participation in the medium allows us to *be* by watching rather than doing. Through existential pornography, we are given leave to participate in death's ritual construction without actually having to enact it, or, more precisely, we are given leave to enact it on the screen rather than on the street. If this is the case then death has not disappeared in the postmodern, merely changed its medium. As we have already heard Barthes point out: 'Death must be somewhere ... if it is no longer in religion, it must be elsewhere; perhaps in the image' (2000, p. 92). The postmodern deathbed, in line with other phenomena of postmodernity, exists in a reality that somehow encompasses both the screen and the street as equally valid modes of being. Could it be that the over-determined portrayal of the modern deathbed on television is not merely a reaction to our exclusion from the deathbed in real life, the repressed resurfacing in mediated form, but *is* ritual sublimated onto the TV screen, and as such makes possible the replacement of the violence of the ER with the violence of *ER*?

I think not. Despite postmodern polemics; representation and reality, though increasingly blurred, remain distinct categories. Though television and film's portrayal of the contemporary deathbed can be extremely moving and even instructive, it is not the same as being there. The televised 'pornography of death', with its slippages of reality and representation, is no more likely to replace the experience of the deathbed than the dirty movie is likely to replace sex. Indeed, for pornography to function as pornography that line between representation and reality, however thin, cannot disappear. Just as pornography's content requires the transgression of certain defined boundaries of decency, so its form requires the transgression of a maintained boundary between representation and the real. Violation of the borders of representation and reality, performance and enactment, life and death ensures the continued existence of each of these necessary but fragile fantasies. Furthermore, whatever postmodernity is or is not, whatever it may or may not do, it is limited by the physical mortality of its vehicle, the human body. In the end, we fuck and die not on television but (usually) in bed.

Television tragedy, no matter how vividly represented and enthusiastically received, remains representation. Ritual, though itself a mode of performance, does not. Ritual crosses the line between representation and reality to breed its own reality. Ritual is lived. Ritual transgresses borders and confounds categories so that we might live the irrational. Pornography gives us illicit pleasure by threatening the collapse of boundaries, but it never quite carries out that threat. If media death is to be construed as a valid form of mourning, which I believe it can be, then it is not because it replaces deathbed ritual but rather because it opens the doors to it, not just on the screen but on the street, not just on *ER* but in the ER. The symbiotic relationship between therapeutic discourse and the secular ritual of CPR is made complete by its representation in the media. The television screen becomes the transcendent source of images giving meaning to the act. It is the fantastical coincidence of death on television that makes the powerful effect of CPR in the ER possible. The real is represented so that the represented might become real. The 'exploitation' of death by the media has been crucial to the re-incorporation of the spectator into the real-life death drama. The man and woman on the street have followed the Steadicam through the doors of the ER to take their places at (and on) the deathbed.

Being there

Until very recently, the invasive and violent nature of the medical procedures involved in resuscitation – IVs, catheters, ET tubes, electric shocks, blood, broken ribs, and so on – was considered too traumatic for the layperson.

> Allowing family members in during a critical treatment period not only hinders medical care but will also scare the hell out of them.... There will be plenty of time for the family to peek in and offer moral support after the patient has been stabilized. (Gibbs and Ross, 1997, p. 80)

The standard medical line was, 'You don't want to remember him that way.' Spectators got in the way, carried on hysterically, gave you two patients to treat instead of one – or so it was assumed. Further, there was a concern over litigation. The ordered chaos that is the resuscitation attempt might be misconstrued as error, not to mention that real mistakes would be open to public scrutiny. It seemed better to keep the public and the family on the other side of the door. So, death becomes invisible. Loss occurs *in absentia*. We end up not only mourning the loss of the person, but our absence from the moment that took them from us. Loss becomes haunted by absence.

Based on a growing belief that the trauma of witnessing and participating in resuscitative efforts may be less than the trauma of passive ignorance, there has been a move on the part of emergency department staff to allow family into the resuscitation room while the resuscitation is in progress.

> A growing number of hospitals and institutions, most often following a local 'grassroots effort' by emergency and critical care nurses, have started programs to ask family members whether they wish to be in the same room with the patient during the resuscitation attempts. Accompanied by a calm, experienced social worker or nurse, families can view the professional efforts made by medical personnel attempting to save their loved one. Afterward they rarely ask the recurring question that so often accompanies an unsuccessful resuscitation attempt: Was everything done? (American, 2000, p. I.12)

Follow-up studies, examining the feelings of family members allowed to witness or participate in resuscitative attempts, showed positive responses with up to 94 per cent stating they would wish to participate again in a similar situation (Doyle et al., 1987, p. 673; Hanson and Straser, 1992, p. 105; Williams, 1993, p. 478; Eichhorn et al., 1996, p. 59; Barratt and Wallis, 1998, p. 109). This movement of the family towards the deathbed has been going on quietly and informally for at least 15 years, but has accelerated over the last five and has now been formalized in the AHA's *Guidelines 2000*. The following question-and-answer exercise is from the *ACLS Provider Manual* (2001):

> You are in the ED assisting in a resuscitation attempt for a normothermic patient who was transported in asystolic cardiac arrest. You are providing a trial of BLS and ACLS. The patient has been successfully intubated, and you have confirmed proper tube placement. IV access has been obtained. Which of the following interventions would be most likely to have the greatest therapeutic effect at this time?
>
> a) Ask the family if they would like to present during the resuscitation attempt.
> b) Administer escalating doses of epinephrine.
> c) Administer fibrinolytics to treat a possible myocardial infarction.
> d) Administer an empiric defibrillatory shock of 200 J ....
>
> The correct answer is a). This scenario documents what is likely to be an unsuccessful resuscitative effort – the patient has failed to respond to a course of BLS and ACLS and has no hypothermia. Unless additional mitigating factors are identified and reversed, this patient is unlikely to survive. Whenever possible, family members should be offered the option of being present during resuscitation. This is particularly important when your resuscitative efforts are unlikely to be effective: under these conditions, the needs of the family members should be strongly considered. Although family presence can be potentially beneficial in many resuscitative situations, the strongest evidence of benefit has been documented in studies of family members following the death of a loved one. Family members who were given the option of being present during the resuscitation attempt showed less anxiety and depression and more constructive grief behavior than family members who were not given the option. (Cummins, 2001, pp. 122, 238)

Worries over family members being unable to handle the violence, 'indelicacy' and indignity of the resuscitative scenario have proven to be unfounded. Problems with family members fainting, interfering or being psychologically traumatized have not surfaced. Increased litigation has not occurred; indeed, it has dropped (Doyle et al., 1987, p. 673; Hanson and Straser, 1992, p. 105; Williams, 1993, p. 478). The blood of the sacrificial lamb is shed for the redemption of all, but it is also on the hands of all. The guilt engendered by sacrifice stains both the community and the individual, but is washed away in the cathartic act of purification. At a very crude level, sacrifice ablates the need for retribution.

The exclusion produced by the medicalization of death is thus, to some extent, being reversed by changes within the protocol that was, to a large extent, responsible for it. Training in CPR, the placing of AEDs in the hands of laymen and the introduction of the family into the resuscitation room bring the layperson closer and closer to the deathbed. This reincorporation of the spectator is a consequence of changes within the healthcare system that the protocol itself helped set in motion. Resuscitative protocols to a great extent spawned the emergency medical system that performs them, and it is the protocol's concept of the chain-of-survival that is now shaping that segment of healthcare. Practitioners in that system – paramedics, emergency department nurses and physicians – having taken over the protocol (in practice, if not yet formally, from cardiology) are in a position to recognize the need for family participation. Emergency medicine's growing power as a specialty, based on its expertise with and knowledge of resuscitative protocols (both their strengths and weaknesses), has perhaps given it the confidence to open the doors of the resuscitation room to the gaze of the public.[7]

What may prove to be as significant change in resuscitative protocols as the use of AEDs, the demotion of external cardiac compression, the repression of mouth-to-mouth or the promulgation of advance directives is the admittance of the family into the resuscitation room. While a therapeutic protocol aimed at the re-equilibration of physiological parameters does not require an audience, ritual most certainly does. When CPR fails to save life, its performance, offering tangible evidence of death, becomes the initial act in mourning's construction of loss. Exclusion of survivors from the deathbed uncouples the act of dying from the act of mourning; it deprives loss of both context and content. There is no point in performing elaborate ritual acts in the absence of the congregation for whose sake those acts are done. It is now beginning to be realized that, regardless of how peaceful or pain-filled, how dignified or demeaning, how appropriate or inappropriate the death, survivors should not be excluded from the deathbed, or what have they survived? Loss need not be compounded by absence. No one should die alone.

The performance of CPR as both protocol and ritual, though extremely problematic, does not negate medical technology or therapeutic discourse. As a protocol, CPR is good for what it is good for – primarily witnessed ventricular fibrillation and various forms of respiratory arrest. As a ritual, CPR does not operate in a vacuum. Ritual supports and is supported by therapeutic discourse. Ritual gives discourse content. Without this content, discourse becomes an endlessly recursive analysis of its own formal structure. When people tell me of their father's death or their mother's funeral, they do not start with an analysis of their grief; rather they tell me what happened. It is in this reconstruction of the lived death that therapeutic discourse originates. Whether it is in the subdued glow of the hospice bedroom or the bright lights of the ER, to be present is to act. There is, in a sense, no possibility of mourning any but the death that we ourselves create. 'Man makes his pain... as he makes his mourning' (Canguilhem, 1991, p. 97).

> *On Wednesday night, this 16-year-old kid, on some stupid dare, climbed a high-tension pylon. He brushed one of the live wires. There was a brilliant flash and he was blasted backwards into the sky. He would surely have fallen to his death had not his pant leg caught on a projection and held him, hanging, 40 feet above the ground. His friends ran for help and eventually the fire department got him down and brought him to the emergency room. His injuries were unusual. There was a small entry burn on the lateral surface of his left knee with a larger exit wound on the medial surface of the same knee. Then the current must have arced across, because there was another entrance wound on the medial surface of the right knee with the final exit wound out his right palm. The path of the electrical current was easy to follow for the flesh along the its route was pale and firm to the touch – like cooked meat. This is a third degree electrical burn. It is not dramatic looking because the tissue damage occurs from the inside out. Deep in the limbs, electrical energy is converted to heat. There is no charring, unless the clothes catch fire, and this had not happened. The current had not traversed his heart, so he had not died from a cardiac arrhythmia,*

nor had it traversed the brain, so he was still conscious and talking. He was in little pain, as in this type of deep burn the nerves are destroyed along with the other tissues. It is important to understand that the clinical state of the patient in the period immediately following this type of injury is deceptively stable, but it is deception; they can deteriorate rapidly. We got two peripheral IV's and a central line established. Did x-rays. Inserted a catheter and n/g tube. Sent off bloods. Gave tetanus toxoid. Cleaned and dressed the small entrance and exit burns. His pressure was good, but, knowing things would change dramatically within the next four to six hours, I started pouring IV saline into him. I explained that this was a serious injury and that we were going to have to transfer him to the burn centre 50 miles away. He was awake, alert, oriented, in no pain, still a little drunk, and only beginning to realize that this was 'some kind'a big fuckin' deal'. We tried to contact his parents, who, it turned out, were out of town. It was now four in the morning, quiet, no other patients in my section of the department. I sat down and waited with him for the transport ambulance to arrive. I don't remember much of what was said, the usual stupid stuff that adults patronize teenagers with – family, school, sports. He was on the high school basketball team. After about ten minutes conversation slowed. He turned to me and asked, 'Am I going to die?' I swallowed, and during that moment a storm of arguments for and against telling him blew through my head. I don't think I decided on any of them; I just looked at him and said, 'Yes.' We sat quietly for a moment, then he began to tell me about how when he was kid (God! When he was a kid!) and it was late at night and he'd had a nightmare and couldn't go back to sleep, his dad used to sit in the dark with him and tell him a story. Then lowering his voice began to murmur, recite, rap – whatever:

Once upon a time there be three bears.
A poppa bear, a momma bear, a baby bear.
One morning their breakfast be too hot,
so they go for a walk in the deep dark forest.
Happen by the house there come a little girl with golden hair.
Her name, Goldilocks. She lost.
She see this house, and she come to the door.
On it she knock, and she say,
'Yoohoo, I am a lost little girl, may I come in.'
She hear nothing. The forest quiet. The house quiet.

So she open the door, slowly, slowly, and she peek inside.
She look to the left; she look to the right.
She see no one.
So in she come on tippy tippy toe.
On the table she see breakfast.
First she go to poppa bear's chair.
She sit down and taste the oatmeal.
'Ooo, Ooo,' she say, 'This here oatmeal, is too hot.'
Then she go to momma bear's chair.
She sit down and taste the oatmeal.
'Ooo, Ooo,' she say, 'This here oatmeal, is too cold.'
Then she go to baby bear's chair.
She sit down and taste the oatmeal.
'Ah ha,' she say, 'This here oatmeal, is just right.'
And she ate it up.
Then she is one very tired girl.
So she goes tippy tippy toe upstairs and she find three beds.
First she go to poppa bear's bed and she lie down.
'Ooo, Ooo,' she say, 'This here bed, is too hard.'
Then she go to momma bear's bed and she lie down.
'Ooo, Ooo,' she say, 'This here bed, is too soft.'
Then she go to baby bear's bed and she lie down.
'Ah ha,' she say, 'This here bed, is just right.'
And she lie down. She go to sleep.
Now, the bears come back from their walk in the deep dark forest.
Poppa bear he sniff and snuff with his big brown nose and he say,
'Someone in our house.'
And momma bear she put her head in the door, and she say
'Someone eat our breakfast.'
And baby bear he run to his bowl and he say,
'Someone eat my breakfast all up.'
And momma bear she go up the stairs on her big brown feet and she say,
'Oh, oh, Someone been in my bed.'
And baby bear he run into the room and he say,
'Ah ha, Someone in my bed.'
And the three bears come and they stand round the bed.
They see this little golden girl.
And baby bear, he push her and he say,
'What you doin' in my bed?'
And Goldilocks, she sit up,

and she look round,
and she see three bears,
and her eyes get so big,
and she jumps out of that bed,
and she runs down the stairs,
and through the kitchen,
and out the door,
and into the deep dark woods.
And poppa bear say 'Who that?'
and momma bear say 'Where she go?'
and baby bear say 'I want breakfast.'
So they went downstairs, and momma bear made pancakes,
and poppa bear and baby bear eat them with honey.
   The ambulance transport arrived. He thanked me as he was being wheeled out. He died Saturday morning.

Postscript

The paradigms of the death-with-dignity and the hi-tech death are, in the end, idealized fantasies. They are tropes, the former nostalgic and the latter heroic, used by those unexposed to the realities of the deathbed. The numbers of particular deaths that fit the ideal pattern of either paradigm are few and far between. There are a lucky few in palliative and hospice care who, due to the nature of their illness and the sophistication of the particular healthcare system in which they are situated, are open to the benefits of narcotics and therapeutic discourse, but they are limited in number. There are also a lucky few in ambulances, ERs and ICUs brought back to lives they desperately want to live. However, most deaths are somewhere between these two ideal extremes. At this point, I have no further argument to offer, only personal observation. I don't know that I would call very many of the thousand or so deaths I have seen 'good' – whether in the ER or on the palliative care ward. Some were; most weren't. Though death may come as a 'blessed release' from indignity, dependence and pain, it is a virtue made of necessity. If there were some other option, most of us would take it. Most deaths, regardless of the paradigm followed, are messy experiences filled with terror and awe, though strangely, all that being said, seldom as bad as we imagine.[8]

   In this book, I have portrayed, rather crudely, what appears to be a battle between those who seek to revive the body through CPR and those who seek to revive death through the death-with-dignity.

However, the apparent conflict between the death-with-dignity and CPR is not nearly as oppositional as it is made to appear. There is conflict and there is no question that this conflict results in perplexity on the theoretical level and suffering in real life. Nevertheless, the two paradigms are also complementary. Each is as necessary as the other. Each is appropriate for what it is appropriate for. Both the cancer patient and the victim of the car crash deserve an appropriate death, whether in a darkened room or the back of an ambulance. In fact, in the real world, both paradigms act in concert as often as they do in opposition, competing and cooperating in an attempt to negotiate life and death to fulfil the needs of both the living and the dead. There is as much cause for comfort as for concern in their ambivalent relationship.

I have undertaken to throw some light on a few of the many factors, besides scientific fact, that influence deathbed behaviour. CPR, positioned as it is at the deathbed, straddling life and death, science and religion, the public and the private, is not just a straightforward therapeutic technique, but a complex cultural phenomenon that is both scientific protocol and secular ritual. However, in the very process of proving my point about ritual, I undermine the phenomenon itself, for enchantment explained is enchantment no longer. As tempted as I am to allow the irrational its inevitable place at the deathbed, as a physician, as a representative, agent and consumer of science, I am obliged to resist that urge. Science, and medicine in particular, needs to recognize the presence of the irrational and its collusion with it. My hope is that I have gone some way in demonstrating that what some see as the culpable promotion of CPR by modern medicine is less the result of malicious intent or uncaring attitude, or even medicine's hidden political and economic agendas (though these do figure), than of factors intrinsic to the methodologies of both religion and science, which are not as disparate as either would wish. Protocol and ritual are so inextricably linked that it is not possible to enact one without performing the other. If the protocols of science are to be accessed at the deathbed, then they must make allowance for the atavism of ritual without succumbing to it. No easy task.

It is disappointing that I have no set formula for a good death, that the best I seem to be able to offer is a superficial pragmatism that recommends we continue striving towards a rational deathbed, matching the death-with-dignity and hi-tech death with the pathophysiological processes for which each is most appropriate; while admitting, at the same time, that such happy conjunctions are rarely possible and that, in many cases, the irrational and ritual must be accepted. When the

Conclusion: Modern Living/Modern Dying 243

CPR protocol does eventually go, it will be, as it was in the past, not merely because of its empirical failings and clinical inefficacies but because it is displaced by something not only more practically efficacious but more psychologically and socially fit for the changing cultural conditions in which it finds itself. Whatever those may be, the protocol that comes into being to better fulfill the therapeutic remit of saving life will still have to take on the ritual tasks of purging the body of life and life of the power of death.

> *In high school, I had a summer job working as a porter in the ER of a large city hospital. In that ER, we had two large, tiled, resuscitation rooms, one beside the other, separated by a small utility room. The utility room was where the instruments were cleaned and sterilized by the service aides, mostly East European immigrant women. It was also where the porter sat awaiting calls. The doors to the two resuscitation rooms were always open and, thus, the aide standing at the sink could easily see into each of them. Olga, had stood at that sink for over 20 years, ever since arriving in Canada after the Second World War. I was sitting behind her on a high stainless-steel stool watching her wash instruments, when they brought in a Code. As they flopped him onto the trauma table, she leaned forward a little and screwing up her eyes looked into the room. All that could be seen of the patient were the soles of his feet. 'This one, he'll die,' she said and went back to washing. I stood in the door, watching the doctors and nurses fly back and forth, intrigued and a little frightened. When all the hollering and drama was over and he was dead, they left, and Olga and I went in to clean up. To avoid looking at or going near the body, I began to pick up the bloody gloves and green cotton tray wrappers that lay strewn about the tiled floor. I asked how she knew he would die. 'The feet. I can tell by the feet.' I was too intimidated by the presence of the dead man to ask more, and keeping my back to the body, I continued to tidy. Olga washed the body while murmuring something in Polish. When she had done, she called me over to help wrap it. Jesus! I had to touch it! Seeing my hesitation, she began telling me how exactly it should be done. She chattered on and on, while I heaved the dead flesh back and forth and she tucked and wrapped. 'Some of these nurses; they are girls; they know nothing ... You must wrap like so and so and so ... There is a right way and a wrong way. Why be so lazy to do wrong?' We were done. I left the room and must have looked pretty pale, as the Head*

Nurse sent me off on coffee break. I went outside and sat under a linden tree. It was in bloom, small, white flowers, with a distinctive, sweet perfume. I looked up through the bright green leaves to a sky intensely blue. I was so happy. Now, years later, the scent of linden blossom brings back that remembered joy and thoughts of death.

Notes

Introduction

1. Poster advertising *Bringing Out the Dead*, 1999. Directed by Martin Scorsese, starring Nicholas Cage.
2. ER = Emergency room. The term 'Emergency Room' or 'ER' is not well favoured within medicine. The preferred term is 'Emergency Department' or 'ED'. The terms 'Emergency Ward', 'Casualty' and 'Accident and Emergency' ('A & E)' are also used. I have no intention of entering this debate. I use the term 'Emergency Room' or 'ER' because it is the term favoured by the public and the media.
3. British medical drama set in an Accident and Emergency department first broadcast in 1986.
4. Throughout this book I shall be using official acronyms for various techniques and procedures, for example CPR, ACLS, ECC, and so on. They are shorthand for long, often clumsy, descriptive phrases. More importantly, acronyms are an integral part of the culture of resuscitation.
5. These are narratives of dying told by those forced to face their own mortality due to terminal disease (de Hennezel, 1998; Hawkins, 1990; Flanagan, 2000). The growing genre of the confessional pathography, in both popular non-fiction and in the medical literature, deserves more than this passing allusion. See Seale, 1998, pp. 31–2, 202; and Walter, 1994, pp. 126–8.
6. Under rubrics such as 'Room for a View' or 'Change of Shift'.

1 Death-with-Dignity: The Fantasy

1. I use the term 'paradigm' in Thomas Kuhn's sense: that of a typical example to be replicated or followed – that is, a 'concrete puzzle-solution' employed as a model or exemplar, where the exemplar chosen implies a consensus of theory, method, language, standards of judgment and goals across a particular community (1996, pp. 174–210).
2. 'Hi-tech' is used less for its denotation of shiny machinery, though the machines certainly are there, than for the connotation of modernity it carries within popular culture. As will become evident in the book, technology and its 'height', though playing an important role in what I am labelling the hi-tech death, is only one aspect of that mode of death and not necessarily the most important one. Rather than burden the term 'hi-tech' with too fine an analysis, it is perhaps best that the reader simply keep in mind the images and emotions that were generated by the scene from *Bringing Out the Dead*, which opened the 'Introduction'.
3. Throughout the following discussion I will treat the two paradigms – the death-with-dignity and the hi-tech death – as they are treated in much of the academic literature, that is, as distinct entities in opposition to each

other. For the purposes of analysis, this polarization is useful, but I caution the reader to keep in mind that, in real life, these lines are not as neatly drawn. Few deaths are entirely one or the other.
4 Death is understood by the medic and to an ever-increasing extent by the general populace as a biological event. Modern medicine's exploration of death seldom ventures outside the body into the world and on towards the heavens. However, social scientists refer to three 'modes' of death: biological, social and ontological (or, if one prefers, spiritual) (Houlbrooke, 1989, p. 148; J. Davies, 1994, p. 26; Walter, 1994, p. 116; Seale, 1998, p. 7). These roughly correspond to the vital triad of body, mind and soul, which are the reified manifestations of, respectively, the physical vehicle of being, the consciousness of being and the existential concept of being.
- Biological death is the irreversible loss of the capacity for life, that is, loss of biological function.
- Social death can be said to commence at the moment when the concept of death, an abstract generalization, is given substance by being applied personally, thus affecting social relations. It starts with the fatal diagnosis and results in the realization that the individual so identified is dying and should be treated as such. It is complete at the point where the dying or deceased individual drops out of social relations, that is, when they are accepted as having lost the ability to act on and be acted upon by others.
- Ontological or spiritual death is that point at which all modes of being cease to be recognized. It is extinction. It is the fall into the abyss, where that-which-was no longer is – no longer exists even as spirit or memory.

Each culture's concept of death is synthesized from its own fluctuating mix of biological reality, social structure and ontological belief, and its own particular mix of body, mind and soul. The deathbed is an attempt to triangulate the border between life and death by bringing into congruence the somatic, the social and the ontological. Different cultures at different stages in their histories achieve congruity in different ways. This congruence does not necessarily mean temporal co-incidence, though it may.
5 Today, more than 80 per cent of people in the United States die in institutions, in contrast to less than 50 per cent 50 years ago and less than 15 per cent a century ago (McCue, 1995, p. 1039). It is estimated that two-thirds of the British currently die in hospital (Walter, 1994, p. 13). Twenty per cent of deaths in the US occur in the ICU (Prendergast, Claessens and Luce, 1997, p. 1).
6 Cancer deaths account for about 25 per cent of deaths in the West and HIV-related illness for about 0.5 per cent (Leading).
7 Of the 2 million people who die annually in the US, about 200,000 die under hospice care (Timmermans, 1999, p. 21).
8 Over the years the specifics of Kübler-Ross's five-step process of dying (denial, anger, bargaining, depression and acceptance) have been much criticized, much amended and even discredited. Nevertheless, the idea of desirable and undesirable psychological states – whether the progression be linear, circular or intermittent – continues to drive therapeutic discourse centered around grief.
9 I shall not be addressing the important issue of euthanasia. The topic is too large and too complex to bring into a discussion of sudden death and

resuscitative protocols, other than to point out that the AHA, in its latest resuscitative guidelines (*Guidelines 2000*), acknowledges that euthanasia (in the somewhat attenuated form of the doctrine of 'double effect') remains a possibility at many deathbeds.

> Patients in the end stage of an incurable disease, whether responsive or unresponsive, should have care that ensures their comfort and dignity. Care is provided to minimize suffering associated with pain, dyspnea, delirium, convulsions and other terminal complications. For such patients it is ethically acceptable to gradually increase the dosage of narcotics and sedatives to relieve pain and other symptoms, even to levels that might concomitantly shorten the patient's life. (American, 2000, pp. I.12–I.22)

10 It is possible to construe therapeutic discourse as a form of ritual. I refer readers to Seale's discussion of this (1998, pp. 197–8). However, one needs to be careful in stretching the bounds of 'ritual'. Both therapeutic discourse and ritual express core values, shape power relations, determine status and may be cathartic; however, their methods are very different. Therapeutic discourse relies on words, ritual on acts. Discourse translates behaviour into feelings; ritual, feelings into acts. Discourse is comparatively private; ritual public. Discourse trades on meaning; ritual on symbol (Walter, 1994, p. 137).

11 Unfortunately, the anthropological literature does not always bear this out. It is considered quite 'natural' in some societies to expose infants, strangle the sick or bury the elderly alive (Barley, 1995, p. 200). Such instances of nostalgia for the past and uncritical valorizations of 'nature' are usually treated as suspect by historians. Was death ever better? How? For whom? Why? And, if it is worse now, how, for whom, and why? Caution should always be exercised over an uncritical recourse to Nature as a justification. The terms 'natural' and 'unnatural' death are thrown around quite freely in the literature on death and dying. Walter points out the difficulties inherent in the naturalization of a particular mode of death: 'The vision of the good death being natural has considerable attractions. It implies that attaining the good death is relatively easy – all you have to do is absent yourself from alienating modern institutions and you can let nature and the family take over' (1994, pp. 113–15). Nostalgic naturalization ignores the possibility that dying in a wattle-and-daub hovel covered in your own excrement was not unusual for much of history and remains a possibility in much of the Third World today. Not that this is any more or less natural than dying well cared for by your extended family, it just points out that dangers of valorizing a norm by labeling it as natural.

2 Cardiopulmonary Resuscitation: The Protocol

1 Recommendations have since changed to a 15:2 sequence of 2 breaths followed by 15 chest compressions, for both single-rescuer and two-rescuer adult CPR. The sequence reverts to 5:1 when an artificial airway is in place (Hazinski, Cummins and Field, 2000, p. 2).
2 Defibrillation = the electrical shock that reverses fibrillation by depolarizing the conducting system of the heart. It causes all the heart's muscle cells

to contract at the same instant, halting the heart's chaotic activity. The myocardial cells become synchronized in identical electrical states, giving the heart's own pacemaker a chance to resume coordinated control of the heart's rhythm.

3. EMS = Emergency Medical Services. These are pre-hospital care services, replacing the prior category of ambulance services. EMS personnel who respond to medical emergencies may be first-, second- or third-tier responders, depending on the EMS system. They may be trained in ACLS or BLS. All should be capable of performing defibrillation. Emergency medical technician (EMT) usually denotes BLS training. Paramedic or EMT-P usually denotes ACLS training.

4. The use of life expectancy at birth, though a common epidemiological index, is problematic. High infant and child mortality rates in earlier eras and presently in developing countries skew this figure downward. More specific, though more difficult to come by, are measures of mortality for specific age groups. John Graunt, in his famous *Natural and Political Observations* of 1662, calculated that 64 per cent of all individuals born in London survived to the age of six years; 40 per cent to the age of 17 and 3 per cent to the age of 67. Those who survived the hazardous childhood years had a reasonable chance of reaching middle age; however, mortality at every stage of life was higher than it is today. Most people died before the age of 60 and only a small minority were left to die in old age (Houlbrooke 1998, 8–9, 22).

5. While most of us do express the wish to 'go quickly', it is on our own terms, that is, painlessly, in sleep as elderly men or women. The good death is seldom fantasized as being within the next hour on the point of a knife blade or the grill of a truck.

6. To be fair, Safar goes on to say that: 'Resuscitation applied without judgment and compassion is morally and economically unacceptable. The debilitated elderly patient or the otherwise terminally ill patient with incurable disease, particularly the one with irreversible coma or stupor, should be permitted to die without the imposition of costly and often dehumanizing efforts' (1997, p. 297).

7. Airway manoeuvres are aimed at opening the respiratory tract so as to provide an unobstructed flow of air from the mouth to lungs. In the BLS (Basic Life Support) protocol this is done with the jaw-thrust or chin-lift, and at the more sophisticated level of ACLS (Advanced Cardiac Life Support) by the use of oral/nasal airways, endotracheal intubation or cricothyrotomy/tracheostomy. I shall not deal with 'airway' separate from 'breathing' as airway manoeuvres are preparatory to mouth-to-mouth and share the same therapeutic end. Nor shall I explore intubation, cricothyrotomy and tracheostomy. Though possessing interesting histories and though components of the ACLS protocol, they are not part of the basic CPR protocol as practiced by the lay public.

8. Basic Life Support (BLS) or Basic Cardiac Life Support (BCLS) is the resuscitative protocol taught to the lay public. It includes activation of the emergency medical services (EMS) system, airway manoeuvres, artificial ventilation and chest compression. Since the introduction of automated external defibrillators (AEDs), defibrillation has also become part of BLS.

Advanced Life Support (ALS) or Advanced Cardiac Life Support (ACLS) extends BLS to include technical manoeuvres initiated by trained healthcare personnel, for example: defibrillation, intubation and other airway manoeuvres, intravenous access and the administration of drugs. There is more to advanced resuscitative protocols than the above discussion indicates – surgical airway techniques, mechanical forms of ventilation, drug and fluid administration, cerebral resuscitation, sophisticated monitoring technology, and so on. I choose to limit my discussion to external cardiac compression, mouth-to-mouth and defibrillation because, historically, they are the originary acts of the protocol; therapeutically, they remain the core acts of the ABCD paradigm; and, iconographically, they have become signifiers of the protocol in popular representation.

9 *Guidelines 2000* = The International *Guidelines 2000 for CPR and ECC* is the latest recension of the CPR protocol, as determined by the First International Guidelines Conference on CPR and ECC held in 1999. They update and combine previous recommendations published by the AHA in 1974, 1980, 1986 and 1992; and similar recommendations published by the European Resuscitation Council in 1992, 1996 and 1998. *Guidelines 2000* is the first instance of consensus guidelines coming from these bodies. They have been published by the AHA in a series of documents including: *Circulation 2000*, 102 [Suppl] (American, 2000); *2000 Handbook of Emergency Cardiovascular Care* (Hazinski, Cummins and Field, 2000); *ACLS Provider Manual* (Cummins, 2001); *Heartsaver AED* (American) and a large number of other instructional manuals and documents. Throughout this book, these recent recommendations are referred to generically as coming from *Guidelines 2000*, except where a direct quotation is used.

10 Asystole = cardiac standstill. Asystole is a complete absence of electrical and myocardial activity – the infamous 'flat line' on the ECG. It is often the end result of other untreated or unsuccessfully treated arrhythmias. It seldom responds to treatment and is usually considered a sign of death.
NSR = normal sinus rhythm–the heart's normal rhythm.
PEA = Pulseless electrical activity, when occasional electrical activity in the heart produces no cardiac contraction or pulse. It carries a prognosis almost as dire as that of asystole. It is often secondary to hypoxia caused by respiratory failure, but may also be due to rare mechanical causes such as cardiac tamponade, tension pneumothorax and pulmonary embolism, or to drugs or severe hypovolemia.
VF = ventricular fibrillation, the 'stalled heart', is a state in which the electrical activity of the heart becomes disorganized. The heart no longer beats in a coordinated fashion and its separate muscle bundles contract randomly. No blood is circulated. It is fatal unless quickly reversed. Its most common cause is myocardial infarction resulting from coronary artery disease – a 'heart attack'. It may also be caused by metabolic abnormalities, drug toxicity and hypothermia.
VT = ventricular tachycardia is an abnormally fast heart rate, which often degenerates into ventricular fibrillation. Cause and treatment are similar to that of ventricular fibrillation.

11 ECC system = emergency cardiac care system. The ECC system includes bystander CPR, rapid activation of the EMS system, the EMS system,

emergency departments, intensive care units, cardiac rehabilitation, cardiac prevention programmes, BLS and ACLS training programmes and citizen defibrillation. It is the institutional realization of the 'chain-of-survival'.
12 AED = 'Automated external defibrillators are computerized, low-maintenance, user-friendly defibrillators that analyze the victim's rhythm to determine whether a shockable rhythm is present. When the AED detects a shockable rhythm, it charges, then prompts the rescuer to press a shock button to deliver a shock. These devices are highly accurate... and can significantly reduce the time to defibrillation .... The widespread effectiveness and demonstrated safety of the AED have made it acceptable for use by nonprofessional responders' (American, 2000, p. I.358).
13 Reperfusion is the reopening of the coronary arteries. It may be accomplished by the use of: fibrinolytic drugs ('clot-busters'), cardiac catheterization and percutaneous angioplasty, stent placement (percutaneous coronary intervention: PCI), and/or coronary artery bypass graft surgery (CABG).
14 This outline of CPR is lamentably cursory. It is meant to give the reader the minimum knowledge necessary for the discussion that follows. The best means of acquiring detailed knowledge of the subject is to do a 'CPR-Provider' or 'Heartsaver' course.
15 A number of histories of CPR have been written (Pearson, 1965, p. 8; R. Lee, 1972, p. 418; Jude, 1987, p. 452; Hermreck, 1988, p. 430; Safar, 1989, p. 1; Wallace, 1996; Eisenberg, 1997; Timmermans, 1999). Many of these were written by individuals central to the development of the modern CPR protocol (for example, Safar, Jude, Eisenberg). Some of these have been accused of vested interest, naivety, whiggishness and evangelism. Though there is some validity to such criticism, I have few concerns in employing these sources for historical event and chronology, as they are, for the most part, when cross-referenced to the medical literature, accurate in their detail. More importantly, the attitudes they convey through the language they use is important to the analysis this book will attempt to make. It should be made clear, however, that my use of the data they have collected and the story they tell is not necessarily an endorsement of their conclusions.
16 Kouwenhoven, Jude and Knickerbocker had previously published their article 'Closed-chest Cardiac Massage,' in July 1960 (1960, p. 1064). Nevertheless, the date of the Maryland meeting is usually sanctioned as the 'official' birthday of CPR. Going back a little further, during the siege of Moscow in the winter of 1941–2, Vladimir Negovsky used artificial ventilation, external cardiac compressions and external defibrillation in a resuscitative protocol similar to what we recognize today as CPR (Negovsky, 1988, p. 287). However, his work did not become known in the West until after 1962, and by that time CPR had already become established. Negovsky's work is seldom, unfortunately as here, given the credit it deserves.
17 Stefan Timmermans, *Sudden Death and the Myth of CPR*. Philadelphia: Temple University Press, 1999.
18 Long-term survival is usually defined as survival until discharge from hospital.
19 This will be discussed further in chapter 7. Survival rates for witnessed ventricular fibrillation may even be as high as 74 per cent, if defibrillation is

delivered in less than three minutes (Valenzuela et al., 2000, 1206). However, long-term survival is complicated by the additional problem of neurological damage in the survivors. Again, there is great variation in study results. Some studies claim neurological dysfunction in survivors as low as 5–7 per cent. Others claim that less than 50 per cent of patients return to pre-arrest function (Bedell et al., 1983, p. 569; Longstreth et al., 1983, p. 588). Nichol, in an extensive review, has found that, although deficits may be present in significant numbers of survivors, overall quality of life is seldom affected (1999, p. 517). The large multi-centre OPALS study, though documenting only 4 per cent survival to one year, found that the majority of patients who survived had a good quality of life, and that citizen-initiated CPR was the single modifiable factor associated with this outcome (Stiell, 2003, p. 1939).

20 The majority of the more optimistic early studies have come from one centre, King County-Seattle. Approximately 85 per cent of research articles on CPR in the United States come from a set of only ten research groups (Niemann, 1993, p. 8).

21 The majority of the Advanced Cardiac Life Support (ACLS) protocol deals with complicated drug regimes for treating cardiac arrhythmias, but it should be noted that of the total number of people who survive from cardiac arrest, 85–95 per cent regain spontaneous circulation with no drug treatment, that is, after only CPR and 1–3 defibrillations (Cummins, 2001, p. 78).

22 Research aimed at improving survival rates is ongoing. There are grounds for some optimism, especially in the area of the 'appropriate' application of the protocol. The AHA is attempting an increasingly evidence-based approach with due appreciation for the limitations of the protocol. However, as will be discussed in the arguments that follow, it is not a simple task.

23 The reader is free to accept this assertion as informed opinion or to make up his or her own mind by referring to the references in the text plus: Eisenberg, Bergner and Hallstrom, 1979, Cobb, 1980, p. 31; Meyerberg et al., 1984, p. 1118; Litwin et al., 1987, p. 787; Eisenberg et al., 1990, p. 179; Cummins et al., 1991b, p. 960; David et al., 1993, p. 1578; Larsen et al., 1993, p. 1652; Saklayen et al., 1995, p. 163; Ballew, 1996, p. 39; Safar, 1996, p. 8; Cummins, 1998, p. 490; p. 30; Mosesso et al., 1998, pp. 200, 920; Stratton and Niemann, 1998, p. 449; Leung and Tong, 2000, p. S38.

24 This particular algorithm from the AHA's 1994 *ACLS Manual* has been superseded by the vastly changed 'Tachycardia Overview' in *Guidelines 2000*. The older version is used because it best illustrates the paradigmatic characteristics of a clinical algorithm. The significant changes this algorithm has undergone will be discussed further in chapter 6.

25 Some American states are in the process of enacting legislation that would require certification in ACLS, ATLS and PALS for credentialing of all physicians. What has been labelled 'merit badge medicine' has become such a concern within the profession that the American Board of Emergency Medicine (ABEM), responsible for the training, testing and certification of the specialty in the US, has felt the need to issue a position statement declaring that competence in the specialty is to be based on board certification procedures not on certificates of completion of ACLS, ATLS

and PALS courses (Proctor, 2000, p. 2). Implicit in ABEM's reaction to the unique position resuscitative protocols have gained in law is the fear that adherence to protocol is valued over and has replaced technical expertise and professional judgement. Emergency physicians, cardiologists and trauma surgeons are exactly those people most involved with the development and teaching of resuscitative protocols, and thus exactly those people most likely to recognize the limitations of them, and deviate from same. It is with some alarm that, like the sorcerer's apprentice, they see themselves being overwhelmed by their own formulae.

3 The Royal Humane Society: The Method

1. For convenience, regardless of date, I shall refer to The Institution for Affording Relief to Persons Apparently Dead from Drowning, the Humane Society and the Royal Humane Society as the 'Humane Society'.
2. Hereafter referred to as 'The Method'.
3. Today, the pathophysiology of drowning is reasonably well understood. Submersion results in voluntary apnoea (breath-holding), air hunger quickly develops, and the victim is forced to take an involuntary gasp, which results in a small amount of water entering the upper airway and irritating it. This results in a reflex spasm of the muscles of the larynx which closes off the trachea (laryngospasm). The closed airway prevents both water and air from entering, and soon the oxygen content of the blood drops to levels that result in loss of consciousness. With loss of consciousness, the laryngospasm relaxes and aspiration of larger amounts of water may occur. Most drowning victims aspirate less than 4 ml/kg of water, that is, less than a cup in a 70 kg man (Feldhouse and Knopp, 1988, p. 1062). The usual amounts of water aspirated do not act as a physical barrier to gas exchange. The immediate danger in drowning is the hypoxia produced by the laryngospasm and consequent exclusion of atmospheric air from the lungs. This hypoxia eventually results in neurological injury, secondary cardiac arrest and death. The immediate treatment of drowning is to re-establish respiration and circulation by establishing an airway, rescue breathing and external cardiac compressions, that is, The ABCs of CPR.
4. Goodwyn's experiments actually added little new to the prior work of investigators such as Robert Boyle, Richard Lower, Robert Hooke, John Mayow, Joseph Priestley, William Hewson, Antoine Laurant-Lavoisier and John Hunter. The relation between Priestley's dephlogisticated air (discovered 1774 and called *oxygène* by Lavoisier) respiration and life was generally accepted by the time Goodwyn wrote his essay (see chapter 5). What Goodwyn did was to bring all the evidence together in an organized fashion and publish it so that it might influence therapeutics.
5. Fire damp is methane; choke damp is a mixture of carbon dioxide, carbon monoxide and dust following explosions or fires in mines.
6. The preservative effect of intentionally induced hypothermia is what allows certain cardiac operations to be done when, for technical reasons,

cardiac bypass is not feasible. It is also the basis of recommendations by some for therapeutic cooling following cardiac arrest.

7   The Society's medals portrayed a young boy blowing on the 'torch of life'. The medal was inscribed *LATEAT SCINTILLA FORSAN* ('Perhaps a Spark May Yet Remain').
8   In all quotations in this book, emphasis, whether by capitals, italics, bold print or underlining, is always the original authors'.
9   The amounts of blood taken were usually in the range of 2–8 oz (60–225 ml). The lesser amount being at the upper limit of what might be taken for blood tests today; the greater figure, an amount that would, as a single episode, cause little untoward physiological alteration in most healthy adults. Unfortunately, bleedings were often multiple.
10 Falling blood pressure and deteriorating blood gases perform a similar prognostic function for today's physicians.
11 'Honor follows on neither the rod, nor the purple, nor riches, nor genius, but in the spirit of devotion to the service of the community.'
12 Biblical references to resuscitation were frequently quoted in the Society's literature: 2 Kings 4: 31–5; 1 Kings 17; Mark 5: 22–43; Luke 9: 56; Luke 7 : 1–16; John 11: 1–46. Even today in scientific papers, 'a biblical story is strategically useful as a rhetorical charm for those who dare to trespass the boundary between life and death .... to make resuscitation a morally sanctioned routine' (Timmermans, 1999, p. 33).
13 The equipment provided by the Society usually consisted of a conical ivory tube (nasal airway), bellows, a silver cannula (endotracheal tube), a tobacco smoke fumigator, flexible leather tube (orogastric tube), enema tubes, flannels, a thermometer and medications: 'essence of any aromatic vegetables, as chamomile, or peppermint, and the volatile alkali, and likewise emetics', matches, candles, and twine. Kite had Savigny's Manufactory of Chirurgical Instruments, No. 129, Pall-Mall, London manufactured and offered for sale a 'Pocket Case of Instruments for the Recovery of the Apparently Dead' based on the Society's recommendations (Kite, 1785, p. 20).
14 'He murders, who does not save.'
15 Declarations praising such altruism continue in the AHA's publications:
    ACLS is about saving lives .... ACLS is about restoring life and turning back the catastrophe of sudden death .... ACLS is about people: with 'foreign-body-obstructed trachea' comes a smiling child who insists on running with small toys in her mouth; with 'lungs filled with pulmonary edema' comes a rheumatic young woman with three small children at home; with 'coarse VF' comes a busy executive who forgot to hug his child that morning; with 'profound vascular collapse' comes a grand matriarch whose anxious family is already filling the waiting room. Finally, ACLS is about preparing yourself – preparing yourself to provide the best care possible for the most dramatic and emotional moment of a person's life. We think this book and the ACLS educational materials will prepare you for this moment, if you make the effort and devote the time. After all, the whole thing is about time – and about giving time back to your fellow man. (Cummins, 1994, p. v)

4 Defibrillation: *Scintilla Vitalis*

16 The 'blip' on the ECG that indicates a heartbeat.
17 The connection between electricity and life inspired such fantasies as Mary Shelley's *Frankenstein* (1818).
18 This interesting history has been well documented by Armstrong and Armstrong (1991), Holbrook (1958) and Roth (1981; 1989–90).
19 It can be argued that successful defibrillations had been accomplished prior to this. The case often cited in the literature as the *locus classicus* of defibrillation is that of Catherine Sophia Greenhill (Hawes, 1774, p. 32). This child fell from a window, but there is little likelihood that she suffered ventricular fibrillation as either the cause or result of the fall. More likely is that she had a concussion, and the coincidence of her awakening and the administration of the electrical shock was merely that. However, there were other reports of electricity's use, and Curry, in 1792, points out that cases of apparent death caused by lightning (which does cause ventricular fibrillation) often respond well to the administration of electrical shocks (1815, p. 64). Regardless of prior use of electricity, Beck's case is important because it was the first human case in which electricity was applied with full knowledge of the cause of cardiac arrest and with the explicit purpose of reversing ventricular fibrillation.
20 As Zoll published first, he is usually given credit.
21 The placing of a tube into the trachea, either through the mouth or nose, to assist breathing.
22 *Phone First*: In adults in cardiac arrest the arrhythmia most amenable to reversal is ventricular fibrillation. For them, the most important determinant of survival is time from collapse to defibrillation. Thus, the new recommendation of *Guidelines 2000* is 'Phone first', that is, dial 911 and activate the EMS system to get a defibrillator on the scene before starting CPR.
Phone Fast: In contrast to cardiac arrest in adults, most causes of cardiopulmonary arrest in infants or children (aged 1–8 years) are related to airway or ventilation problems rather than sudden cardiac arrest. In these victims, rescue breathing is essential and should be attempted first, before activation of the EMS system. In children, the rescuer should provide approximately one minute of CPR and then activate the EMS system.
Exceptions to the 'phone first/phone fast rule' include:
1. Submersion/near drowning = phone fast: all ages,
2. Arrest associated with trauma = phone fast: all ages,
3. Drug overdoses = phone fast: all ages,
4. Cardiac arrest in children known to be at high risk for arrhythmias = phone first.
(American, *Guidelines* I.22–I.59)
23 Current American Heart Association guidelines suggest limiting AED deployment to sites with a 20 per cent annual probability of cardiac arrest and cost per QALY gained of $30,000. Examples of where public AEDs would be a good investment, based on a cost of less than $30,000 per QALY gained, include international airports, where cost per QALY gained is estimated to be $13,000, as well as public sports venues, county jails and large

shopping malls. AEDs in locations with exceedingly low cardiac arrest rates, such as hotels, retail stores and restaurants, where cost per QALY gained exceeds $500,000, is unlikely to be cost-effective (Cram, 2003, p. 745).

24 *'Iatro'*: From the Greek for physician (ιατρος). Thus iatromechanism and iatrochemistry were, respectively, mechanical and chemical theories of physiology and therapeutics.

25 A group of researchers, located mainly at Oxford from the late 1640s to the mid-1660s. A number of the, including Robert Boyle, Robert Hooke, Richard Lower, John Mayow and Christopher Wren, were interested in investigating air, respiration and their relation to what it was that was in the blood that gave life to the body (Wear, 1995, 349–51).

26 Vitalism is often said to have originated with Aristotle's refusal to accept either the animism implicit in the idealistic concept of Platonic 'Form', or the Atomists' contention that life could be explained entirely in material terms. If life was not under the direct control of the gods, if it was not the expression of the Platonic Form of Life, if it was not merely the behaviour of a certain kind of matter, then what sort of *thing* was it? Aristotle saw the *psyche*, as a 'vital quality' animating all living things. It was immanent in the organism, neither independent of nor identical with the body. In Aristotle, *psyche* or life is the substantial form of which body is the matter. Importantly, 'substantial' here is *not* in the sense of having substance, but in the sense of being the essential quality that identifies something as being the sort of thing it is. Life, in Aristotle's sense, is the end to which the living process aspires (*De Anima*, II, 2, 14–15). This doctrine stood for almost 2,000 years as one of Galenic medicine's main supports until the Enlightenment charge of tautology was brought against it. The 'substantial form' or 'essential quality' of anything was accused of being a tautology because it was merely the description of a phenomenon, not an explanation. Life is the result of the quality of vitality, the nature of which is to enliven. The Aristotelian doctrine of substantial form was thus accused of being one big circular argument, ending where it began, and, in the process, revealing nothing.

27 At the risk of belabouring the point of tangible imponderability – a thing is tangible if it can be felt, as both the wind and a lump of coal may be. Ponderability denotes 'having weight', but the connotation broadens to include extension and thus shape. Only the lump of coal is ponderable: it has weight, extension and shape; breath, though capable of being 'felt', does not; it is imponderable.

28 The *rete mirabile* is a network of blood vessels at the base of the brain in ungulates. Galen mistakenly believed, on the basis of animal dissection, that it was present in man.

29 Combustion and respiration are, in fact, somewhat different processes; the former explosive and unrestrained, the latter gradual and under meticulous control, but, at their most basic level, both are the oxidation of carbon compounds to carbon dioxide and water, with the resulting release of energy in the form of heat, light and work.

30 The history of the discovery of animal electricity and its development into electrical physiology is presented by Heilbron (1979), Hoff (1977), Schecter (1983), Rowbottom and Susskind (1984).

31 In 1976, the artist Chris Burden electrocuted himself (not fatally) with two bare wires to produce the performance piece documented in the photograph, *Doorway to Heaven*.
32 Though the issue of brain death most frequently involves patients on life support where a decision is being made as to whether or not to continue that support, decisions about resuscitation are also necessary. A related area is that of organ transplantation. It is no accident that transplantation and resuscitative technology have developed side by side. The necessity of keeping bodies alive as preps for donation was an important factor in the reinvigoration of resuscitative protocols in the 1960s.
33 I have not address traditional images of death. Others have more than adequately done so (Ariès, 1981; Guthke, 1999; Kemp and Wallace, 2000).

5 Mouth-to-Mouth: The Lips of a Corpse

1 'Fixed air' or carbonic acid gas were the terms in use for what we now call carbon dioxide.
2 Karl Wilhelm Scheele in Sweden isolated this same gas a year earlier, but Priestley published first and to him credit is usually given.
3 'Vital air' was the term in general use in the English literature at the end of the eighteenth century for Priestley's 'dephlogisticated air' and Lavoisier's '*oxygène*', what we now call oxygen.
4 Gunpowder = nitre (potassium nitrate) + charcoal + sulphur.
5 Similar to the bagging units used in hospitals and ambulances today.
6 We now know this is only true within certain limits. Too high levels of oxygen over prolonged periods can be toxic, as can too low levels of carbon dioxide. Oxygen is not absolutely good, nor carbon dioxide absolutely bad: it is in their proportions that benefit or harm exists.
7 For example:
Marshall Hall Method – involved rolling the victim from stomach to side sixteen times a minute and applying expiratory pressure to the back while prone.
Silvester Method – placed the patient in the supine position and involved alternating traction on the arms and compression of the chest. Its aim was to imitate 'the natural respiratory movements'.
Schafer Method – essentially the Silvester method, but with the patient prone rather than supine.
Holger Nielsen Method – the patient was placed in the prone position, the rescuer kneeling at the patient's head and alternately compressing the upper back and lifting the arms by the elbows:
   Out goes the bad air (while compressing the chest).
   In comes the good (while lifting the elbows).
8 Tidal volume is the quantity of air moved in and out of the lungs in a single breath.
9 IPPV encompasses all forms of ventilation in which gases are blown into the lungs by positive pressure. It thus includes mouth-to-mouth, bellows ventilation, bag-valve-mask ventilation, intubation and most (though not all) forms of mechanical respirators. One would have thought that the

development of inhaled anaesthesia, beginning in the late eighteenth century and advancing through the nineteenth would have supported IPPV's claim to a place in resuscitative protocols. Nevertheless, during the nineteenth and the first half of the twentieth centuries, the importance of anaesthesia to resuscitative protocols was less in the ventilation techniques that might be transferred from the anaesthesia to life-saving, than in the opportunities that the complications of general anesthesia, primarily chloroform-induced cardiac arrest, gave for the development of defibrillation and cardiac compression techniques (Macewen, 1880, p. 122; Waters et al., 1933, p. 196).

10 We need to beware the 'enormous condescension of posterity' (a phrase used by E. P Thompson [1991, p. 12] in quite a different sense). Explanations that ascribe errors of the past to ignorance and the inadequacies of the historical moment assume that we have access to a wisdom and sophistication absent in the past. Certainly, we do work from a much larger knowledge base and use more refined methodologies, but the logic, if not the detailed methodology, of what we term the scientific method was as well known to the natural philosopher of the seventeenth century as it is to the scientist of the twentieth, and there were, no doubt, the same number of wise men and fools then as there are now. We should take care in too hastily condemning the sins of prior generations – in accusing individuals of carelessness and systems of primitiveness. The same pitfalls in the scientific method that trapped our predecessors lay in wait for us.

11 There have been only 15 reports of CPR-related infections published between 1960 and 2000 (American, 2000, pp. I.22–I.59). These are anecdotal reports of mouth-to-mouth transmitting *Helicobacter pylori* (Figura, 1996, p. 1342), *Mycobacterium tuberculosis* (Heilman, 1965, p. 1035), meningococcus (Feldman, 1972, p. 1107), *herpes simplex* (Finkelhor and Lampan, 1980, p. 650), shigella (Todd and Bell, 1980, p. 331), streptococcus (Valenzuela et al., 1991, p. 90), salmonella (Ahmad 1990, 787) and *Neisseria gonorrhoea* (Mejicano and Maki, 1998, p. 813). These are all single reports, with the exception of herpes simplex (cold sores) of which there were three reports. The risk of contracting an infectious disease through mouth-to-mouth is so low as to be almost, albeit not quite, nil.

12 There is some evidence that ventilation may not be necessary in the first 6–10 minutes after cardiac arrest. However, this based on only a few studies and is enormously controversial (Hallstrom, 2000. p. N190; Hallstrom et al., 2000, p. 1546; Groh et al., 2000, p. 815; Kern, 2000, p. N186).

13 Though disgust too takes historically and culturally specific forms, and though one must be careful about making universal claims, it is hard to imagine a culture in which disgust, in some form, is not present (Miller, 1997; C. Turner, 2000).

14 Before travelling too far along this abstract route, I should point out that, although I shall be arguing for the symbolic construction of concepts such as contagion, we should be in no doubt as to the reality of *Mycobacterium tuberculosis* or HIV. They are real things, spread by real contact, causing real disease. The deaths they cause are anything but symbolic effect. However, objects of science, such as the bacterium and the virus, though ontologically distinct realities, are also symbolic and linguistic objects.

15 Purity, I take as meaning that nothing of the outside is inside; integrity, that nothing of the inside is outside. More or less the same thing viewed from opposite sides of the line of being. For an object to exist or 'be', in both the ontological and epistemological senses, it must have and maintain a certain degree of individuality and distinctiveness. It must maintain its borders by maintaining its purity and integrity.

16 As mentioned in chapter 2, rates of bystander CPR vary from 10–50 per cent. As will be discussed in chapter 7, CPR is perhaps realized more frequently as a heroic fantasy than in dutiful action.

6 External Cardiac Compression: Beating a Dead Horse

1 In the 1940s and 1950s, open chest cardiac massage did come to be used on hospital wards for cardiac arrest, but it was always an exceptional procedure. Today, thoracotomy's main use is as the ultimate act in the 'trauma arrest'.

2 This is a confusing area. Most flow studies use animal models. There are considerable differences in response between healthy animals put into experimental arrest and ill human beings in spontaneous arrest. The latter usually faring more poorly than the former.

3 It is not possible in this book to give a detailed discussion of experimental evidence for and against the effectiveness of external cardiac compression. In my opinion, the case for significant effect in the clinical arrest situation is extremely weak. Readers wishing to decide for themselves should see the articles cited in the text plus: Ames et al., 1983, p. 219; Devita, 2001, p. 58; Abramson, 1998, p. 110; Safar et al., 1996, p. 105; Stiell, 1996, p. 1417; Little and Cairns, 1999, p. S90; Berg et al. 2001, p. S26.

4 Defibrillation, though on much firmer empirical and theoretical ground than either manual ventilatory techniques or external cardiac compression, is, as has been pointed out, far from universally successful (see chapter 4). Currently, much effort is being invested in increasing the efficacy of defibrillation – AEDs, high energy, low energy, stacked shocks, pre-CPR, post-CPR, monophasic wave form and biphasic wave form variants.

5 Electroencephalograms, brain scans and the like are used to determine brain death, but these usually only come into play in the comparatively infrequent situations of irreversible coma or vegetative state.

6 This is not to say that criteria of death, such as the flat line on the ECG or the electrical silence of the EEG, do not remain important, from both a scientific and symbolic point of view, but they do remain suspect unless confirmed by the absence of response. The EEG criterion for brain death is bilateral absence of cortical *response* to median somato-sensory- *evoked* potentials. The flat line on the ECG is usually accepted as such only *after* attempts at defibrillation (American, 2000, pp. I.12–I.22).

7 In this Bloch acknowledges his debt to Victor Turner's elaboration of Arnold van Gennep's 'rites of passage' (van Gennep, 1960; V. Turner, 1969). These rites of passage are a three-stage process in which there is a separation from the old status (pre-liminal), a period of transition in which a change in identity occurs (liminal), and then a reincorporation into the

new status (post-liminal). If we think back to chapter 5, we may remember that the process of contagion was also characterized by a similar movement of transgression, transformation and aggressive return.

8 The process of identification is, in Freudian terms, part of the construction of the self. In identifying with others, we internalize them and make them a part of our own ego structure. Thus, we necessarily invest ourselves in other people, whom we might be said to love. When they are lost to us through death, their loss is experienced as loss of self. We grieve not only the disappearance of the other person but also the loss of that part of ourselves that was constructed from the other person (Freud, 1984b, pp. 251–67).

9 The questioning of this impulse is almost as old as the impulse itself. It might, arguably, be seen as one of the founding manoeuvres of natural philosophy, what we now think of as the scientific mode of thought. Heraclitus mocked ritual catharsis, comparing those who purge blood with blood to a man who tries to wash off dirt by bathing in mud (fr. 5). Plato makes the same argument in the *Phaedrus*, but concedes the psychological need for catharsis, irrational as it is, as does, most famously, Aristotle in the *Poetics*.

10 This is not to deny the comfort of language in therapeutic discourse or the use of language in ritual. However, ritual uses language in a way very different from that of discursive speech. In ritual, speech is performative, more a verbal act than a form of communication. In ritual, words are less vehicles of meaning than creative agents. The last act of resuscitation, when revival has failed, is to declare the patient dead. Here, the power of performative speech is starkly revealed. Whatever biological death might be, however it is measured, identified and insured, you are not dead until I, the physician, declare you dead.

11 Shen, in his introduction to Timmermans' book, perceives much of the problem with modern death as resulting from an inability to make 'the distinction between saving life and coping with death' (1999, p. 1). Any analysis of the deathbed requires this distinction to be made. However, articulating a distinction is not the same as operating within the phenomenon described. The struggle to save life and the construction of an appropriate death, though perhaps logically distinct, are, if my argument is correct, difficult if not impossible to separate operationally.

12 Luke Davidson (2000) points out that 'feeling like a god' is a dangerously loaded phrase. What exactly does it mean to feel like God? God, or at least His putative attributes, are notoriously historically specific. An analysis of the phrase, as it is used in modernity, should reveal it to be meaningless. We doubt if God is, or if He is what He is, or, even if we do concede the former, what He might feel like, if He does indeed feel. Nevertheless, the phrase is not meaningless, nor is the subjective state it describes unrecognizable. Davidson asks, is it the adrenalin-rush brought on by the frenzied activity of a life-and-death situation? Is it manic self-intoxication brought on by the exercise of power? Is it the madness of the mad scientist, Dr Frankenstein laughing alone in the lab? Is it the hubris of science: a God that cares not for his creation but only for the exercise of power over it? To Luke's accusations, I would have to answer, Yes. It is all these – frenzy, intoxication, madness, power. And that is, perhaps shamefully, my point.

13 There is a great deal more that might be said about death and the erotic. I would refer readers to Bataille (1957), Ariès (1981), Twitchell (1981), Freud (1984a, pp. 275–337), and Stewart (1984).
14 The fundamental aspiration of positivism is to know in order to act, and empiricism's method is to act in order to know. The scientific experiment is the most obvious example of the latter. CPR as an act of revival uses medical knowledge to guide its actions, as a manoeuvre diagnosing death, it acts in order to know.

7   The Media: Getting it Right?

1 Between 1952 and 1995, when *ER* topped the ratings, over 60 doctors' series had aired on prime-time US television (Turow, 1996, p. 1241). With $13 million available for each episode, *ER* is, up to this point, the most expensive drama in the history of television.
2 The fictional hospital where *Casualty* is set.
3 However, that percentage is growing; shows such as *Westwing* and *24 Hours* rely heavily on Steadicam footage. The movie *Russian Ark*, released in April 2003, is the Steadicam's apotheosis: a single, unedited, 90-minute Steadicam shot, encompassing 300 years of Russian history.
4 It can be argued that all realisms are constructions. The form of realism or the form that a realism takes depends upon the norm of reality you have chosen to recognize. All forms of realism are in fact artificial conventions, no matter how carefully they try to mimic 'reality'. The shakiness of the hand-held documentary camera and the steadiness of the Steadicam are both meant to signal 'reality', though in very different ways and for very different purposes. It *is* possible to over-anthropomorphize the effect of the Steadicam. It is a convention. Nevertheless it is a technology that has been chosen for particular phenomenal reasons.
5 In C. S. Peirce's classification of signs, an indexical image or sign is one that partakes of the reality of the thing it represents or signifies. A fingerprint is an indexical sign of the person fingerprinted in that it requires the physical contact of flesh, ink and paper. A photograph is indexical as the physical presence of the object photographed is required to reflect the light that registers on the film as an image. An indexical image implicitly declares the facticity of its content: 'What I portray is what actually happened, because I could not exist unless it did.' The indexicality of the image is taken as a guarantee not only of the object's fact but of the image's truth. What is represented is what was, not what is made by the seeing. However, it can be argued that all forms of artistic 'realism' are constructions. The form that a realism takes depends upon the norm of reality you have chosen to recognize. All forms of representational realism, even photographs and especially cinema and video, are artificial conventions, no matter how carefully they attempt to document 'reality'. Capturing this image and not another, the position of the camera, the framing of the subject, and so on are all decisions made by the photographer in his or her construction of the image. Likewise, the viewer has as many options when deciding what see and how to view it. It is, obviously, possible to over-emphasize the index-

icality of photography, film and video, especially in these days of digital manipulation and special effects. Nevertheless, the rhetoric of 'seeing is (as) believing' remains powerful.
6 The United States is not the only producer of and market for medical dramas. In the UK the success rate of resuscitation in medical dramas during the 1980s and 1990s was around 25 per cent, less out of line with real-life rates. There are many other major differences between the UK and US (and I dare say between other countries) in the portrayal of medicine on television, however, that is another book (Tunstall-Pedoe et al., 1992, p. 1347; P. Gordon, Williamson and Lawler, 1998, p. 780).
7 There is a conflation here of CPR and trauma resuscitation – of ACLS and ATLS. ACLS and ATLS are not the same thing, though both are resuscitative protocols and there is considerable overlap, especially in the initial ABC stages of each. However, in the public's imagination, the two are usually perceived as one and the same.
8 Tragic flaw, surprising discovery, reversal of fortune, building tension and release.
9 For an effective example of this, see the 'Hell and Highwater' episode of *ER*, available on the videotape *ER: By Popular Demand* (1995). This is the most popular episode of *ER* ever broadcast and is credited with making George Clooney a star. In it, Dr Ross's heroic saving of one child (from drowning) is balanced by another's tragic death (the result of a motor vehicle accident). This opposition is an enormously effective dramatic device, and can, perhaps, be criticized as cynically manipulative. At the same time, I can assure you, in real ERs, it is a not unheard of occurrence in multiple-victim accidents.
10 Gorer, *The Pornography of Death*, 1955.
11 Motion Picture Association of America rating: PG13 is suggested parental guidance for children under 13 years of age. It is roughly equivalent to the British Board of Film Classification's 12 certificate.

8 Conclusion: Modern Living, Modern Dying

1 0–1 per cent of patients over the age of 70, who receive out-of-hospital CPR, survive to hospital discharge (American, *Guidelines* I.136–I.165; Murphy et al., 1989, p. 199; Taffet et al., 1989, p. 1579).
2 It should be pointed out that this rather discouraging picture is not universal. Advances have been made in rationalizing the management of terminally ill patients in the ICU and on the wards. For patients in multiple-organ failure or with global cerebral ischemia (severe irreversible brain damage due to lack of oxygen) a pro-active approach encouraging the early recognition of poor prognosis and the writing of DNR orders does result in a decrease in length of time spent in ICU, time dying, unnecessary medical interventions and costs (Prendergast, Claessens and Luce, 1997, pp. 1163–7; Campbell and Guzman, 2003, pp. 266–71).
3 In 1996, it was estimated that it cost US $200 to declare a patient dead on arrival at the emergency department, whereas an unsuccessful resuscitation averaged $4,150 (Pasquale et al., 1996, p. 726). If the resuscitation was

successful, then costs increase due to the need for further care (Ebell and Kruse, 1994, p. 640). The cost of CPR per six-month survivor then becomes in the range of $344,314–966,759 (K. Lee, Angus and Abramson, 1996, p. 2046).

4 'Code' is medical slang for a resuscitative episode.
5 Slow heart rate.
6 In a 'resuscitation will', one would be resuscitated only if one had so specified ahead of time, as opposed to an advance directive where one is *not* resuscitated only if one so specifies. The use of a 'resuscitation will' is supported by the Canadian Ethics Committee (Vancouver, 1996a).
7 Beckman reports that as the experience of physicians increases, so too does the likelihood that they will allow parental presence in the resuscitative situation:

Years of post-graduate experience	*Percentage allowing parental presence*
0–5	28.3 per cent
6–10	30.7 per cent
>10	43.9 per cent

There was also a slight (though I would say in the light of my hypothesis, significant) increase from 31.9 per cent to 35.6 per cent of those allowing parental presence, if they thought the outcome of the resuscitation was more likely to be fatal as opposed to non-fatal (Beckman, Moore and Knoop, 1999, p. S63).

8 Readers may be disappointed that something is not said about 'near death experiences'. There is some anecdotal evidence to suggest that the last moments of life are not nearly the torment we imagine them to be. In most deaths, there does seem to be a point reached where struggle ceases and a sort of calm ensues. Investigation into the possible psycho-physiological factors involved indicate that this may be due to the release of neurotransmitters called endorphins, a sort of internal narcotic, producing a feeling of well-being and some relief from pain. I refer readers to discussions in this area: Basford, 1990; Kellehear, 1993, pp. 148–56; Nuland, 1994, pp. 129–36, Greyson, 2000, pp. 460–3; van Lommel et al, 2002, p. 2039.

References

Abramson, N. 'Brain Resuscitation', *Emergency Medicine: Concepts and Clinical Practice*, ed. Peter Rosen. St. Louis: Mosby, 1998. 107–19.

Ahmed, F. et al. 'Transmission of Salmonella via Mouth-to-Mouth Resuscitation', *Lancet* 335 (1990): 787–8.

Albury, W. 'Ideas of Life and Death', *Companion Encyclopedia of the History of Medicine*, eds. W. Bynum and R. Porter. London: Routledge, 1993. Vol. 1, 249–80.

Ames, A. et al. 'Pathophysiology of Ischemic Cell Death. I. Time of Onset of Irreversible Damage: Importance of the Different Components of the Ischemic Insult', *Stroke* 14 (1983). 219.

American Heart Association. 'Standards for Cardiopulmonary Resuscitation (CPR) and Emergency Cardiac Care (ECC)', *JAMA* 227 Suppl (1974): 796–868.

—— *Advanced Cardiac Life Support*. Dallas: American Heart Association, 1994.

—— *Heartsaver AED*. Dallas: American Heart Association, 1999.

—— *Heart and Stroke Statistical Update*. Dallas: American Heart Association, 2002.

—— 'Emergency Cardiovascular Care', *American Heart Association*. (2002): Online: http://www.americanheart.org/presenter.jhtml?identifier=1200000. Accessed 27 March 2003.

American Heart Association and National Academy of Sciences–National Research Council. 'Cardiopulmonary Resuscitation: Statement by the Ad Hoc Committee on Cardiopulmonary Resuscitation of the Division of Medical Sciences, National Academy of Science National Research Council', *JAMA* 198 (1966): 372–9.

American Heart Association in collaboration with International Liaison Committee on Resuscitation. 'Guidelines 2000 for Cardiopulmonary Resuscitation and Emergency Cardiovascular Care: International Consensus on Science', *Circulation* 102 (suppl I) (2000) CD-ROM. Dallas: American Heart Association, 2000.

Angelos M. et al. 'Flow Requirements in Ventricular Fibrillation: An In-Vivo Nuclear Magnetic Resonance Analysis of the Left Ventricular High-Energy Phosphate Pool', *Ann Emerg Med* 34 (1999): 583–8.

Annas, G. 'Death by Prescription', *JAMA* 331 (1994): 1240–3.

Ariès, P. *The Hour of Our Death*, 1977, trans. H. Weaver. Oxford: Oxford University Press, 1981.

Armstrong, D. and E. Armstrong. *The Great American Medicine Show*. New York: Prentice Hall, 1991.

Arnold, K. *Doctor Death: Medicine at the End of Life*. London: Wellcome Trust, 1997.

Arnold, M. 'Dover Beach', *The Golden Treasury*, ed. F. Palgrave. London: Collins, 1954. 406.

Babbs, C. 'Hemodynamic Mechanisms in CPR: A Theoretical Rationale for Resuscitative Thoracotomy in Non-Traumatic Cardiac Arrest', *Resuscitation*. 15 (1987): 37–50.

Bachelard, G. *Water and Dreams: An Essay on the Imagination of Matter*, 1942, trans. Edith R. Farrell. Dallas: Dallas Institute Publications, 1983.

Baer, N. 'Cardiopulmonary Resuscitation on Television: Exaggerations and Accusations', *NEJM*. 334 (1996): 1604–5.

Baker, A. 'Artificial Respiration: the History of an Idea', *Medical History*. 15 (1971), 336–51.

Bakhtin, M. *Rabelais and His World*, trans. H. Iswolsky. Bloomington: Indiana University Press, 1984.

—— 'Contemporary Vitalism', *The Crisis in Modernism: Bergson and the Vitalist Controversy*, 1926, trans. C. Byrd, eds. F. Burwick et al. Cambridge: Cambridge University Press, 1992. 75–97.

Ballew, K. A. 'Active Compression-Decompression CPR for Cardiac Arrest Did Not Improve Survival or Neurologic Outcomes', *ACP J Club* 125 (1996): 39.

Barley, N. *Grave Matters: A Lively History of Death around the World*. New York: Henry Holt & Co., 1995.

Barratt, F. and D. Wallis. 'Relatives in the Resuscitation Room: Their Point of View', *J Accid Emerg Med* 15 (1998): 109-11.

Barthes, R. *Camera Lucida*, 1980, trans. R. Howard. London: Vintage, 2000.

Bartlett, A. *Discourse on the Subject of Animation*. Boston: Thomas and Andrews, 1792.

Basford, T. *Near-Death Experiences: An Annoted Bibliography*. New York: Garland Publishing, 1990.

Bataille, G. *Visions of Excess: Selected Writings, 1927–1939*, Trans. A. Stoekl. Minneapolis: University of Minnesota Press, 1985.

—— *Eroticism*. 1957, Trans. M. Dalwood. Marion Boyars: London, 1987.

Batcheller, A. et al. 'Cardiopulmonary Resuscitation Performance of Subjects Over Forty is Better Following Half-Hour Video Self-Instruction Compared To Traditional Four-Hour Classroom Training', *Resuscitation* 43 (2) (2000): 101–10.

Bath Humane Society, Instituted in the Year 1805. Bath: W. Meyler, 1806.

Baudrillard, J. *Symbolic Exchange and Death*, 1976, trans. I. Grant. London: Sage, 1993.

Baumann, Z. *Mortality and Immortality*. Cambridge: Polity, 1992.

Beck, C. and D. Leihnenger. 'Reversal of Death in Good Hearts.' *Journal of Cardiovascular Surgery* 3 (1962): 357.

Beck, C., W. Pritchard and H. Feil. 'Ventricular Fibrillation of Long Duration Abolished by Electric Shock', *JAMA* 135(15) (1947): 985–6.

Beck, C. et al. 'Death after a Clean Bill of Health', *JAMA* 174 (1960): 133–5.

Becker, L., D. Smith and K. Rhodes. 'Incidence of Cardiac Arrest: A Neglected Factor in Evaluating Survival Rates', *Ann Emerg Med* 22 (1993): 86–91.

Becker, L. et al. 'Outcome of CPR in a Large Metropolitan Area: Where Are the Survivors?' *Ann Emerg Med* 20 (1991): 355–61.

—— 'A Reappraisal of Mouth-to-Mouth Ventilation during Bystander-Initiated Cardiopulmonary Resuscitation', *Circulation* 96 (1997): 2102–12.

—— 'The Impact of Television Public Service Announcements On the Rate of Bystander CPR.' *Prehospital Emergency Care* 3 (1999): 353-6.

Beckman, A., G. Moore and K. Knoop. 'Should Parents Be Present? Physician Perception of Parental Presence during Emergency Department Procedures', *Ann Emerg Med* 34 (1999): S63.

Bedell, S. et al. 'Survival after Cardiopulmonary Resuscitation in the Hospital', *NEJM* 309(10) (1983): 569–76.
Belling, C. 'Reading the Operation', *Literature and Medicine* 17 (1998): 1–23.
Benson, D. 'Recent Advances in Emergency Resuscitation', *Maryland State Medical Journal*. 36 (1961): 398–411.
Berg, R. et al. 'Chest Compressions and Basic Life Support-Defibrillation', *Ann Emerg Med* 37(4) (2001): S26–S35.
—— 'Automated External Defibrillation Versus Manual Defibrillation for Prolonged Ventricular Fibrillation: Lethal Delays of Chest Compressions before and after Countershocks', *Ann Emerg Med* 42(4) (2003): 458–67.
Bichat, X. *Physiological Researches on Life and Death*, 1800, trans. F. Gold. London: Richardson and Lord, 1827.
Blank-Reid, C. and L. Kaplan. 'Video Recording Trauma Resuscitations: A Guide to System Set-up, Personnel Concerns, and Legal Issues', *Journal of Trauma Nursing* 3(1) (1996): 9–12.
Bloch, M. *Prey into Hunter*. Cambridge: Cambridge University Press, 1992.
Blouin, D. and S. Moore. 'Time to Recurrent Ventricular Tachycardia or Ventricular Fibrillation after Defibrillation', *Ann Emerg Med* 34 (1999): S17.
Bondeson, J. *Buried Alive: The Terrifying History of Our Most Primal Fear*. New York: W. W. Norton & Co., 2001.
Bonnin, M. et al. 'Distinct Criteria for Termination of Resuscitation in the Out-of-Hospital Setting', *JAMA* 270 (1993): 1457–62.
Bouchie, F. 'Guy Bee: Camera Operator', *CSULB: Film and Electronic Arts Alumni*. (2 November 1999). Online: http://www.csulb.edu/depts/fea/archives/guybee.htm. Accessed 4 June 2002.
Bradshaw, P. 'Driven round the Bend', *Guardian Weekly*, 13 January 2000: 15.
Braslow, A. et al. 'CPR Training without an Instructor: Development and Evaluation of a Video Self-Instructional System for Effective Performance of Cardiopulmonary Resuscitation', *Resuscitation* 34 (1997): 207–20.
Brenner, B. et al. 'Determinants of Physician Reluctance to Perform Mouth-to-Mouth Resuscitation', *J Clin Epidemiol* 53(10) (2000): 1054–61.
Bringing Out the Dead. Dir. Martin Scorcese, 1999. Videocassette. Paramount, 2000.
Brison, R. et al. 'Cardiac Arrest in Ontario: Circumstances, Community Response, Role of Prehospital Defibrillation and Predictors of Survival', *Can Med Assoc J* 147 (1992): 191–9.
British Heart Foundation. 'News', *British Heart Foundation* (2001). Online: http://www.bhf.org.uk/. Accessed 7 July 2001.
Brodie, B. *The Works of Sir Benjamin Collins Brodie*, ed. C. Hawkins. Vol. 1. London: Longman, Roberts, & Green, 1865.
Bromley, R. *A Sermon Preached Before the Humane Society at St. Andrew's, Holborn*. London: Rivington, 1782.
Brown, C. et al. 'The Effects of Graded Doses of Epinephrine on Regional Myocardial Blood Flow during Cardiopulmonary Resuscitation in Swine', *Circulation* 75 (1987): 491–7.
——. 'A Comparison of Standard-Dose and High-Dose Epinephrine in Cardiac Arrest Outside Hospital', *NEJM* 327 (1992): 1051–5.
Brown, D. 'Americans Move to Put Heart Machines in Public Places', *Guardian Weekly* 14–20 October 1999: 33.

Brown, R. 'Yesterday's Zero'. Fifth International Conference on Death, Dying and Disposal. Goldsmith's College, London. 8 September 2000.
Bunch, T. et al. 'Long-term Outcomes of Out-of-Hospital Cardiac Arrest after Successful Early Defibrillation', *N Engl J Med* 348 (2003): 2626–33.
Burden, C. 'Interview with Chris Burden at the Royal Academy of Fine Arts, Stockholm.' *Artnode*. 5 February 1999. Online: http://www.artnode.se/burden/. Accessed 10 April 2000.
Burkert, W. *Homo Necans*. London: University of California Press, 1983.
Burwick, F. and P. Douglass. 'Introduction', *The Crisis in Modernism*, ed. F. Burwick. Cambridge: Cambridge University Press, 1992. 1–11.
Bynum, W. *Science and the Practice of Medicine in the Nineteenth Century*. Cambridge: Cambridge University Press, 1994.
Caffrey, L. et al., 'Public Use of Automated External Defibrillators' *NEJM* 347(16) (2002): 1242–7.
Campany, R. 'Xunzi and Durkheim as Theorists of Ritual Practice', *Readings in Ritual Studies*, ed. Ronald Grimes. Upper Saddle River: Prentice Hall, 1996. 86–103.
Campbell, D. 'Hollywood Braces itself for Violent End', *Guardian Weekly*, 13 June 1999: 7.
Campbell, M. and J. Guzman. 'Impact of a Proactive Approach to Improve End-of-Life Care in a Medical ICU', *Chest* 123(1) (2003): 266–71.
Canguilhem, G. *The Normal and the Pathological*, trans. C. Fawcett and R. Cohen. New York: Zone, 1991.
Carel, H. 'At His Majesty's Service: Death as Transcendence in Freud and Heidegger'. Fifth International Conference on Death, Dying and Disposal. Goldsmith's College, London. 10 September 2000.
CDC (Center for Disease Control). 'Leading Causes of Death Reports', *WISQARS*. Online: http://webapp.cdc.gov/sasweb/ncipc/leadcaus10.html. Accessed 3 April 2004.
Chesterton, G. K. *Heretics*, 1905. New York: John Lane, 1919.
Cobb, L., J. Werner, and G. Trobaugh. 'Sudden Cardiac Death. I. A Decade's Experience with Out-of-Hospital Resuscitation; II. Outcome of Resuscitation Management and Future Directions. *Modern Concepts of Cardiovasc Dis* 49 (1980): 31–42.
Cobb, L. et al. 'Community Cardiopulmonary Resuscitation', *Annu Rev Med* 31 (1980): 453–62.
Coleman, E. *A Dissertation on Suspended Respiration, from Drowning, Hanging, and Suffocation*. London, 1791.
Cooper, D. 'Minireview: Mouth-to-Mouth Resuscitation: Influence of Alcohol on Revival of an Old Technique', *Life Sciences*. 16 (1975): 487–500.
Cork, R. 'The Critic's View: *The New Anatomists*'. *Wellcome Trust* (2000). Online: http://www.wellcome.ac.uk/en/old/new_anatomists/MISexhTWOanaCRT.ht ml. Accessed 23 December 2000.
Cousins, M. 'The Ugly', *AA Files*. 28 (1994): 61–4.
Cram, P., S, Vijan and A. Fendrick. 'Cost-effectiveness of Automated External Defibrillator Deployment in Selected Public Locations', *J Gen Intern Med* 18 (2003): 745–54.
Crayford, T., R. Hooper and S. Evans. 'Death Rates in Characters in Soap Operas on British Television: Is a Government Health Warning Required?' *BMJ* 515 (1997): 1649–52.

Cullen, W. *Letter to Lord Cathcart, President of the Board of Police in Scotland, Concerning the Recovery of Persons Drowned and Seemed Dead: Aug 8, 1774.* London: J. Murray, 1776.
Culley, L. et al. 'Public Access Defibrillation in Out-of-Hospital Cardiac Arrest. A Community-Based Study', *Circulation* 109 (2004): p. S1524.
Cummins, R. *Advanced Cardiac Life Support.* Dallas: American Heart Association, 1994.
—— 'Resuscitations from Pulseless Electrical Activity and Asystole: How Big a Piece of the Survivors' Pie?' *Ann Emerg Med* 32 (1998): 490–2.
—— *ACLS Provider Manual.* Dallas: American Heart Association, 2001.
Cummins, R. et al. 'Survival of Out-of-Hospital Cardiac Arrest with Early Initiation of Cardiopulmonary Resuscitation', *Am J Emerg Med* 3 (1985): 114–19.
—— 'Improving Survival from Sudden Cardiac Arrest: the "Chain of Survival" Concept: A Statement for Health Professionals from the Advanced Cardiac Life Support Subcommittee and the Emergency Cardiac Care Committee, American Heart Association', *Circulation* 83 (1991a): 1832–47.
—— 'Recommended Guidelines for Uniform Reporting of Data from Out-of-Hospital Cardiac Arrest: the Utstein Style', *Circulation* 84 (1991b): 960–75.
Cunningham, R. 'The Cause of Death from Industrial Electrical Currents', *New York Medicine Journal* (1899): 618–22.
Curry, J. *Observations on Apparent Death from Drowning, Hanging, Suffocation by Noxious Vapours, Fainting Fits, Intoxication, Exposure to the Cold, &c. &c. and an Account of the Means to be Employed for Recovery, to which are added, the Treatment Proper in Cases of Poison; with Cautions and Suggestions Respecting Various Circumstances of Sudden Danger,* 1792. London: E. Cox and Son. 1815.
Danforth, L. *The Death Rituals of Ancient Greece.* Princeton: Princeton University Press, 1982.
Danzl, D. 'Accidental Hypothermia', *Emergency Medicine: Concepts and Clinical Practice,* ed. Peter Rosen. St. Louis: Mosby, 1998. 963–86.
d'Aquili, E. and C. Laughlin. 'Neurobiology of Myth and Ritual', *Readings in Ritual Studies,* 1979, ed. Ronald Grimes. Upper Saddle River: Prentice Hall, 1996. 132–45.
Darwin, C. *The Expression of the Emotions in Man and Animals,* 1872. London: HarperCollins, 1998.
David, J. and P. Prior-Willeard. 'Resuscitation Skills of MRCP Candidates', *BMJ* 306(6892) (1993): 1578–9.
Davidson, L. Letter to author. 13 November 2000.
Davies, D. *Death, Ritual and Belief.* London: Cassell, 1997.
Davies, J. 'Introduction', *Ritual and Remembrance: Responses to Death in Human Societies.* Ed. Jon Davies. Sheffield: Sheffield Academic Press, 1994.
Davis, E., J. McCrorry and V. Mosesso. 'Institution of Police Automated External Defibrillation Program: Concepts and Practice', *Prehosp Emerg Care* 3 (1999): 60–5.
de Hennezel, M. *Intimate Death.* trans. Carol Janeway. New York: Time Warner, 1998.
De Maio, V. et al. 'Cardiac Arrest Witnessed by Emergency Medical Services Personnel: Descriptive Epidemiology, Prodromal Symptoms, and Predictors of Survival', *Ann Emerg Med* 35 (2000): 138–6.

Devita, M. 'The Death Watch: Certifying Death Using Cardiac Criteria', *Progress in Transplantation* 11(1) (2001): 58–66.

Dickens, C. *Nicholas Nickleby*, 1839. Oxford: Oxford University Press, 1990.

Diem, S., J. Lantos and J. Tulsky. 'Cardiopulmonary Resuscitation on Television – Miracles and Misinformation', *NEJM* 334(24) (1996): 1578–82.

Dill, D. 'Manual Artificial Respiration', *U.S. Armed Forces Medical Journal*. 3(2) (1951): 171–84.

—— 'Symposium on Mouth to Mouth Resuscitation', *Journal of the American Medical Association*. 167(3) (1958): 317–19.

Dodds, E. *The Greeks and the Irrational*. Berkeley: University of California Press, 1951.

Douglas, M. *Purity and Danger*. London: Routledge, 1966.

Doyle, C. et al. 'Family Participation during Resuscitation: An Option', *Ann Emerg Med*. 16(6) (1987): 673–5.

Durkheim, E. *The Elementary Forms of Religious Life*, 1912, trans. K. Fields. New York: Free Press, 1995.

Dworkin, A. *Pornography: Men Possessing Women*. New York: Perigee, 1981.

Easton, J. 'Mouth-to-Mouth Ventilation's Role in CPR Questioned'. 16 September 1997. Online: http://www.uchospitals.edu/news/1997/19970916-mtm-cpr.html. Accessed 2 April 2001.

Ebell, M. and J. Kruse. 'A Proposed Model for the Cost of Cardiopulmonary Resuscitation', *Medical Care* 32(6) (1994): 640–9.

Eichhorn, D. et al. 'Opening the Doors: Family Presence during Resuscitation', *J Cardiovasc Nurs* 10(4) (1996): 59–70.

Einthoven, W. et al. 'On the Direction and Manifest Size of the Variations of Potential in the Human Heart and on the Influence of the Position of the Heart on the Form of the Electrocardiogram', *Am Heart J* 40 (1950): 163–211.

Eisenberg, M. 'Cardiac Resuscitation in the Community: Importance of Rapid Provision and Implications for Program Planning', *JAMA* 241 (1979): 1905–7.

—— *Life in the Balance: Emergency Medicine and the Quest to Reverse Sudden Death*. New York: Oxford University Press, 1997.

Eisenberg, M., L. Bergner and A. Hallstrom. 'Paramedic Programs and Out-of-Hospital Cardiac Arrest, I: Factors Associated with Successful Resuscitation', *Am J Public Health* 69 (1979): 30–8.

Eisenberg, M., M. Copass and A. Hallstrom. 'Treatment of Out-of-Hospital Cardiac Arrest with Rapid Defibrillation by Emergency Medical Technicians', *NEJM* 302 (1980): 1379–83.

Eisenberg, M. et al. 'Out-of-Hospital Cardiac Arrest: Improved Survival with Paramedic Services', *Lancet* 1 (1980): 812–15.

– 'Cardiac Arrest and Resuscitation: A Tale of 29 Cities', *Ann Emerg Med* 19 (1990): 179–86.

Eisenburger, P. and P. Safar. 'Life Supporting First Aid Training of the Public–Review and Recommendations', *Resuscitation* 41(1) (1999): 3–18.

Elam, J., E. Brown and J. Elder. 'Artificial Respiration by Mouth to Mask Method: A Study of the Respiratory Gas Exchange of Paralyzed Patients Ventilated by Operator's Expired Air', *NEJM* 250 (1954): 749–54.

Eliade, M. *The Sacred and the Profane*, trans. W. Trask. San Diego: Harcourt Brace & Co., 1957.

Elias, N. *The Loneliness of the Dying*, trans. E. Jephcott. Oxford: Basil Blackwell, 1985.

'ER: Room for Emergency.' *iafrica*. Online: http://entertainment.iafrica.com/tv/archives/3310.htm. Accessed 10 May 2002.

Feldhouse, K. and R. Knopp. 'Near Drowning', *Emergency Medicine: Concepts and Clinical Practice*, ed. Peter Rosen. St. Louis: Mosby, 1998. 1061–6.

Feldman, H. 'Some Recollections of the Meningococcal Disease: The First Harry F. Dowling Lecture', *JAMA*. 220 (1972): 1107–12.

Figura, N. 'Mouth-to-Mouth Resuscitation and Helicobacter Pylori Infection', *Lancet* 347 (1996): 1342.

Finkelhor, R. and J. Lampman. 'Herpes Simplex Infection following Mouth-to-Mouth Resuscitation', *JAMA* 243 (1980): 650.

Fisher, H. *Resuscitation in Medical Physics*, ed. Otto Glasser. Chicago: Year Book Publishers, 1944. 1241–54.

Flanagan, B. *The Pain Journal*. Los Angeles: Semiotext(e)/Smart Art Press, 2000.

Fong, J. *Inside 'ER'*. 7 August 2000. Online: http://www.emedhome.com/archives-data.cfm?ID=news080700&Type=news. Accessed 3 May 2003.

Fothergill, J. 'Observations on a Case Published in the Last Volume of the Medical Essays, &c. of Recovering a Man Dead in Appearance, by Distending the Lungs with Air', *A Complete Collection of the Medical and Philosophical Works of John Fothergill*, 1744. Ed. John Elliot. London: Robinson, 1782: 110–19.

Fothergill, A. *A New Inquiry into the Suspension of Vital Action in the Cases of Drowning and Suffocation*. Bath: S. Hazard, 1795.

—— *An Address to the King and Parliament of Great-Britain, On Preserving the Lives of the Inhabitants*. London: Dodsley, 1783.

Foucault, M. 'Introduction' to GeorgesCanguilhem, *The Normal and the Pathological*, trans. Carolyn R. Fawcett. New York: Zone Books, 1991. 6–20.

Freud, S. 'On the Psychical Mechanisms of Hysterical Phenomena: Preliminary Communication', *The Standard Edition of the Complete Psychological Works of Sigmund Freud*, 1893, ed. James Strachey, trans. James Strachey. Vol. 2. London: Hogarth Press, 1955. 3–17

—— 'Negation.' *The Standard Edition.*. Vol. 19. London: Hogarth Press, 1961. 235–9.

—— 'Beyond the Pleasure Principle', *On Metapsychology*, 1920, ed. Angela Richards, trans. James Strachey. London: Penguin Books, 1984a. 276–337.

—— 'Mourning and Melancholia.' *On Metapsychology*, 1917, ed. Angela Richards, trans. James Strachey. London: Penguin Books, 1984b. 251–67.

—— 'Civilization and Its Discontents', *Civilization, Society and Religion*, 1930, ed. Angela Richards, trans. James Strachey. London: Penguin Books, 1985a. 251–340.

—— 'Thoughts for the Times on War and Death', *Civilization, Society and Religion*, 1915. ed. Angela Richards, trans. James Strachey. London: Penguin Books, 1985b. 57–89.

—— 'Totem and Taboo', *The Origins of Religion*, 1913, ed. Angela Richards, trans. James Strachey. London: Penguin Books, 1985c. 43–159.

'From What Will We Die in 2020?' Editorial. *Lancet* 349 (1997): 1263.

Gallagher, E., G. Lombardi and P. Gennis. 'Effectiveness of Bystander Cardio-pulmonary Resuscitation and Survival Following Out-of-Hospital Cardiac Arrest', *JAMA* 274(24) (1995): 1922–5.

Gibbs, H. and A. Ross. *The Medicine of ER, or, How We Almost Die*. London: Flamingo, 1997.

Giddens, A. *Modernity and Self-identity*. Cambridge: Polity Press, 1991.
Gill, S. and J. Fox. *The Dead Good Funerals Book*. Ulverston: Welfare State International, 1997.
Gombeski, W. et al. 'Impact on Retention: Comparison of Two CPR Training Programs', *Am J Public Health* 72 (1982): 849–52.
Goodwyn, E. *The Connexion of Life with Respiration*. London: J. Johnson, 1788.
Gordon, A. et al. 'Manual Artificial Respiration', *JAMA* 14 (1950): 1447–52.
Gordon, A. et al. 'Critical Survey of Manual Artificial Respiration', *JAMA* 147 (1951): 1444–53.
Gordon, P., S. Williamson and P. Lawler. 'As Seen on TV: Observational Study of Cardiopulmonary Resuscitation in British Television Medical Dramas', *BMJ* 317 (1998): 780–3.
Gorer, G. 'The Pornography of Death'. *Death, Grief, and Mourning*, 1955. New York: Doubleday, 1965. 192–9.
The Governors of the Newcastle Dispensary. Proposal for Recovering Persons Apparently Dead by Drowning and Suffocation from Other Causes. Newcastle: Hodson, 1789.
Green, T. 'Heart Massage as a Means of Restoration in Cases of Apparent Sudden Death', *Lancet* ii (1906): 1707–4.
Greene, K. 'ER–Another Day, Another Trauma', *Motion Picture Editors Guild Newsletter*. September 1997. Online: http://www.editorsguild.com/newsletter/SepOct97/morgan.html. Accessed 12 May 2002.
Greyson, B. 'Dissociation in People Who Have Near-Death Experiences: Out of Their Bodies or Out of Their Minds?' *Lancet* 355(9202) (2000): 460–3.
Grim, P. *Just Here Trying to Save a Few Lives*. New York: Warner Books, 2000.
Groh, W. et al. 'Cardiopulmonary Resuscitation by Chest Compression Alone', *NEJM* 343 (2000): 815–17.
Gruman, G. 'Ethics of Death and Dying: Historical Perspective', *Omega* 9 (1978–9): 203–37.
Gubar, S. and J. Hoff, eds. *For Adult Users Only: the Dilemma of Violent Pornography*. Bloomington: Indiana University Press. 1989.
Guild of Television Cameramen. 'Steadicam Masterclass Transcript', *The Guild of Television Cameramen*. Online: http://www.gtc.org.uk/mainsite/newsview/tvshowtr.htm. Accessed 12 May 2002.
Guthke, K. *The Gender of Death: A Cultural History in Art and Literature*. Cambridge: Cambridge University Press, 1999.
Guthrie, W. *Aristotle: An Encounter*. Cambridge: Cambridge University Press, 1981.
Guyer, B., J. Marti and M. MacDorman. 'Annual Summary of Vital Statistics–1996', *Pediatrics* 100(6) (1997): 905–18.
Hake, T. 'Studies on Ether and Chloroform from Prof. Schiff's Physiological Laboratory', *Practitioner* 12 (1874): 241.
Hallstrom, A. 'Dispatcher-assisted "Phone" Cardiopulmonary Resuscitation by Chest Compression Alone or with Mouth-to-Mouth Ventilation', *Crit Care Med* 11 Suppl (2000): N190–2.
Hallstrom, A. et al. 'Cardiopulmonary Resuscitation by Chest Compression a Alone or with Mouth-to-Mouth Ventilation', *NEJM* 342(21) (2000): 1546–53.
Hanson, C. and D. Straser. 'Family Presence during Cardiopulmonary Resuscitation: Foote Hospital Emergency Department's Nine-Year Perspective', *J Emerg Nurs*. 18 (1992): 104–6.

Harris, T. 'How Steadicams Work', *Howstuffworks*. Online: http://entertainment.howstuffworks.com/steadicam4.htm. Accessed 12 May 2002.

Hawes, W. *The Plan of an Institution for Affording Relief to Persons Apparently Dead, from Drowning and Also for diffusing a general Knowledge of the manner of treating Persons in a similar critical State, from various other Causes; Such As Strangulation by the Cord, Suffocation by noxious Vapours, &c. &c.* London: Hawes, 1774.

—— *An Address to the Public on Premature Death and Premature Internment*. London: 1778.

—— *Royal Humane Society the Annual Report 1796*. London: Rivington, 1797.

Hawkins, A. H. 'Constructing Death: Three Pathographies about Dying', *Omega* 22(4) (1990): 301–17.

Haynes, B. et al. 'A Statewide Early Defibrillation Initiative Including Laypersons and Outcome Reporting', *JAMA* 266(4) (1991): 545–7.

Hazinski, F., R. Cummins and J. Field. *2000 Handbook of Emergency Cardiovascular Care*. Dallas: American Heart Association, 2000.

Heilbron, J. *Electricity in the Seventeenth and Eighteenth Centuries: A Study in Early Modern Physics*. Berkeley: University of California Press, 1979.

Heilman, K. and C. Muscheheim. 'Primary Cutaneous Tuberculosis Resulting from Mouth-to-Mouth Respiration', *NEJM* 273 (1965): 1035–6.

'Hell and Highwater', *ER: By Popular Demand*. Dir. C. Chulack. Prod. M. Crichton. 1995. Videocassette. Warner Home Video, 1997.

Henry, J. *The Scientific Revolution and the Origins of Modern Science*. London: Macmillan Press, 1997.

Hermreck, A. 'The History of Cardiopulmonary Resuscitation', *American Journal of Surgery* 156 (1988): 430–6.

Hertz, R. 'A Contribution to the Study of the Collective Representation of Death', *Death and the Right Hand*, eds. R. Needham and C. Needham. New York: Free Press, 1960.

Hew, P. et al. 'Reluctance of Paramedics and Emergency Medical Technicians to Perform Mouth-To-Mouth Resuscitation', *J Emerg Med* 15(3) (1997): 279–84.

Hoff, H., 'Galvani and the Pre-Galvanian Electrophysiologists', *Annals of Science* I (1977): 157–72.

Holbrook, H. *The Golden Age of Quackery*. New York: Macmillan, 1958.

Houlbrooke, R. *Death, Religion and the Family in England 1480–1750*. Oxford: Clarendon Press, 1998.

Homans, P. *The Ability to Mourn*. Chicago: University of Chicago Press, 1989.

Honigman, B. and J. Armstrong. 'Life and Death', *Emergency Medicine: Concepts and Clinical Practice*, ed. Peter Rosen. St. Louis: Mosby, 1998. 197–212.

Horowitz, B. and L. Matheny. 'Health Care Professionals' Willingness to do Mouth-to-Mouth Resuscitation', *West J Med* 167(6) (1997): 392–7.

Hotz, H. Interview. Cedars-Sinai Medical Center. 15 December 2001.

Houlbrooke, R. *Death, Ritual, and Bereavement*, ed. R. Houlbrooke. London: Routledge, 1989.

Humane Society. *Reports of the Humane Society Instituted in the year 1774 for the Recovery of Persons Apparently Drowned for the Year 1776*. London: Humane Society, 1777.

—— *Reports of the Humane Society Instituted in the year 1774 for the Recovery of Persons Apparently Drowne. for the Years 1779 and 1780*. London: Humane Society, 1781.

—— *Reports of the Humane Society Instituted in the year 1774 for the Recovery of Persons Apparently Drowned for the Years 1783 and 1784*. London: Dodsley and Cadell, 1785.

Hunter, J. *The Surgical Works of John Hunter*, ed. James Palmer. Vol. III. London: Longman, 1837.

Hurlitz, J. et al. 'Resuscitation on Europe: a Tale of Five European Regions', *Resuscitation* 41 (1999): 121–31.

Huyler, F. *The Blood of Strangers*. London: Fourth Estate, 2000.

Ibsen, B. 'The Anaesthetist's Viewpoint on the Treatment of Respiratory Complications in Poliomyelitis during the Epidemic in Copenhagen, 1952', *Proc R Soc Med* 47 (1954): 72.

Illich, I. *The Limits to Medicine: Medical Nemesis: the Appropriation of Health*. Harmondsworth: Penguin Books, 1976.

Jameson, F. *Postmodernism: or, the Cultural Logic of Late Capitalism*. London: Verso, 1991.

Johns, R. and D. Cooper. *Chemical Corp Medical Laboratory Report No. 761*. Edgewood, Md: Army Chemical Center, 1957.

Johnson, A. *An Account of Some Societies at Amsterdam and Hamburg for the Recovery of Drowned Persons*. London, 1773.

Jude, J. 'Origins and Development of Cardiopulmonary Resuscitation', *The History of Anaesthesia*, ed. T. Boulton and R. Atkins. International Congress and Symposium Series, No. 134. New York: Parthenon, 1987: 452–64.

Jude, J., W. Kouwenhoven and G. Knickerbocker. 'Cardiac Arrest: Report of Application of External Cardiac Massage on 118 Patients', *JAMA* 178 (1961): 1063–70.

Kant, I. *The Critique of Judgement*, 1790, trans. James Creed Meredith. Oxford: Clarendon Press, 1978.

Karch, S. et al. 'Response Times and Outcomes for Cardiac Arrests for Las Vegas Casinos', *Amer J Emerg Med* 16 (1998): 249–53.

Kaye, W. and M. Mancini. 'Retention of Cardiopulmonary Resuscitation Skills by Physicians, Registered Nurses, and the General Public', *Crit Care Med* 14 (1986): 620–2.

Keith, Sir A. 'Three Hunterian Lectures on the Mechanism Underlying the Various Methods of Artificial Respiration Practised Since the Foundation of The Royal Humane Society in 1774', *Lancet* i (1909): 745–9, 825–8, 895–9.

Kellehear, A. 'Culture, Biology, and the Near-Death Experience: A Reappraisal', *Journal of Nervous and Mental Disease* 181(3) (1993): 148–6.

Kellerman, A., B. Hackman and G. Somes. 'Predicting the Outcome of Unsuccessful Prehospital Advanced Cardiac Life Support', *JAMA* 270 (1993): 1433–6.

Kemp, M., and M. Wallace, eds. *Spectacular Bodies*. Berkeley: University of California Press, 2000.

Kern, K. 'Cardiopulmonary Resuscitation without Ventilation', *Crit Care Med.* 11 Suppl. (2000): N186–9.

King, L. *The Philosophy of Medicine: The Early Eighteenth Century*. Cambridge, Mass.: Harvard University Press. 1978.

Kipnis, L. 'Pornography.' *The Oxford Guide to Film Studies*, eds. J. Hill and P. Gibson. Oxford: Oxford University Press, 1998. 153–7.

Kirchheimer, S. 'Value of AEDs in Public Questioned', *Medscape Medical News* (2003): Online: http://wwwmedscape.com/viewarticlew465457. Accessed 4 April 2004.

Kite, C. *Description of a Pocket Case of Instruments for the Recovery of the Apparently Dead*. London, 1785.

—— *An Essay on the Recovery of the Apparently Dead*. London: Dilly, 1788.

Klinkenborg, V. 'The Finish Line', *The New Yorker*. 28 February 1994: 92.

Kouwenhoven, W. and D. Hooker. 'Resuscitation by Countershock', *Electrical Engineering* (1933): 475–7.

Kouwenhoven, W., J. Jude and G. Knickerbocker. 'Closed Chest Cardiac Massage', *JAMA* 173 (1960): 1064–7.

Kouwenhoven, W. et al. 'Closed Chest Defibrillation of the Heart', *Surgery* 42 (1957): 550–61.

Kristeva, J. *Powers of Horror: An Essay on Abjection*, trans. Leon Roudiez. New York: Columbia University Press, 1982.

Kübler-Ross, E. *On Death and Dying*, 1968. London: Tavistock and Routledge, 1973.

Kuhn, T. *The Structure of Scientific Revolutions*, 1962. Chicago: University of Chicago Press, 1996.

Lacan, J. *The Seminar of Jacques Lacan, Book II: The Ego in Freud's Theory and in the Technique of Psychoanalysis, 1954–1955*, ed. Jacques-Alain Miller, trans. Sylvia Tomaselli. Cambridge: Cambridge University Press, 1988.

Laplanche, J. and J. Pontalis. *The Language of Psychoanalysis*. London: Karnac, 1973.

Lapus. 'About the Steadicam Jr.', *raisnaimaging*. Online: http://www.rasnaimaging.com/people/lapus/steadi.html. Accessed 27 March 2003.

Larsen, M. et al. 'Predicting Survival from Out-of-Hospital Cardiac Arrest: a Graphic Model', *Ann Emerg Med* 22 (1993): 1652–8.

Lathrop, J. *A Discourse before the Humane Society in Boston delivered on the Second Tuesday of June, 1787*. Boston: Ruffel, 1787.

Laurent, D. 'AHA Re-examines Value of Mouth-to-Mouth Ventilation in Cardiopulmonary Resuscitation', *Emergenza2000*. September 1997. Online: http://www.emergenza2000.it/articoli/12_01/dic_02.htm. Accessed 2 April 2001.

Lee, K., D. Angus and N. Abramson. 'Cardiopulmonary Resuscitation: What Cost to Cheat Death?' *Critical Care Medicine* 24(12) (1996): 2046–52.

Lee, R. 'Cardiopulmonary Resuscitation in the Eighteenth Century: A Historical Perspective on Present Medical Practice', *Journal of the History of Medicine and Allied Sciences* 72 (1972): 418–33.

Lesch, J. *Science and Medicine in France: The Emergence of Experimental Physiology, 1790–1855*. Cambridge, Mass.: Harvard University Press, 1984.

Leung, L. and H. Tong, 'Prehospital Resuscitation of Out-of-Hospital Cardiac Arrest in Hong Kong', *Ann Emerg Med* 35 (2000): S38.

Lévi-Strauss, C. 'The Sorcerer and His Magic', *Structural Anthropology Volume I*. 1958, trans. C. Jakobson and B. G. Schoepf. London: Basic Books, 1963. 173–85.

—— *The Savage Mind*, 1962. Chicago: the University of Chicago Press. 1966.

Levinas, E. *God, Death, and Time*, trans. Bettina Bergo. Stanford: Stanford University Press, 2000.

Levine, S. *Who Dies? An Investigation of Conscious Living and Conscious Dying.* Bath: Gateway, 1988.

Levy, A. Goodman and T. Lewis. 'Heart Irregularities Resulting from the Inhalation of Low Percentages of Chloroform Vapour, and Their Relationship to Ventricular Fibrillation', *Heart* 3 (1911): 99.

Little, C. and C. Cairns. 'Restoration of Cerebral Blood Flow Does Not Restore Function after Brain Ischemia', *Ann Emerg Med* 34 (1999): S90.

Litwin, P. et al. 'The Location of Collapse and its Effect on Survival from Cardiac Arrest', *Ann Emerg Med* 16 (1987): 787–91.

Lloyd, G., ed. *Hippocratic Writings.* Harmondsworth: Penguin Classics, 1978.

Lombardi, G. et al. 'Outcome of Out-of-Hospital Cardiac Arrest in New York City: The Pre-Hospital Arrest Survival Evaluation (PHASE) Study', *JAMA* 271(9) (1994): 678–83.

Longrigg, J. *Greek Rational Medicine from Alcmaeon to the Alexandrians.* London: Routledge, 1993.

Longstreth, W. T. Jr. et al. 'Neurologic Recovery after Out-of-Hospital Cardiac Arrest', *Ann Intern Med* 98 (1983): 588–92.

Lown, B. 'Cardioversion of Arrhythmias (I)', *Modern Concepts of Cardiovascular Diseases* 33. Dallas: American Heart Association, 1964. 863–8.

Macewen, W. 'Clinical Observations on the Introduction of Tracheal Tubes by the Mouth Instead of Performing Tracheotomy or Laryngotomy', *BMJ* 2 (1880): 122–4 and 163–5.

Mackinnon, C. *Only Words.* Cambridge, Mass.: Harvard University Press, 1993.

Macpherson, R. *Dissertation on the Preservative from Drowning and Swimmers Assistant.* London: J. Murray, 1783.

Mah, S. *Steve's TV Page.* Online: http://www.dimensional.com/~smah/tv.html. Accessed 4 June 2002.

Malinowski, B. 'The Role of Magic and Religion', *Reader in Comparative Religion*, 1931, eds. W. Lessa and E. Vogt. Evanston, Ill.: Row Peterson, 1962. 97.

— *Magic, Science and Religion*, 1948. London: Souvenir Press, 1974.

Mannis, M. and R. Wendel. 'Transmission of Herpes Simplex during Cardiopulmonary Resuscitation Training', *Compr Ther* 10 (1984): 15–17.

Markert, R. and M. Saklayen. 'Cardiopulmonary Resuscitation on Television', *NEJM* 335 (1996): 1605–7.

Massachusetts Humane Society. *Method of Treatment.* Boston: Massachusetts Humane Society, 1788.

McCue, J. 'Special Communication: the Naturalness of Dying', *JAMA* 273(13) (1995): 1039–43.

McWilliam, J. 'Cardiac Failure and Sudden Death', *BMJ* 5 (1889a): 6–8.

—— 'Electrical Stimulation of the Heart in Man', *BMJ* 16 (1889b): 348–50.

Mead, G. and C. Turnbull. 'Cardiopulmonary Resuscitation in the Elderly: Patients' and Relatives' Views'. *J Med Ethics* 21 (1995): 39–44.

A Medical Practitioner. *A Treatise on Vital Suspension.* London: Rivington and Sons, 1791.

Mejicano, G. and D. Maki. 'Infections Acquired during Cardiopulmonary Resuscitation Estimating the Risk and Defining Strategies for Prevention', *Ann Intern Med* 129 (1998): 813–28.

Melanson, S. and K. O'Gara. 'EMS Provider Reluctance to Perform Mouth-to-Mouth Resuscitation', *Prehospital Emergency Care* 4(1) 2000: 48–52.

Mendelsohn, E. *Heat and Life*. Cambridge, Mass.: Harvard University Press, 1964.
Mercier, T. Lecture. CME Associates. 12 December 2001.
Meyerberg, R.J. et al. 'Outcome of Resuscitation from Bradyarrhythmic or Asystolic Prehospital Cardiac Arrest', *J Am Coll Cardiol* 4 (1984): 1118–22.
Miller, I. *The Anatomy of Disgust*. Cambridge, Mass.: Harvard University Press, 1997.
Mims, C. *When We Die*. London: Constable Robinson, 1999.
Mitford, J. *The American Way of Death*. Harmondsworth: Penguin Books, 1963.
Morocco, M. Interview. Warner Brothers Studios. 19 December 2001.
Mosesso, V. The Most Neglected Tool in EMS: The Clock', *Ann of Emerg Med* 22(8) (1993): 1311–12.
Mosesso, V. et al. 'Use of Automated External Defibrillators by Police Officers for Treatment of Out-of-Hospital Cardiac Arrest', *Ann Emerg Med.* 32 (1998): 20–7.
Mulvey, L. 'Visual Pleasure and Narrative Cinema', *Screen* 16(3) (1975): 6–18.
Murphy, D. et al. 'Outcomes of Cardiopulmonary Resuscitation in the Elderly', *Annals of Internal Medicine* 111 (1989): 199–205.
Murphy D. et al. 'The Influence of the Probability of Survival on Patient's Preferences Regarding Cardiopulmonary Resuscitation', *NEJM* 330 (1994): 545–9.
Negovsky, V. 'Fifty Years of the Institute of General Reanimatology of the USSR Academy of Medical Sciences', *Crit Care Med* 16 (1988): 287–91.
Neumar, R. and K. Ward. 'Cardiopulmonary Arrest', *Emergency Medicine: Concepts and Clinical Practice*, ed. Peter Rosen. St. Louis: Mosby, 1998. 35–60.
Neve, M. 'Conclusion', *The Western Medical Tradition: 800 BC to AD 1800*, ed. L. Conrad et al. Cambridge: Cambridge University Press, 1995. 477–94.
Newton, I., *Principia*, 1687, trans. Andrew Motte, 1729. *The Principia*, 18 March 1998. Online: http://members.tripod.com/~gravitee/. Accessed 29 March 2003.
Nichol, G. et al. 'Potential Cost-effectiveness of Public Access Defibrillation in the United States', *Circulation* 97 (1998): 1315–20.
Nichol, G. et al. 'A Cumulative Meta-analysis of the Effectiveness of Defibrillator Capable Emergency Medical Services for Victims of Out-of-Hospital Cardiac Arrest', *Ann Emerg Med* 34 (1999): 517–25.
Nichol G. et al. 'Cost Effectiveness of Defibrillation by Targeted Responders in Public Settings', *Circulation* 108 (2003): 697–703.
Niemann, J. 'Study Design in Cardiac Arrest Research: Moving from the Laboratory to the Clinical Population', *Annals of Emergency Medicine* 22 (1993): 8–9.
Niemann, J. et al. 'Immediate Countershock versus CPR before Countershock and a Five-Minute Ventricular Fibrillation (VF) Arrest Swine Model', *Ann Emerg Med* 34 (1999): S4.
Nilsson, E. 'On Treatment of Barbiturate Poisoning. A Modified Clinical Aspect', *Acta Med Scand* 253 Suppl (1951): 1.
Nuland, S. *How We Die: Reflection's on Life's Final Chapter*. New York: Alfred A. Knopf, 1994.
OED (*The Oxford English Dictionary*). Second edition. CD-ROM. Oxford: Oxford University Press, 1992.

Olson, D. et al. 'EMT-defibrillation: The Wisconsin Experience', *Ann Emerg Med* 18 (1989): 806–11.
Onians, R. *The Origins of European Thought about the Body, the Mind, the Soul, the World, Time, and Fate.* Cambridge: Cambridge University Press, 1951.
Page, R. et al. 'Use of Automated External Defibrillators by a U.S. Airline', *NEJM* 343(17) (2000): 1210–16.
Pantridge, J. and J. Geddes. 'A Mobile Intensive-Care Unit in the Management of Myocardial Infarction', *Lancet* ii (1967): 271–3.
Paradis, N. A. et al. 'Simultaneous Aortic, Jugular Bulb, and Right Atrial Pressures during Cardiopulmonary Resuscitation in Humans: Insights into Mechanisms', *Circulation* 80 (1989): 361–8.
Pasquale, M. et al., 'Defining "Dead on Arrival": Impact on a Level 1 Trauma Center', *Journal of Trauma* 41(4) (1996): 726–30.
Pearson, J. *Historical and Experimental Approaches to Modern Resuscitation.* Springfield, Ill: Charles C. Thomas, 1965.
Pell, J. 'The Debate on Public Place Defibrillators: Charged but Shockingly Ill Informed', *Heart* 89 (2003): 1375–6.
Pell, J. et al. 'Effect of Reducing Ambulance Response Times on Deaths from Out-of-Hospital Cardiac Arrest: Cohort Study', *BMJ* 322 (2001): 1385–8.
Pepe, P. et al. 'ACLS – Does It Really Work?' *Ann Emerg Med* 23 (1994): 1037–41.
Physician, A. *A Physical Dissertation on Drowning.* London: Jacob Robinson, 1746.
Porter, D. *Health, Civilization and the State.* London: Routledge, 1999.
—— Interview. UCSF. 10 October 2003.
Porter, R. 'Religion and Medicine', *Companion Encyclopedia of the History of Medicine*, ed. W.F. Bynum and R. Porter. Vol. 2. London: Routledge, 1993. 1449–68.
—— 'The Eighteenth Century', *The Western Medical Tradition: 800 BC to AD 1800*, eds. L. Conrad et al. Cambridge: Cambridge University Press, 1995. 363–476.
—— *The Greatest Benefit to Mankind. A Medical History of Humanity form Antiquity to the Present.* London: Fontana, 1999.
Prendergast, T. and J. Luce 'Increasing Incidence of Withholding and Withdrawal of Life Support from the Critically Ill', *Am J Respir Crit Care Med.* 155 (1997): 1–2.
Prendergast, T., M. Claessens and J. Luce. 'A National Survey of End-of-Life Care for Critically Ill Patients', *Am J Respir Crit Care Med* 158 (1998): 1163–7.
Prevost, J. and F. Battelli. 'On Some Effects of Electrical Discharges on the Hearts of Mammals', *Compt Rend Acad Sci* 129 (1899): 1267.
Priestley, J. *Additions to the History and Present State of Electricity, with Original Experiments.* Second edition. London: J. Johnson, 1772.
Proctor, J. 'Merit Badge Medicine', *ACEP News* June 2000: 1–2.
de Réamur, R. A. F. *Notice in Order to Give Help to Those Believed to be Drowned*, 1740, trans. L. Brown. Los Angeles: K. Garth Huston Jr., 1990.
Rensin, D. 'Young Doctors in Love', *TV Guide*, 1995. Online: http://www.angelfire.com/ny4/JuliannaMargulies/int9.html. Accessed 8 February 2002.
Robiscek, F. and L. Littman. 'The First Reported Case of External Heart Massage', *Clinical Cardiology* 6 (1983): 569–71.
Reports of the Society Instituted in the year 1774, for the Recovery of Persons Apparently Drowned. London, 1775.

Rohde, E. *Psyche*. 1893, trans. W. Hillis. Eighth edition. London: Kegan Paul, 1925.
Roth, N. 'Good Vibrations: Abram's Oscilloclast and the Instrumental Cure', *Medical Instrumentation* 15 (1981), 383–4.
—— 'Electrical Knowledge and the Pursuit of Happiness', *Medtronic News* (1989–90).
Rousseau, G. 'The Perpetual Crisis of Modernism and the Traditions of Enlightenment Vitalism: With a Note on Mikhail Bakhtin', *The Crisis in Modernism: Bergson and the Vitalist Controversy*, eds. Frederick Burwick and Paul Douglass. Cambridge: Cambridge University Press, 1992. 15–63.
Rowbottom, M. and C. Susskind. *Electricity and Medicine: History of Their Interaction*. San Francisco: San Francisco Press. 1984.
Royal Humane Society. *Reports of the Royal Humane Society for 1787, 1788, 1789*. London: Cadell, Becket, Robson, Hookham, Dilly, Johnson, and Robinsons, 1790.
—— *Annual Report of the Royal Humane Society for the Recovery of the Apparently Drowned for the Year 1812*. London: J. Nichols and Son, 1812.
—— *Case of Resuscitation by His Imperial Majesty The Emperor of Russia*. London: Nichols, Son, and Bentley. 1814.
—— *The Seventy-Fifth Annual Report of the Royal Humane Society for the Recovery of the Apparently Drowned for the Year 1849*. London: Compton and Ritchie, 1849.
Rubin, R. 'Who's Afraid of Mouth-To-Mouth?' 23 January 1998. Online: http://more.abcnews.go.com/sections/living/RubinReport/rubinreport_13.html. Accessed 2 April 2001.
Safar, P. 'Ventilatory Efficacy of Mouth-to-Mouth Artificial Respiration', *JAMA* 167 (1958): 335–41.
—— 'Failure of Manual Artificial Respiration', *J Appl Physiol* 14 (1959): 84–8.
—— *Advances in Cardiopulmonary Resuscitation*. New York: Springer-Verlag. 1977.
—— 'History of Cardiopulmonary-Cerebral Resuscitation', *Cardiopulmonary Resuscitation*, eds. William Kaye and Nicholas Bircher. New York: Churchill Livingston, 1989. 1–53.
—— 'On the History of Modern Resuscitation', *Crit Care Med* 24(2) Suppl. (1996): 3S–11S.
Safar, P., T. Brown and W. Holtey. 'Ventilation and Circulation with Closed-Chest Cardiac Compressions in Man', *JAMA* 176 (1961): 574–6.
Safar, P., L. Escarraga, and F. Chang. 'Upper Airway Obstruction in the Unconscious Patient', *J Appl Physiol* 14 (1959): 760–4.
Safar, P., L. Escarraga and J. Elam. 'A Comparison of the Mouth-to-Mouth and Mouth-to-Airway Methods of Artificial Respiration with the Chest-Pressure Arm-Lift Methods', *NEJM* 258 (1958): 671–7.
Safar, P. et al. 'Resuscitative Principles for Sudden Cardiopulmonary Collapse', *Diseases of the Chest* 43 (1963): 34–49.
– 'Improved Cerebral Resuscitation from Cardiac Arrest with Mild Hypothermia Plus Blood Flow Promotion in Dogs', *Stroke* 27 (1996): 105–13.
Saklayan, M, H. Liss and R. Markert. 'In-hospital Cardiopulmonary Resuscitation: Survival in 1 Hospital and Literature Review', *Medicine* 74 (1995): 163–75.
Saunders, C. *Beyond the Horizon*. London: Dartman, Longman & Todd, 1990.

Schecter, D. 'Early Experience with Resuscitation by Means of Electricity', *Surgery* 69 (1971): 360–72.
—— *Exploring the Origins of Electrical Cardiac Stimulation*. Minneapolis: Medtronic, 1983.
Scheller, J. 'Angels of ER', *US Magasine* (May 1966): Online: http://www.angelfire.com/md/shipper/CAROLandDOUGaUS96.html. Accessed 22 March 2002.
Schneider, A., D. Nelson and D. Brown. 'In-hospital Cardiopulmonary Resuscitation: a 30-year Review', *J Am Board Fam Pract* 6 (1993): 91–101.
Schonwetter, R. et al. 'Educating the Elderly: Cardiopulmonary Resuscitation Decisions before and after Intervention', *J Am Geriatr Soc* 39 (1991): 372–7.
—— 'Resuscitation Decision Making in the Elderly: the Value of Outcome Data', *J Gen Intern Med* 8 (1993): 295–300.
Seale, C. *Constructing Death: the Sociology of Dying and Bereavement*. Cambridge: Cambridge University Press, 1998.
Silver, R. *Casualty: Behind the Scenes*. London: BBC Worldwide, 1998.
Silvester, H. 'A New Method of Resuscitating Still-Born Children, and of Restoring Persons Apparently Drowned or Dead', *BMJ* (1858): 576–9.
Smith, W. *Religion of the Semites*. London: Adam and Charles Black, 1894.
Snell, B. *The Discovery of the Mind: the Greek Origins of European Thought*. Oxford: Basil Blackwell, 1953.
Stephenson, H. Jr., L. Reid and J. Hinton. 'Some Common Denominators in 1200 Cases of Cardiac Arrest', *Ann Surg* 137 (1953): 731–44.
Stewart, G. *Death Sentences: Styles of Dying in British Fiction*. Cambridge, Mass.: Harvard University Press, 1984.
Stiell, I. 'Modifiable Factors Associated with Improved Cardiac Arrest Survival in a Multicenter Basic Life Support/Defibrillation System: OPALS Phase I Results. Ontario Prehospital Advanced Life Support', *Annals of Emerg Med* 33(1) (1999): 44–50.
Stiell, I. et al. 'The Ontario Trial of Active Compression–Decompression Cardiopulmonary Resuscitation for In-Hospital And Prehospital Cardiac Arrest', *JAMA* 275 (1996): 1417–23.
—— 'Improved Out-of-Hospital Cardiac Arrest Survival through an Inexpensive Optimization of an Existing Defibrillation Program: OPALS Study Phase II', *JAMA* 281 (1999): 1175–81.
—— 'Health-Related Quality of Life is Better for Cardiac Arrest Survivors Who Received Citizen Cardiopulmonary Resuscitation', *Circulation* 108 (2003): 1939–44
Stoker, B. *Dracula*, 1897. Harmondsworth: Penguin Books, 1993.
Stratton, S. and J. Niemann. 'Outcome from Out-of-Hospital Cardiac Arrest Caused by Nonventricular Arrhythmias: Contribution of Successful Resuscitation to Overall Survivorship Supports the Current Practice of Initiating Out-of-Hospital ACLS', *Ann Emerg Med* 32 (1998): 448–3.
Struve, C. *A Practical Essay on the Art of Restoring Suspended Animation*, 1801. Albany, NY: Whiting, Backus & Whiting, 1803.
Stults, K. et al. 'Prehospital Defibrillation Performed by Emergency Medical Technicians in Rural Communities', *NEJM* 310 (1984): 219–23.
Sudnow, D. *Passing on the Social Organisation of Dying*. Englewood Cliffs: Prentice Hall, 1967.

SUPPORT Principal Investigators. 'A Controlled Trial to Improve Care for Seriously Ill Hospitalized Patients: The Study to Understand Prognosis and Preferences for Outcomes and Risks of Treatments', *JAMA* 274(20) (1995): 1591–8.
Sweeney, T. et al. 'EMT Defibrillation Does not Increase Survival from Sudden Death in a Two-Tiered Urban–Suburban EMS System', *Ann Emerg Med* 31 (1998): 234–40.
Taffet, G. et al. 'In-hospital Cardiopulmonary Resuscitation', *JAMA* 261 (1989): 1579–82.
Temkin, O. *Galenism: Rise and Decline of a Medical Philosophy*. Ithaca and London: Cornell University Press, 1973.
Tercier, J. 'From Aer to Air: the Kiss of Life', *Critical Quarterly*, 44(1) (2002): 1–24.
Thompson, E. P. *The Making of the English Working Class*, 1963. London: Penguin Books, 1991.
Timmermans, S. *Sudden Death and the Myth of CPR*. Philadelphia: Temple University Press, 1999.
Todd, K. et al. 'Randomized, Controlled Trial of Video Self-Instruction versus Traditional CPR Training', *Ann Emerg Med* 31 (1998): 364–9.
—— 'Simple CPR: a Randomized, Controlled Trial of Video Self-Instructional Cardiopulmonary Resuscitation Training in an African American Church Congregation', *Ann Emerg Med* 34 (1999): 730–7.
Todd, M.A. and J. S. Bell. 'Shigellosis from Cardiopulmonary Resuscitation', *JAMA* 243(4) (1980): 331.
Tossach, W. 'A Man Dead in Appearance, Recovered by Distending the Lungs with Air', *Medical Essays and Observations*. Fourth edition. Vol. 5. Part II. Edinburgh: Hamilton, Balfour & Neil, 1752. 108–11.
Troy, A. 'Cardiopulmonary Resuscitation on Television'. *NEJM* 335 (1996): 1605–7.
Tunstall-Pedoe, H. et al. 'Survey of 3765 Cardiopulmonary Resuscitations in British Hospitals (The BRESUS Study): Methods And Overall Results', *BMJ* 304 (1992): 1347–51.
Turner, C. 'The Disgusting'. Diss. University of London, 2000.
Turner, V. *The Ritual Process*. London: Routledge, 1969.
Turow, J. 'Television Entertainment and the US Health-care Debate', *Lancet* 347(9010) (1996): 1240–3.
Twitchell, J. *The Living Dead: A Study of the Vampire in Romantic Literature*. Durham, NC: Duke University Press. 1981.
Vancouver Hospital and Health Sciences Centre. *This Is Not ER: The Facts about Cardiopulmonary Resuscitation*. 1996a.
—— *Policy/Guidelines on Resuscitative Interventions*. May 1996b.
—— *Ethics Committee Report on the Evaluation of the Cardiopulmonary Resuscitation Policy/Guidelines Introduced in 1996*. 1998.
Valenzuela, T. et al. 'Transmission of "Toxic Strep" Syndrome from an Infected Child to a Firefighter during CPR', *Ann Emerg Med.* 20 (1991): 90–2.
—— 'Rapid defibrillation by non-traditional responders: The Casino Project.' *Acad Emerg Med.* 5 (1998): 414–15.
—— 'Outcomes of Rapid Defibrillation by Security Officers after Cardiac Arrest in Casinos', *N Engl J Med* 343 (2000): 1206–9.

van Alem, A. et al. 'Use of Automated External Defibrillator by First Responders in Out-of-Hospital Cardiac Arrest: Prospective Controlled Trial' *BMJ* 327(7427) (2003): 1312.
van Gennep, Arnold. *The Rites of Passage*, 1909, trans. M. Vizedom and G. Caffee. Chicago: University of Chicago Press, 1960.
van Lommel, P. et al. 'Near Death Experience in Survivors of Cardiac Arrest: A Prospective Study in the Netherlands', *Lancet* 358(9298) (2002): 2039–45.
van Walraven, C. et al. 'Do Advanced Cardiac Life Support Drugs Increase Resuscitation Rates from In-Hospital Cardiac Arrest?' *Ann Emerg Med* 32 (1998): 544–53.
van Walraven, C. et al. 'Validation of a Clinical Decision Aid to Discontinue In-Hospital Cardiac Arrest Resuscitations', *JAMA* 285 (2001): 1602–6.
Vukov, L. et al. 'New Perspectives on Rural EMT Defibrillation', *Ann Emerg Med* 17 (1988): 318–21.
Walker, A. et al. 'Cost Effectiveness and Cost Utility Model of Public Place Defibrillators in Improving Survival After Prehospital Cardiopulmonary Arrest', *BMJ* 327 (2003): 1312–16.
Wallace, M. A *History of Resuscitation*, 29 October 1996. Online: http://www.hartfirstrsponse.org.uk/CPRhistory.html. Accessed 29 April 2004.
Wallack, E. and G. Bingle. 'Cardiopulmonary Resuscitation on Television', *NEJM* 335 (1996): 1605–7.
Walter, T. *The Revival of Death*. London: Routledge, 1994.
Waterhouse, B. *On the Principle of Vitality. A Discourse delivered in the First Church in Boston, Tuesday, June 8, 1790, before the Humane Society of the Commonwealth of Massachusetts*. Boston: Thomas and John Fleet, 1790.
Waters, R. et al. 'Endotracheal Anesthesia and its Historical Development', *Anesth Analg* 1 (1933): 196.
Waugh, E. *The Loved One: An Anglo-American Tragedy*, 1948. London: Penguin Books, 2000.
Wear, A. 'Early Modern Europe: 1500–1700', *The Western Medical Tradition: 800 BC to AD 1800* eds. L. Conrad et al. Cambridge: Cambridge University Press, 1995. 215–361.
White, R., D. Hankins and T. Bugliosi. 'Seven Years' Experience with Early Defibrillation by Police and Paramedics in an Emergency Medical Services System', *Resuscitation* 39 (1998): 145–51.
Williams, M. Letter. 'Family Presence during Resuscitation', *Journal of Emergency Nursing* (1993): 478–9.
Willich, A. *Lectures on Diet and Regimen*. London: Longman, Hurst, Rees, & Orme. 1809.
Zoll, P. et al. 'Termination of Ventricular Fibrillation in Man by Externally Applied Electric Countershock', *NEJM* 254 (1956): 727–32.

Index

A & E (accident and emergency department), *see* emergency room
A & E, 215
ABCDs of resuscitation, 25–31, 47, 65, 103, 191, 228, 248–9, 252, 261
Abdilgard, 67
ABEM *see* American Board of Emergency Medicine
ACEP, *see* American College of Emergency Physicians
ACLS *see* Advanced Cardiac Life Support Acronyms, 245
Acute care medicine, 37
Advanced Cardiac Life Support, 24, 27, 28, 30, 32, 33, 35, 38, 42, 97, 101, 102, 103, 123, 141, 142, 185, 223, 226, 227, 228, 236, 245, 248, 249, 250, 251, 252, 253, 261
Advanced directives, 3, 184, 224, 227–9, 232, 237, 262
Advanced Trauma Life Support, 27, 175, 228, 251–2, 261
Aldini, Giovanni, 119
Algorithms, 38–42, 45, 227
  asystole, 223
  grieving, 19
  ILCOR Universal Algorithm and Comprehensive ECC Algorithm, 38
  image, 39
  ritual, 164, 179
  tachycardia, 39, 227–8, 251
  unity, 39
ALS (advanced life support), *see* advanced cardiac life support
AEDS, *see* automated external defibrillators
Aer, 112–13, 151
Aesthetic
  distance, 214
  effect, 198, 205
  experience, 214, 216

Agitations, 62, 65-6, 118, 155
Agon, 209
AHA *see* American Heart Association
Air, 112–14, 132–4, 138–9, 152–3, 157
Airports, 105, 254
Airway manoeuvres, 25, 27, 31, 142, 248–9
Alexander II, Tsar, 86
Ambulance, 2, 30,
  chain-of-survival, 47–8
  defibrillators, 101–2
  emergency medical services, 248
  response time, 35
American Board of Emergency Medicine, 103, 252
American College of Emergency Physicians, 103
American Heart Association, 24, 25, 27, 31–2, 37–9, 45, 101–2, 103, 105, 141–2, 183, 191, 224, 236, 247, 249, 251, 253, 254
American Medical Association, 135, 136
American Red Cross, 31, 32, 135, 136
American Way of Death, The, 15
Anagnorisis, 209
Analogy, 163–4, 211, 230
Anaesthesia
  intermittent positive pressure ventilation, 256–7
  ventricular fibrillation, 99–100, 157–8, 257
Anima, 108–10, 116
Animism, 107–8, 146, 255
Animus, 109–10, 116
Antiarrhythmics, 102, 227
Apnoea, 252
Apoplexy, 52–3, 71, 117, 130, 155
Apothecaries, 50, 82
Argenterius, 114
Ariès, Philippe, 3, 10–15, 37, 210, 256, 260

Aristotle
  Aristotelian qualities, 107, 110
  catharsis, 259
  physiology, 113, 130
  soul, 113, 255
  substantial form, 255
Armed Forces Conference on Artificial Respiration and Nerve Gas Poisoning, 190
Army, 136, 190
Arnold, Ken, 22
Arrest, see cardiac arrest
Arrhythmias, 29, 99, 227–8, 249, 251, 254
Asphyxia, 52–4, 71, 77, 117, 133, 155
Asystole, 29, 34, 58, 99, 223, 236, 249
ATLS, see advanced trauma life support
Atomism, 106, 255
Atrial fibrillation and flutter, 227
Automated external defibrillators, 31, 101–5, 248, 250, 254–5
Autonomy, 19, 185, 222, 229
Avis pour donner du secours a ceus l'on croit noyez, 51, 128

Bacchic dance, 180
Baer, Neil, 198, 206
Bagging-unit, 141–2, 256
Baglivi, Georgio, 107
Bakhtin, Mikhail, 145
Barthes, Roland, 178, 210, 233
Barthez, Paul-Joseph, 117
Basic Life Support, 27, 28, 30–3, 38–9, 226, 248
  ACLS, 249–50
  AEDs, 101–6
  EMTs, paramedics, 248
  instruction, 191
  mouth-to-mouth, 141
Bataille, George, 145, 260
Battelli, Frederic, 99
Baudrillard, Jean, 15, 22
Baumann, Zygmunt, 15
Baywatch, 196
BCLS (Basic Cardiac Life Support) see Basic Life Support
Beck, Claude, 100, 101, 254

Being, 146, 178, 216–17
Belling, C., 207
Bellows, 51, 53, 61–2, 64–5, 127, 132–4, 253, 256
Ben Casey, 193
Bequests, 12, 82
  Humane Society, 82
  romantic death, 12
Bergson, Henri, 120
Bichat, Xavier, 119, 167, 178, 210, 216
Black, Joseph, 116, 130, 132
Blair, James, 128
Bloch, Maurice, 164, 166, 171–2, 181, 183, 258
Bloodletting, 53, 69, 70–2, 160–2, 169, 253
BLS see Basic Life Support
Boas, Franz, 201
Body, the
  contagion, 146–8
  death, 246
  disgust, 145, 148–52
  female, 213
  mechanism, 106–8
  ritual, 17
  transplant, 256
  violence and the, 66–5, 242–3
  vitalism, 108–10
Boerhaave, Hermann, 108, 115
Borelli, Giovanni, 107
Boyle Robert, 106, 111, 116, 130, 252
Bradycardia, 228
Brain death, brain, 28, 35, 106, 121, 123, 256, 258
Breath
  cardiac arrest, 28
  contagion and infection, 139, 150–4
  last, 20, 233
  life-force, 110, 111–14, 127, 129, 138–9
  mouth-to-mouth ventilation, 25
  resuscitation, 25, 27, 103, 127, 141, 247, 252
  signs of death, 56, 58, 167
  tangible imponderability, 67
  valorization, 132–3
Brigham and Women's Hospital, 196

Bringing Out the Dead, 1–2, 179, 181, 219–20, 245
British Heart Foundation, 28
Brodie, Benjamin, 70, 133–4
Bronchotomy, 51
Brown, John, 117
Brown, T., 31
Bruhier, Jean-Jacques, 51, 57
Buchan, William, 129
Buffy the Vampire Slayer, 189–90
Bull, Frederick, 82
Bynum, William, 72, 160, 193

CABG, *see* coronary artery bypass graft
Cage, Nicholas, 245
Caloric, 111, 115, 119–20
Camera
 death, 217
 indexicality, 260
 pornography, 213–14
 Steadicam, 199, 201–3, 205, 235, 260
 technique, 201–3, 205, 211, 260
Campanella, Thomas, 114
Cancer, 14, 25, 246
Carbon dioxide, 112, 116, 132, 135, 139, 151–2, 252, 255, 256
Carbon monoxide, 252
Carbonic acid gas, 130–2, 256
Cardiac arrest
 anaesthetic-induced, 99, 256–7
 cardiac, 28–30, 52–8
 deaths from, 26
 primary, 28–30, 35, 52, 168, 208
 respiratory, 28, 29, 35, 249, 252
 secondary, 28, 29, 35, 249, 252
 treatment, *see* cardiopulmonary resuscitation
Cardiac Arrest Survival Act, 103
Cardiac compression, *see* external-cardiac-compression
Cardiac rhythms, 25, 27, 29, 33, 34, 41–2, 58, 99, 100, 223, 227, 228, 230, 248, 249, 250, 251, 254
Cardiopulmonary resuscitation, 24–48
 ABCDs, 25, 27–31
 airway manoeuvres, 25, 27, 31, 142, 248–9

birth, 31, 50, 136, 191, 158, 250
bystander performance, 25, 33, 35, 46, 141, 145, 159, 191, 249, 258
certification and competence, 191, 196, 250, 251–2
complications, 31, 159, 221–5
costs, 105, 254, 261–2
CPR-as-protocol, 163, 177, 184, 221, 228, 229, 232
CPR-as-ritual, 176–84, 221–38
development, 31–2
efficacy, 2, 25–6, 33–7, 104–5, 158–60, 162, 186, 222, 229
expectations, 33–4, 36, 61, 206–8, 217
family presence, 235–8, 262
future, 226–8
'golden period', 28, 33, 35, 100, 102, 104, 251
Guidelines 2000, 28, 33, 38, 42, 102, 121, 123, 127, 141, 142, 159, 160, 223, 226, 227, 232, 236, 247, 249, 254
history, 31–2
images, 36, 184, 217–18, 234
in-hospital, 46
indications, 254
instruction, 32, 35, 42, 102, 190–1, 196, 221, 249, 250, 251–2
lay participation, 30, 31, 36, 42, 44, 101, 103, 139, 186, 221, 235, 237
manuals, 31, 32, 38, 236, 249, 251
media, 186, 190–212
myth, 33–7
out-of-hospital, 2, 25, 104, 168, 261
protocol, 24–48, 103, 254
representations, 30, 36, 48, 61, 184, 186, 189–212, 215, 217, 222, 224, 228, 229, 230, 234, 249, 258
rescuers and responders, 3, 4, 43, 44, 100, 102, 103, 105, 132, 134, 136, 138, 140, 141, 142, 151, 152, 179, 182, 183, 185, 186, 190, 217, 221, 222, 230, 248, 250, 254

284 *Index*

Cardiopulmonary resuscitation – *continued*
  survival rates, 2, 25, 32, 33–6, 46, 100, 104, 160, 206–9, 224, 250, 251, 261
Cardiovascular disease, 26
Carnot, Lazare, 115
Cartesian dualism, 107, 109
Case Western Reserve University, 100
Casualty, 2, 61, 194, 195, 198, 199, 208, 209, 215, 260
Casualty department, *see* emergency room
Catharsis
  family participation, 237
  murder, 175–6, 220
  psychological violence, 172–4
  ritual, 180–1, 247, 259
Cathartics, 72
Cavendish, Henry, 116, 130, 132
Cerebral congestion, 53, 155
Cerebral cortical
  blood flow, 158–9
  response, 258
Chadwick, Edwin, 139
Chain-of-survival, 30–1, 45–8, 94, 228, 237, 254
Chaplains, 20
Chest compression, *see* external-cardiac-compression
Chesterton, G. K., 154, 185
Chicago Hope, 193
Children
  CPR, 140, 254
  Humane Society protocol, 49, 56, 80–1
  mouth-to-mouth, 136, 140–1
  physiology, 81
  television representation, 207
  victim and sacrifice, 80–1, 141, 180, 261
Chin-lift, 248
Chloroform, 99, 157, 257
Choke-damp, 54, 252
Cholera, 139
Cinader, Robert, 192
Cinema, *see* media
Circulation
  ABCDs, 25–7
  adequacy, 35–6
  cardiac arrest, 28–9
  diagnosis of death, 106, 167, 220
  external-cardiac-compression, 156–7
  theories, 65, 107, 115
  William Harvey, 53, 107
City Hospital, 18, 93
Clear-shock-clear, 2, 98, 121, 123
Closed-chest-compression, *see* external-cardiac-compression
Clergy, 20, 82, 84
Clooney, George, 194, 261
Clowes, William, 49
Cobb, Leonard, 31
Cogan, Thomas, 50, 51
Cold, *see* hypothermia
Coleman, Edward, 70
Coma, 258, 248
Combustion, 114–16, 130–1, 255
Condemnation
  bellows, 134
  bloodletting, 71
  folk practice, 154–6
  CPR and hi-tech death, 10–11, 21–2, 37, 185, 211–12, 221–6, 231–2
  mouth-to-mouth, 132–3, 137–8
  pornography, 212–15
  slow-code, 226
Consciousness, 28, 52, 53, 56, 58, 108, 109, 167, 252
Consolidated Electrical Company of New York, 99
Constructing Death: The Sociology of Dying and Bereavement, 5
Construction
  being, 149–50
  community and society, 17, 46–8, 76, 92, 163, 165, 176, 182, 222
  death, 21, 23, 26, 48, 172, 178, 182–4, 216, 230, 233, 237
  humanity, 89–91
  life, 48, 176–8, 216–17
  reality, 260
  self, 17–18, 20, 92, 148, 185, 222, 259
Contagion, 138–43, 146–8, 150–3, 157, 171, 257, 259
Contagionism, 138–9
Coronary artery

blood flows, 158
bypass graft, 250, 253
disease, 28, 38, 249
reperfusion, 250
Corpse
  contagion, 146–8
  death, 246
  disgust, 136, 138, 144–5, 148–52, 151–2
  fear, 150–1, 167, 170
  return to life, 57
  ritual, 17, 72, 172
  violence and, 66–7, 85, 155–6, 166–70, 174–5, 181–5, 242–3
Costs
  automated external defibrillators, 103, 105, 254–5
  ER episode, 260
  resuscitation, 26–2
Coulomb, Charles, 119
CPR, *see* cardiopulmonary resuscitation
Crawford, John, 116
Crichton, Michael, 195
Cricothyrotomy, 248
Critical care medicine, 47
Cullen, William, 70, 117, 133
Curry, James, 161, 254

d'Etoiles, Leroy, 134
Darwin, Charles, 145
Davidson, Luke, 82, 259
Davies, Douglas, 14, 16
Davy, Humphrey, 115, 119
De Generatione, 110
De humani corporis fabrica, 127
de La Mettrie, Julien Offray, 107, 108
de Réamur, René-Antoine Ferchault, 51, 57, 128
De Viribus Electricitatis in Motu Musculari Commentarius, 118
Death
  absolute, 54–60
  allegory, 211
  apparent, 54–60, 108, 118, 254
  appropriate, 169, 182–3, 242, 259
  asymbolic, 210
  bad, 3, 11, 185, 242
  biological, 11–13, 20, 22, 246, 259
  brain, 28, 35, 106, 121, 123, 256, 258
  certificate, 13
  clinical, 41–2, 56
  coincidence, 12, 13, 20, 233–4, 246
  consciousness, 11
  cost, 261–2
  causes, 25–6
  death-with-dignity, 2, 3, 9–24, 123, 185–6, 193, 206, 222–5, 232–3, 241–2, 245, 247, 248
  declaration, 167, 169, 259, 261
  denial, 3, 15–16, 20–2, 36–7, 164–6, 176, 206, 207, 208, 209, 212
  euphemism, 211
  fear, 21, 138, 150–1, 167, 170, 184
  good death, 10, 12, 14–15, 185, 233, 241, 242, 247, 248
  hi-tech death, 2, 3, 10, 241, 242, 245
  indignity, 206, 221, 222, 242
  institutional, 246
  invisibility, 13, 21–2, 166, 210
  living dead, 51–61, 67, 99, 167
  medicalization, 13, 15–16, 21, 101, 185, 210, 221, 237
  ontological, 11–13, 20, 232–3, 246
  premature or sudden, 24, 26, 32, 75, 166
  representations, 2, 22, 23, 106, 193, 199, 210–12, 215–17, 233–4, 256
  signs, 51, 54–8, 59, 60, 67, 79, 106, 167–70, 184, 220, 260
  sleep, 12, 19, 232
  social, 11–13, 20, 22, 246
Deathbed
  'Death of Self', 11
  exclusion, 102, 197, 221, 234, 237–8
  fantasies, 3, 10, 26, 61, 241
  history, 11–13
  'Invisible', 13, 21–2
  psychological features, 3, 10, 15, 20, 23, 92, 142, 152, 153, 164, 166, 171, 172–4, 221–3, 225, 228, 243, 246, 259
  rationalization, 3, 16, 20, 222, 224, 226–8, 232–3, 242, 261

Deathbed – *continued*
'Remote', 12
'Romantic', 12, 14
spiritual, 3, 10, 18, 221, 222, 225, 246
'Tame', 11
Death-with-dignity, 2, 3, 9–24, 123, 185–6, 193, 206, 222–5, 232–3, 241–2, 245, 247, 248
Defibrillation, 97–123
AEDS (automated external defibrillators), 31, 101–5, 248, 250, 254–5
costs, 105
efficacy, 25, 102–5, 251, 258
external, 100
history, 98–101, 254
Humane Society, 68, 254
internal, 100
protocol, 254
Dehumanization, 36, 181–4, 222, 231–2, 248
Democritus, 106
dénouement, 209
Department of Defense, 136
Department of Health, 105
Department of Justice, 210
Dephlogisticated air, 131, 252
Derrida, Jacques, 149
Descartes, René, 107, 108, 109, 115, 117, 120
Dethardingius, 51
Diderot, Dennis, 117
Diem, S., 206
Diogenes, 112, 113
Dionysus, 180, 181
Disgust, 138, 143–6, 147–52, 257
Dissertations sur l'incertitude des signes de la mort, 51, 57
DNR orders, *see* do not resuscitate orders
Doctors
at deathbed, 3, 12, 13, 23, 73
fear of infection, 139–40
as hero, 193–4, 201, 212, 260
as priest, 162–3, 184, 201, 225, 226, 242
representations, 193, 198, 215
Dodds, E. R., 181

Do not resuscitate orders, 3, 224, 225, 261
Douglas, Mary, 149
Driesch, Hans, 120
Dr. Kildare, 193
Drowning, 51–4
as cause of death, 26
experiment, 131
folk therapies, 154
hypothermia, 58–61
The Institution for Affording Relief to Persons Apparently Dead from Drowning, 50, 252
Method for the Restoration of the Apparently Dead, 61–74
pathophysiology, 155, 252
secondary cardiac arrest, 29
television, 207, 261
Du Bois-Reymond, Emil, 119
Durkheim, Emile, 174, 181, 182

ECC, *see* emergency cardiovascular care
ECG, EKG, *see* electrocardiogram
Ecstasy, 150, 178–81, 183, 230–1
ED, *see* emergency department
EEG, *see* electroencephalogram
Einstein, Albert, 119
Einthoven, Willem, 122
Eisenberg, Mickey, 46, 137, 250
Eisenburger, P., 191
Elam, James, 135, 136, 158, 190, 192
Élan vital, 120
Electricity, 116–19
animal, 66, 108, 110–11, 116–19, 255
diagnostic use, 66–7
defibrillation, 98–101
electromagnetism, 119
history, 98–101, 116–19, 254
Humane Society, 63, 66–8
images, 10, 106, 121–3, 177, 190, 229, 254
irritability, 116–19
life, 106
therapeutic use, 67–8
vitalism, 108–11, 118–19
Electrocardiogram, 29, 122, 223, 249, 254, 258

Electrocution, 38, 99, 256
Electroencephalogram, 38, 106, 121, 123, 258
Eliade, Mircea, 181
Elias, Norbert, 3, 15
ELS, *see* emergency life support
Embrocations, 50, 69
Emergency cardiovascular care, 30, 32, 38, 245, 249
Emergency department, *see* emergency room
Emergency life support, 29, 31, 32
Emergency medical services, 30, 46, 47, 101–3, 224, 248, 249, 254
Emergency medical technicians, 1–2, 30, 47, 48, 97, 101, 143–4, 154, 179, 185, 189–90, 192, 198, 219, 220, 248
Emergency medicine, 30, 193, 196, 197, 198, 245, 252
Emergency room, 2, 30, 47, 48, 61, 101, 143, 154, 179, 193, 194, 195, 196, 197, 198, 199, 200, 201, 202, 203, 206, 209, 215, 234, 235, 238, 242, 243, 245, 260, 261
Emetics, 69, 133, 253
Empedocles, 113
Empiricism, 37, 225, 260
  empirical observation, 74, 75, 137, 152, 155
  empirical failure, 72, 160, 162, 243
EMS *see* emergency medical services
EMT, *see* emergency medical technicians
Endorphins, 262
Endotracheal intubation, 1, 127, 141, 175, 220, 248, 253, 256
Entelechy, 120
ER, *see* emergency room
ER, 2, 61, 179, 193, 194, 195, 196, 197, 199, 200, 201, 202, 203, 206, 209, 215, 234, 260, 261
Erasistratus of Ceos, 113
Erotics
  CPR, 216, 231
  death, 178–81, 260
  disgust, 149–50
  kiss, 143–5

European Resuscitation Council, 103, 249
Euthanasia, 15, 22, 225, 246–7
Evidence-based medicine, 47, 160, 227, 233, 251
External-cardiac-compression, 154–86
  AHA Ad Hoc Committee on Closed Chest Cardiac Resuscitation, 31
  anaesthetic-induced cardiac arrest, 157, 257
  blood flows, 158–9
  CPR, 2, 25–7, 30–1, 41–2, 247, 248, 249
  defibrillation, 104, 229
  demotion, 33, 141–2, 237
  development, 157–8, 250
  efficacy, 158–60, 258
  film, 191
  Humane Society's Method, 62, 64, 66, 69, 118, 155
  manual-ventilatory techniques, 134, 153, 156, 256
  persistence, 157, 160–2, 174, 222
  ritual, 177, 220–2, 228–9
  survival, 158–60
  terminal paradox, 184–6
  theories, 160–1
  variants, 160
  violence, 156
External Cardiac Massage, 191

Fantasy
  body, 175
  death-with-dignity, 3, 9, 10, 241
  heroic, 258
  immortality, 37, 206
  life, 106, 122, 123, 234
  pornography, 213
  rescue, 81, 183, 231
  revival, 26, 61, 209
  sacrifice, 81, 183, 229, 231
  sudden death, 26, 248
Faraday, Michael, 119
Federal Aviation Administration, 103
Fernel, Jean, 115
Fibrillation, *see* ventricular fibrillation
Film, *see* Media

Fire, 63, 68–9, 109, 110–12, 114–15
  image, 111
  services, 24, 101, 103, 105, 192, 238
Fire damp, 54, 105, 224, 252
First International Guidelines Conference on CPR and ECC, 249
First-responders, 33, 103, 248, 250
Five-step process of dying, 246
Fixed-air, 133, 256
Flat line, 98, 121–3, 189, 194, 258
Flatliners, 2
Fluids, 63, 99, 108, 111, 115, 117, 118, 119, 131
Folk practice, 65, 72, 127, 154–6, 174, 232
Foments, 68
Formless, The, 148–9, 151, 180
Fothergill, Anthony, 64, 68, 117, 131, 132
Fothergill, John, 51, 71, 128–9
Fothergillian essay competition, 52, 57, 128, 252
Foucault, Michel, 121
Fox, John, 22
Fracastro, Giralamo, 138
Frankenstein, 121, 254, 259
French Academy of Medicine, 138
Freud, Sigmund, 17, 145, 149, 175, 176, 259, 269
Friction, 49, 51, 55, 61, 65, 67, 68, 69, 118, 137, 155
Frisson, 215–16
Fumigations *see* tobacco
Funerals, 15, 16, 22, 141, 164

Galen, 52, 70, 108, 113, 114, 255
Galvani, Luigi, 118
Galvanism, 199
Galvanometer, 122
Garrick, David, 82
Gas, 112, 130–3
  nerve, 136, 190, 256
Gassendi, Pierre, 106
Gaze
  ambivalent, 150, 216–17
  male, 213
  scientific and medical, 120, 122

Gennep, Arnold van, 258
Germ theory, germs, 138–9, 146–7, 153
Ghosts, 146, 147, 170, 246
Gill, Sue, 21
Glisson, Frances, 117
God
  disappearance, 107, 211, 255
  playing, 179–80, 259
Goldsmith, Oliver, 82
Goodwyn, Edmund, 53, 252
Good death, 10, 12, 14–15, 185, 233, 241, 242, 247, 248
Good Samaritan Laws, 43, 104, 196
Gordon, Archer, 135, 191
Gorer, Geoffrey, 3, 15, 210, 212, 213, 214, 261
Greenhill, Catherine Sophia, 254
Grief, grieving, 15, 17, 19, 23, 165, 174, 232, 236, 246, 259
Guerke, Otto von, 130
Guidelines 2000, 28, 33, 38, 42, 102, 121, 123, 127, 141, 142, 159, 160, 223, 226, 227, 232, 236, 247, 249, 254
Guilt, 150, 167, 172–3, 174, 176, 180, 183, 220, 237

Haller, Albrecht von, 115, 117, 120
Hamartia, 209
Harvey, William, 53, 65, 107, 110, 115, 120
Hawes, William, 50, 84, 117
Heart
  attack, 28, 29, 61, 249
  disease, 25, 29
  electricity, 98–101
  function and physiology, 28, 29, 35, 53, 59, 65, 67, 69, 70, 93, 106, 113–19, 130, 133, 156–9, 247, 249, 262
  heartbeat and pulse, 56, 58, 122, 223, 254
  too good to die, 100
Heartsaver course, 249
Heartstart course, 29, 32
Heat, 69, 107, 110–11, 114–16, 108
Heaven, 11, 113, 170, 177, 211
Heberden, William, 82

Hell, 11, 177
Helmholtz, Hermann von, 115, 119
Helmont, Joan-Baptista van, 110, 115, 130
Heraclitus, 259
Hero
  doctor, 85, 193–4, 212, 217, 261
  paramedic, 179
  rescuer, 152, 186, 190, 220, 228
  victim, 17, 75, 229
Heroic medicine, 3, 74, 152, 182, 222, 226, 228, 241
Hewson, William, 252
Hierophilus of Chalcedon, 113
Hippocrates, 113, 114, 159
Hi-tech death, 2, 3, 10, 241, 242, 245
Hoffa, Moritz, 99, 119
Hoffman, Friedrich, 115
Holtey, W., 31
Hooke, Robert, 116, 132, 252
Hospices
  death in, 246
  founding, 15–16
  St Christopher's Hospice, 15
Hospital
  death in, 2, 11, 13, 165, 185, 210, 235, 246
  resuscitation in, 25, 100–1, 157, 169, 258
Hour of Our Death, The, 11, 15
Humane Society, 49–94
  agitations, 62, 65–6, 118, 155
  annual festival, 82, 87
  Annual Reports, 57, 66, 71, 74–5, 82, 85, 131, 155
  benefactors, 81–3
  bloodletting, 70–2
  children, 80–1
  circulation, 65–6
  see drowning
  drugs, 69–70
  founding, 50
  gold medal, 53, 86
  heat, 68–9
  instruction, 50, 75
  instruments and equipment, 69, 74, 133, 143, 87, 94, 253
  medals, 52, 53, 66, 85, 86, 87, 94, 109, 253
  Method for the Restoration of the Apparently Dead, The, 49, 50–1, 53–4, 60–74, 79, 80, 83–4, 87–8, 89, 91–2, 94, 108, 109, 117, 118, 121, 155, 167, 174, 252
  rescuers, 8, 9, 50, 64, 75, 83–6, 87, 133, 136, 152, 155
  rewards, 50, 52, 53, 55, 66, 84–7, 94, 109, 253
  silver medal, 52
  spectators, 87–9
  stimulation and stimulants, 50, 51, 53, 65, 66, 67, 68, 69, 70, 93, 116, 118, 155, 156
  suicides, 78–80
  ventilation, 64–5
  victims, 52, 61, 73, 75–81, 84, 87, 88, 91, 92, 182, 252
  workmen, 77–8
Humanity, 20, 89–93, 176, 181, 182–4, 186, 214, 231
Humboldt, Wilhelm von, 119
Humours, 70, 113, 160, 161
Hunter, John, 66, 71, 82, 117, 118, 131, 133, 252
Hydrogen, 130
Hypothermia, 58–62
  apparent death, 60
  asphyxia, 52
  children, 81
  CPR, 35, 38, 167, 236
  diagnosing death, 54–5, 60, 167, 236
  drowning, 60
  expectations of revival and resuscitation, 54–5, 60–1, 81, 180
  pathophysiology, 58–9
  premature burial, 60–1
  signs and symptoms, 58
  therapeutic, 252
  treatment, 62, 68, 97–8
  ventricular fibrillation, 58, 249
Hypoxia, 35, 42, 52, 59, 60, 71, 249, 252

Iatrochemistry, 137, 161, 255
Iatromechanism, 52, 53, 70, 107, 160–1, 255

ICU, *see* intensive care unit
ILCOR, International Liaison Committee on Resuscitation, 38
Illich, Ivan, 3, 15, 210
Images, 199, 203–5, 260
 algorithm, 39
 CPR, 36, 184, 217–18, 234
 death, 211, 215–16, 233, 256
 electric, 10, 106, 121–3, 177, 190, 229, 254
 fire, 111
 life, 121
 media, 186, 207
 pornographic, 213–14
 processing, 202
 reality, 210, 211–12
Immaterial substance, 108, 111–21, 123, 255
Immortality, 37, 105, 165, 176, 182, 205, 206
Imperatives
 deathbed, 73, 153, 206, 226, 231
 malevolent, 174
 moral, 216
 ontological imperative, 112
 performative, 230
 social, 222
 technological imperative, 37, 185, 206, 222
 temporal imperative, 83
Imponderables, 108, 111–21, 123, 255
Impurity, 132, 143, 144, 145, 146, 147, 148, 150, 151, 170, 174, 180, 220, 221
Indelicacy, 132, 143–6
Index, indexicality, 204, 211, 215, 260
Indiana University School of Medicine, 193
Individualism, 17–18, 211
Infection
 contagion, 146–7, 171, 175
 mouth-to-mouth and fear, 138–42, 151, 153, 257
Institution for Affording Relief to Persons Apparently Dead from Drowning, *see* Humane Society
Intensive care unit, 2, 30, 43, 47, 101, 102, 161, 197, 210, 225, 233, 246, 261

Intermittent positive pressure ventilation 135–6, 141, 246, 247
Intoxication, 179–83, 230, 259
Intubation, 1, 127, 141, 175, 220, 248, 253, 256
IPPV *see* intermittent positive pressure ventilation
Irritability, 65, 69–70, 116–19, 120, 130, 156, 157, 160

Jaw thrust, 248
Johns Hopkins University, 100
Joule, James Prescott, 115, 119
Journal of the American Medical Association, 31
Jude, James, 31, 157, 158, 191, 192, 250
Jung, Carl, 176

Kant, Immanuel, 146
Kelvin, Lord, 115, 119
Kipnis, Laura, 215
Kircher, Athanasius, 138
Kiss
 disgust, 144, 150
 kiss of death, 150–1
 kiss of life, 150–1
Kite, Charles, 52, 53, 56, 57, 64, 68, 70, 133, 253
Knickerbocker, Guy, 157, 158, 191, 250
Kouwenhoven, William, 31, 100, 157, 158, 191, 192, 250
Kristeva, Julia, 149
Kübler-Ross, Elizabeth, 3, 15, 23, 246
Kuhn, Thomas, 245
Kymograph, 122

Lacan, Jacques, 145, 149
Lack, 149, 205
Language, limits of, 149–50, 178, 180, 211, 214, 216
Laplace, Pierre Simon, 131, 132
Laryngospasm, 52, 53, 155, 252
Lavoisier, Antoine Laurant, 111, 115, 116, 130, 131, 132, 252, 256
Law and litigation, 43, 104, 196, 226, 229, 235, 237, 251
Leeuwenhoek, Anton van, 138
Lessing, Gotthold, 145

Index 291

Lettsom, John Coakley, 50, 71, 129
Levinas, Emmanuel, 183
Levy, Alfred Goodman, 99
Lewis, Thomas, 99
Life
 affirming, 176, 183
 daemon of, 178
 expectancy, 25–6
 kiss of, 150–1
 representation, 85, 106, 12, 123, 215, 253
 spark of, 106
 story, 18
 torch of, 85
Life-force, 65, 66–7, 71, 99, 108, 109–21, 123, 130, 141, 151, 155–6, 167, 178, 211
Life-saving organizations, 32, 135, 191, 192
Life-soul, 110
Lightning, 38, 54, 129, 254
Limits to Medicine, The, 15
Living wills, 3, 184, 224, 227–9, 232, 237, 262
Loneliness of the Dying, The, 15
Louis, Pierre, 71
Loved One, The, 15
Lown, Bernard, 100
Ludwig, Karl, 99, 119, 122

Machin, Barbara, 209
Magnetism, animal, 108, 111, 117, 119
Malinowski, Bronislaw, 21
Manual ventilatory techniques, 127, 134–5, 153, 156–7, 160, 174
Marcus Welby MD, 193
M*A*S*H, 193
Massachusetts General Hospital, 195
Massachusetts Humane Society, 91
Matteucci, Carl, 119
Maxwell, James, 111, 115, 119
Mayer, Julius, 115, 119
Mayow, John, 116, 130, 132, 252
McWilliam, John, 99
Mechanism, 52, 65, 106–8, 109, 110, 115, 117, 130, 155, 160, 255
Medals, 52, 53, 66, 85, 86, 87, 94, 109, 253
Media, The, 189–218

CPR, 2–3, 36, 123, 179, 186, 190–210, 218
death, 2, 3, 22, 106, 121, 123, 209–11
documentary, 190–2, 196–7, 204, 260
entertainment, 193–4, 197, 204–5, 206–7
images in, 186, 207
indexicality, 204, 211, 215, 260, 261
instruction, 190–1, 195–6, 217, 203–4
medical drama, 189–210, 245, 260, 261
pornography, 213–14, 217–18, 234
propaganda, 190–2
reality, 194–204, 215–17, 217–18
ritual, 234
UK, 261
Walter Reed Movie Group, 190
Medical Center, 193
Medicalization, 13, 15, 21, 101, 185, 210, 221, 237
Methane, 252
Method, The, 49, 50–1, 53–4, 60–74, 79, 80, 83–4, 87–8, 89, 91–2, 94, 108, 109, 117, 118, 121, 155, 167, 174, 252
Méthode numérique, 71
MI, *see* myocardial infarction
Miasmas, 132, 139, 147
Microscope, 138, 193
Midwives, 127
Mines, 51, 77, 128, 135, 252
Mise en scène, 179
Mitford, Jessica, 15
MMV, *see* mouth-to-mouth ventilation
Mnemonic device, 27, 39, 41, 127, 164, 191, 204
Monitor, cardiac, 106, 121,122, 123, 177, 190, 249
Monro II, Alexander, 133
Montpelier vitalists, 117
Morgagni, Giovanni, 120
Morgues, mortuaries, 13, 19, 58, 170, 210
Morocco, Mark, 195, 196, 200, 201
Mortality and immortality, 15

292 Index

Mourning, 10, 15–17, 20, 22, 165, 170, 173, 221, 232, 234, 235, 237–8
Mouth, 138–9, 143–6, 149–53
Mouth-to-mask ventilation, 141–2
Mouth-to-mouth ventilation, 124–53
   aversion, 138–53, 156, 157
   biblical precedent, 127
   condemnation, 94, 132–3, 137–8
   contagion, 146–7
   CPR, 25, 27, 31, 36, 41, 101, 127, 135–6, 248, 249
   disgust, 138, 148–50
   downgrading, 33, 104, 141–2, 227–9, 237, 257
   film, 190, 191, 218
   first case report, 127–9
   history, 119, 127–33, 152–3, 158
   Humane Society protocol, 3, 50, 51, 53, 64–5, 127–9
   indelicacy, 143–6
   infection, fear, 139–43, 257
   intermittent positive pressure ventilation, 256
   kissing, 144–5
   ritual and symbolic import 42, 151–3, 157, 177–9, 184, 219–21
   valorization, 132–3, 137–9, 150–3
Mouth-to-nose ventilation, 135, 142
Murder, 174, 175–6, 183–4, 220
Myocardial infarction, 29, 236, 249
Myth, 162, 164, 170, 177, 184, 212, 221, 231

NALS *see* Neonatal Advanced Life Support
Narratives, 17, 18, 39, 121, 184, 194, 199, 202, 204, 205, 211, 212, 221, 245
National Academy of Sciences-National Research Council, 31, 135, 136
National Health Service, 199
National Lifeboat Institution, 135
National Research Council Ad Hoc Conference on Cardiopulmonary Resuscitation, 31
Negovsky, Vladimir, 250
Neonatal Advanced Life Support, 27, 228

New England Journal of Medicine, 192
Nerve gas, 136, 190
Nerves, nervous system, 27, 28, 53, 65, 66, 69, 114, 115, 116, 117, 118, 119, 121, 160, 167
Neurological damage, 251, 252
Neve, Michol, 161
Newton, Isaac, 115, 116, 137
NHS, *see* National Health Service
Nichol, G., 251
Nielson, Holger Louis, 135
Nightingale, Florence, 139
Nitre, 130, 131, 256
Nitro-aerial particles, 130
Nitrogen, 112, 116, 130
Nobili, Leopoldo, 119
Normal sinus rhythm, 100, 230, 249
Nostalgia, 121, 241, 247
NSR *see* normal sinus rhythm
Nuland, Sherwin, 19
Nurses, 3, 20, 23, 100, 185, 198, 226, 235, 237

Obscenity, 205, 212, 214
Oceanic Feeling, 176
Ohm, Georg, 119
Open-chest-cardiac-massage, 100, 157, 258
Omnipotence, 147–8, 179
On Death and Dying, 15
One-shot-sequence, 202–3
OPALS study (Ontario pre-hospital advanced life support study), 34, 251
Opium and narcotics, 2, 12, 13, 14, 20, 54, 73, 79, 225, 241, 247
Oreibasia, 180
Organicism, 108, 109, 120
Orgia, 180
Orsted, Hans Christian, 119
Oxford group, 107, 255
Oxygen, 27, 28, 29, 59, 112, 116, 129, 132–3, 135, 151, 152, 158, 231, 252, 256, 261
Oxygène, 115, 130, 131, 252

Palliative care, 3, 14, 16, 185, 210, 233, 241, 242
PAD, *see* public access defibrillation

PALS *see* Pediatric Advanced Life Support
Paracelsus, 110, 115, 127
Paramedics, 1–2, 30, 47, 48, 97, 101, 143–4, 154, 179, 185, 189–90, 192, 198, 219, 220, 248
Passing On: The Social Organization of Dying, 15
Pasteur, Louis, 138, 139
Pathography, 3, 245
PEA, *see* pulseless electrical activity
Pechlin, Johann Nicholas, 57
Pediatric Advanced Life Support, 27, 228, 252
Peirce, C. S., 260
PCI *see* percutaneous coronary intervention
Percutaneous coronary intervention, 250
Performatives, 92, 230, 259
Peripeteia, 209
Phaedrus, 180, 181, 259
Pharmakos, 173
Phlogiston, 111
Photography, 204, 210, 211, 213, 215, 256, 260–1
Physicians, *see* doctors
Pingo, Thomas, 85
Pitcairne, Archibald, 115
Planck, Max, 119
Plato, 113, 181, 255, 259
Pneuma, 108, 112–13, 130, 151
Poetics, 259
Poison
  cause of death, 29, 38, 166, 190
  expired breath, 132–3, 138–9, 151, 152
Police, 27, 103, 105, 211
Pornography
  condemnation, 212–14
  of death, 15, 210–17
  defence, 214
  existential, 215–17, 233–4
  images, 210–14
Pornography of Death, 15, 120, 210, 212, 232, 260, 261
Positivism, 37, 120, 121, 185
Postmodernism, 18, 205, 211, 214, 233, 234

Pratt, Rev., 90, 182
Praxagoras, 113
Pre-hospital care, 30, 46, 47, 101–3, 224, 248, 249, 254
Premature burial, 51–61, 67, 99, 167, 247
Prevost, Jean Louis, 99
Priests, 12, 13, 20, 73, 163
Priestley, Joseph, 66, 116, 118, 130, 131, 132, 252, 256
Primary arrest, 28–30, 35, 52, 168, 208
Primem vivens, 67
Principe vital, 117
Principia, 116
Propp, Vladimir, 221
Protocol, 37–48, 162–9
  assessment, 33
  advanced, 249, 252, 261
  conformity, 42–4
  fragmentation, 228
  institutional effects, 47–8, 237
  power, 44–7
  rationalization, 226–8, 242
  ritual, 162–4, 174–5, 181–7, 221–6, 228–31
  unity, 39
  universality, 38–42, 64, 83, 87, 89, 222, 227–8
Psyche, 3, 20, 21, 23, 92, 162, 214
Psyche, 108–13, 151, 255
Psychic-spirit, 114
Psychoanalysis, 16, 173
Pulseless electrical activity, 29, 34, 39, 24, 249
Pulse of Life, The, 191
Public access defibrillation, 103, 105
Pubs, publicans, 84, 87
Purity, purification, 111, 113, 133, 141, 146–8, 150–1, 174, 180, 221, 237, 258
Purgatives, 50, 51, 69
Purgatory, 11

QALY, *see* quality adjusted life year
QRS complex, 106, 122–3
Quality adjusted life year, 105, 254, 255
Quesalid, 201

Index

Rationalism, 12, 19, 76, 90, 131, 132, 137, 180, 211, 226
Reality and representation, 48, 61, 197, 201–2, 203–5, 206, 210–12, 213–17, 230, 233–4, 260
Recherches sur les effets de la saignée, 71
Redemption, 13, 80, 89, 90, 91, 92, 174, 175, 177, 183–5, 220, 221, 222, 230, 231
Re-enactment, 150, 164–5, 174, 213
Reflex, 107, 117, 120
Reification, 110, 112, 120, 170, 177, 246
Religion, 3, 12, 13, 17, 19, 21, 22, 23, 42, 73, 74, 75, 76, 80, 81, 82, 87, 93, 107, 110, 114, 162, 163, 164, 168, 178, 210, 226, 233, 242
Reperfusion, 30, 250
Representations
  CPR and resuscitation, 30, 36, 48, 61, 184, 186, 189–212, 215, 217, 222, 224, 228, 229, 230, 234, 249, 258
  death, 2, 22, 23, 106, 193, 199, 210–12, 215–17, 233–4, 256
  disgust, 145
  life, 85, 106, 123, 215, 253
  medicine, 195, 198, 261
  reality, 48, 61, 197, 201–2, 203–5, 206, 210–12, 213–17, 230, 233–4, 260
Repression, 181
  death, 20–1, 165–6, 210–12, 234
  desire, 212–13
  history, 184
  mouth-to-mouth, 33, 94, 104, 132–3, 137–8, 141–2, 156, 157, 227–9, 237, 257
  violence, 153, 174, 231
Res cogitans, 107, 109
Rescue 911, 215
Rescue Breathing, 190
  see mouth-to-mouth
Res extensa, 107
Respiratory
  failure, 29, 35, 36, 79, 228, 238, 248, 249
  physiology, 52–4, 65, 107, 115, 116, 130–2, 137, 152–3, 255
  sign of death, 55, 56, 59, 72, 167
Resuscitation, *see* cardiopulmonary resuscitation
Resuscitators of America, 31, 101, 102
Respiratory arrest, 28, 29, 35, 249, 252
Rete mirabile, 114, 255
Revivalism, 16, 18, 19, 232
Rewarming, 50, 51, 60, 68–9, 86, 93, 118
RHS, *see* Royal Humane Society
Ritual, 162–86
  CPR, 46–7, 215–16, 220–5, 226, 231–2, 238, 242
  denial of death, 13, 20–1, 164–6
  disappearance, 13, 17–18, 22–3, 73, 168, 210–12
  erotics, 178–81
  funerary, 14, 19, 141
  life, 176–8, 215–16
  mechanism, 150, 166–76, 178–81, 220–1, 258–9
  media, 217–18, 222–6, 233–4
  myth, 161–2
  participation in, 232–9
  protocol, 3, 162–4, 184–7, 226–31
  religious, 11–13
  rites of passage, 170–2, 258
  therapeutic discourse, 16–18, 247, 259
  violence, 150, 166–76, 181–4, 185, 231–2
Rockefeller Institute, 99
Romanticism, 153
Ross, Doug, 212, 261
Royal Charter, 50
Royal College of Surgeons, 133
Royal Humane Society, *see* Humane Society
Royal Life Saving Society, 32, 135
Royal Mint, 85
Rumford, Count, 115
Russell, Thomas, 91
Russian Ark, 260
Rutherford, Daniel, 116, 130, 132

Sacrifice, 81, 150, 152, 170–3, 176–8, 180, 182–3, 184, 220–1, 222, 229, 230–1, 237
Safar, Peter, 31, 136, 158, 183, 190, 191, 192, 248, 250
Saunders, Cicely, 3, 15–16
Savigny, J. H., 133, 253
Scapegoat, 173–4
Scheele, Karl Wilhelm, 256
Scorsese, Martin, 245
Scrobiculus cordis, 55–6
Scrubs, 215
Seale, Clive, 5, 21, 162, 165, 182, 245, 247
Seattle, King County, 25, 31, 36, 46, 101, 192, 102, 251
Second National Conference on Standards for CPR and Emergency Cardiac Care, 31
Secondary arrest, 28, 29, 35, 249, 252
Secularism, 12, 13, 15, 60, 61, 73, 74, 90, 91, 92, 171, 173, 177, 205, 211, 221, 234, 242
Seguin, Marc, 116
Self, 17, 18, 92, 143, 146, 147, 148, 149, 150, 151, 152, 166, 170, 173, 174, 179, 180, 183, 185, 214, 216, 217, 222, 259
Sex, 15, 181, 193, 194, 212–14, 215, 234
Shamanism, 163, 181, 201
Shelley, Mary, 254
Shen, Bern, 259
Signification, 184, 215–16, 249, 260
60 Minutes, 192
Slow code, 226
SmithKline French, 191
Social structure, 47–8, 81, 165, 183, 232, 246
Socrates, 180
Soul, 11, 12, 13, 22, 23, 73, 107, 108, 109, 110, 112, 113, 114, 117, 141, 146, 148, 151, 163, 166, 167, 170, 174, 175, 177, 178, 181, 205, 221, 246
Spectatorship, 22, 87–9, 179, 197, 210, 212, 213–14, 234–8
Spirit, 108, 110, 113, 114, 115, 122

Spirits, 146, 147, 170, 246
St. Elsewhere, 193
Stahl, George Ernst, 108
Steadicam, 199, 201–3, 205, 235, 260
Stevenson, John, 107
Story arcs, 194, 198, 199, 209
Sublimation, 111–12, 120–1
Substantival vitalism, 108–21, 123, 178, 216, 255
Sudden Death and the Myth of CPR, 36, 250
Sudnow, David, 15
Suffering, 14, 16, 21, 73, 76, 85, 166, 205, 230, 242, 247
Suicide, 26, 52, 76, 77, 78–80, 81
Surgeon-apothecaries, 50, 82
Surgeons, 50, 82, 100, 193, 252
Symbol, 15, 41–2, 92, 122, 145, 146, 149–50, 151–3, 162–4, 164–6, 167, 170–2, 173, 175–6, 180, 184–5, 211–12, 220–1, 222, 225, 229–30, 232, 247, 257
Symbolic Exchange and Death, 15

Tachycardia
 algorithm, 40, 227–8, 251
 ventricular, 29, 34, 39, 227, 249
Tangibility, 111–12, 115, 255
Technological imperative, 37, 185, 206, 222
Telesius, 114
Television *see* media
Terminal therapeutics and terminal paradox, 71–2, 106, 169, 184–6
Thales, 99
Thermon, 113
Thompson, E. P., 257
Thomson, J. J., 115, 119
Thoracic pump, 159–60
Thoracotomy, 157, 258
Thymos, 109
Tidal volume, 256
Timmermans, Stefan, 3, 5, 36, 105, 161, 231, 232, 250, 259
Tissot, Samuel, 129

Index

Tobacco enemas and fumigations, 50, 62, 69, 70, 101, 118, 133, 155, 253
Torch, 66, 109
Torricelli, Evangelista, 130
Tossach, William, 127–8
Totenweib, 170
Tracheostomy, tracheotomy, 51, 127, 248
Transcendence, transcendent, 11, 45, 73, 90, 92, 107, 108, 109, 110, 114, 116, 163, 168, 171, 172, 173, 175, 177, 178, 179, 180, 181, 182, 211, 216, 218, 221, 230, 232, 234
Transgression, 143–51, 175, 178, 181, 213–14, 216, 220–1, 234, 259
Transplantation, 256
Trauma, 175, 261
 cause of death, 26, 29, 208
 television, 61, 206–8
Trauma, 215
Traumatic excess, 123, 178, 211, 212, 216
Turner, Chris, 149
Turner, Viktor, 258

Ultimum moriens, 67
University of California Davis Medical Centre, 139
University of Glasgow, 105
Utstein criteria, 34

Vaublanc, Grenot, 91
Ventilation
 artificial, 27, 53, 64–5, 68, 127–37
 Bain Method, 134
 bellows, 51, 53, 61–2, 64–5, 127, 132–4, 253, 256
 Bowles Method, 134
 condemnation of techniques, 134, 137–8, 154–6
 folk practice, 154–6
 Holger Nielson Method, 134, 135, 256
 Howard Method, 134
 intermittent positive pressure, 135–6, 141, 246, 247
 Laborde Method, 134
 Leroy Method, 134
 manual ventilatory techniques, 127, 134–5, 153, 156–7, 160, 174
 mouth-to-mouth, *see* mouth-to-mouth ventilation
 Marshall Hall method, 134, 256
 necessity, 228–9, 257
 Pacini Method, 134
 recommendations, 247–8
 Schafer Method, 134, 135, 256
 Schultze Method, 134
 Schroeder Method, 134
 Schuller Method, 134
 Silvester Method, 134, 135, 256
Ventricular fibrillation, 29, 33, 34, 38, 44, 53, 58, 59, 68, 99–100, 104, 106, 119, 157–8, 159, 168, 191, 228, 230, 238, 247, 249, 250, 254, 257
Ventricular tachycardia, 29, 34, 39, 227, 249
Verisimilitude, 195, 198, 204–5, 215
Vesalius, Andreas, 114, 120, 127
VF, *see* ventricular fibrillation
V-Fib, *see* ventricular fibrillation
Video
Vis vitae see life-force
Violence
 corpse, 66–7, 85, 155–6, 166–70, 174–5, 181–5, 242–3
 CPR, 10, 36, 123, 174, 220, 230, 231–2
 deathbed violence, 153, 156, 157, 166–86, 220–1, 230, 231–2
 folk therapy, 66, 155
 Humane Society protocol, 156
 media, 194, 213–17, 234
 psychological, 172–4
 rebounding, 171–2
 ritual, 150, 166–76, 181–4, 185, 231–2
Vital air, 131, 132
Vital force, 65, 66–7, 71, 99, 108, 109–21, 123, 130, 141, 151, 155–6, 167, 178, 211
Vital functions, 28, 29, 35, 53, 56, 65, 118, 130, 156, 246
Vitalism, 52, 53, 60, 66, 71, 107–21, 123, 155–6, 177–8, 216, 229, 255
Vital signs, 56, 167

Viviani, Vincenzo, 130
Void, 123, 149–50, 176, 178, 216–17
Volatiles, 69, 155, 253
Volta, Alessandro, 118
Voyeurism, 209, 211, 213, 214, 215
VT, *see* ventricular tachycardia

Walls, Ron, 196
Walsh, John, 66
Walraven, C. van, 34
Walter Reed Movie Group, 190
Walter, Tony, 16, 17, 18, 232, 247

Warner Brothers, 199
Waterhouse, Benjamin, 132
Watermen, 77, 84, 152
Watkinson, Dr., 85
Waugh, Evelyn, 15
Webb, Jack, 192
Westwing, 260
Whytt, Robert, 117
Williams, Linda, 215
Willis, Thomas, 116

YMCA, 135